Pediatric ECG Holter

Due to the brief nature of arrhythmias, which may not be seen during the short recording periods of a typical ECG, Holter monitoring enables physicians to make more informed decisions on cardiac patients. This book is a case-by-case instructional exercise on interpreting Holter monitorings in the pediatric setting. The cases illustrate the wide range of pediatric arrhythmias that are most commonly observed. Pediatric cardiologists, pediatricians, and pediatric arrhythmologists will develop the ability to analyze Holter ECGs in children of diverse ages.

Key Features:

- Covers various cardiac conditions, from supraventricular tachycardia, to long QT syndrome and cardiac pacemakers

- Uses real-life examples with patient history to enhance the learning experience of students and medical professionals

- Trains professionals to discern arrhythmias from electrical artifacts found during a Holter examination

- Educates clinicians to determine the appropriate timing for referring a patient for arrhythmogenic consultation or ablation procedures

Pediatric ECG Holter
A Case-Based Approach to Interpretation

Edited by
Cismaru Gabriel
Cecilia Lazea
Simona Cainap

CRC Press
Taylor & Francis Group
Boca Raton London New York

CRC Press is an imprint of the
Taylor & Francis Group, an **informa** business

Designed cover image: Cismaru Gabriel

First edition published 2026
by CRC Press
2385 NW Executive Center Drive, Suite 320, Boca Raton FL 33431

and by CRC Press
4 Park Square, Milton Park, Abingdon, Oxon, OX14 4RN

CRC Press is an imprint of Taylor & Francis Group, LLC

ISBN: 978-1-032-89872-8 (hbk)
ISBN: 978-1-032-89871-1 (pbk)
ISBN: 978-1-003-54504-0 (ebk)

DOI: 10.1201/9781003545040

Typeset in Palatino
by SPi Technologies India Pvt Ltd (Straive)

Contents

Preface

One cannot become a skilled surgeon solely through theoretical knowledge without practical experience. Understanding the theory of Holter ECG interpretation is insufficient; medical students are capable of learning it too. However, to become a competent practitioner, it is essential to connect theory with practice.

This book addresses pediatricians who use Holter ECG to monitor their patients. Whether they are pediatric cardiologists or pediatricians working in the Intensive Care Unit or the Emergency Department, they will come across Holter-type examinations or ECG monitor traces during their bedside activity. On the other hand, the book offers detailed descriptions of electrophysiological mechanisms that arrhythmologists can employ to improve their understanding of pediatric cardiac arrhythmias.

From a pragmatic perspective, we selected a uniform book format for all chapters. It begins with a real-life clinical case, presents the relevant Holter ECG images, succeeded by a final analysis of the recording. The subsequent section of each case is the Discussion section, which covers the theoretical framework related to the specific case, concluding with an instructive final image. This methodology was used for each of the 30 cases presented in the book, enabling the reader to assess their practical interpretation of the traces prior to verification at the end of the chapter. This method is the most advantageous for young doctors eager to master the complexities of electrocardiography. This book was conceived from the very beginning with a strong educational objective.

Only a limited number of pediatric arrhythmologists exist in Europe, and they gather at European conferences focused on arrhythmology or pediatric cardiology. This book was produced through the participation of young pediatric arrhythmologists who aimed to share their expertise by selecting interesting clinical examples from their practice. This clinical case book was conceived through our friendship. Due to the disparate monitoring instruments and interpretation softwares utilized in various countries, the format of the Holter will differ in each chapter. All of the chapters share a similarity: the expertise of the clinician who analyzed the ECG data, which in all cases was a clinician who focuses on arrhythmia disorders. We acknowledge that the book has errors. How could it not be, having been developed by clinicians instead of arrhythmia specialists? We await your feedback and suggestions at the editors' email address to improve the subsequent editions of the book. Your comments will render you authors of the improved edition.

We extend our gratitude to all our arrhythmologist colleagues for their trust in contributing to our book project, and we anticipate continuing our collaboration on additional cases for an upcoming collection of pediatric arrhythmia cases.

The authors. January 4, 2025.

Editor Biographies

Dr. Cismaru Gabriel is an adult and pediatric cardiologist who specializes in cardiac arrhythmias. He gained his EHRA Certification in Invasive Cardiac Electrophysiology in 2019 and his EHRA Certification in Cardiac Implantable Electronic Devices in 2021. During his daily medical activity he implants loop recorders for pediatric patients with syncope or suspicion of arrhythmias, and performs electrophysiological studies and catheter ablation for different types of arrhythmias. He also implants pacemakers in children with bradyarrhythmias and defibrillators for primary or secondary prevention of sudden cardiac death. He is also a Lecturer in the Cardiology Department of the University of Medicine and Pharmacy Iuliu Hatieganu Cluj-Napoca.

Cecilia Lazea is an associate professor and a pediatric cardiologist at Emergency Paediatric Hospital Cluj-Napoca, Romania. She graduated from University of Medicine and Pharmacy "Iuliu Hatieganu" Cluj-Napoca in 1996 and has trained in Paediatrics and Paediatric Cardiology. She benefited from research grants awarded in France in 2000 and 2009, one of them being in the field of Medical Genetics. She has been working in the Paediatric Cardiology Department of her current hospital since 2003. Her medical activity consists in taking care of the hospitalized patients with cardiovascular diseases and arrhythmia, medical advice and consultation of the patients with arrhythmias in the Emergency Department and Paediatric Intensive Care Unit and follow-up visits of the patients with cardiovascular diseases in the Outpatient Clinic. She has extensive experience in pediatric arrhythmia, and she has read a significant number of pediatric ECG Holter monitoring and paediatric ECGs during her current medical activity on the Paediatric Cardiology Department. She is also experienced in the genetic basis and molecular analysis of a large variety of arrhythmias and genetic cardiovascular diseases in children.

Simona Cainap is an Associate Professor of Pediatrics at the "Iuliu Hatieganu" University of Medicine and Pharmacy Cluj-Napoca. She is a specialist in Pediatric Cardiology and her current position is as a consultant in Clinic No. 2 of the Pediatric Cardiology Department. In 2012, she was awarded an Erasmus scholarship to study at the Zentrum für Angeborne Herzfeler und Diabeteszentrum NRW Bad Oeynhausen, Germany. She has published articles on congenital heart diseases and pediatric cardiac arrhythmias and has conducted pediatric screenings for children with congenital diseases during her involvement in the POSDRU and HORIZON 2020 European projects, resulting in the collection of extensive databases that have been utilized in numerous publications in the field of pediatric arrhythmias.

Contributors

Gabriela Abrudan
Emergency Clinical Hospital
Neonatology II Department
Cluj-Napoca, Romania

Sorin Andreica
Neonatology, Mother and Child Department
"Iuliu Hatieganu" University of Medicine and
    Pharmacy
and
Neonatology Department
Regina Maria Hospital
Cluj-Napoca, Romania

Marie Bartos
Pediatric Heart Centre
Queen Silvia Childrens Hospital
Gothenburg, Sweden

Bogdan Caloian
Cardiology Department
Rehabilitation Hospital
and
4th Department of Internal Medicine
"Iuliu Hatieganu" University of Medicine and
    Pharmacy
Cluj-Napoca, Romania

Andrei Cismaru
Research Center for Functional Genomics,
    Biomedicine and Translational Medicine
"Iuliu Hatieganu", University of Medicine and
    Pharmacy
Cluj-Napoca, Romania

Ioana Ciuca
Prevent Clinic
Alba Iulia, Romania

Iulia Ciobotariu
Department of Cardiology
Carol Davila Central Military Universitary
Emergency Hospital
Bucharest, Romania

Alexandra Cocoi
Pediatric Clinic No 1
Cluj-Napoca Children's Emergency Clinical
    Hospital
Cluj-Napoca, Romania

Horatiu Comsa
Cardiology Department
Rehabilitation Hospital
and
4th Department of Internal Medicine
"Iuliu Hatieganu" University of Medicine and
    Pharmacy
Cluj-Napoca, Romania

Radu Andrei Dan
Laboratory of Interventional
    Cardiology
Carol Davila Central Military Universitary
    Emergency Hospital
Bucharest, Romania

Corina Diaconescu
Department of Cardiology
Carol Davila Central Military Universitary
Emergency Hospital
Bucharest, Romania

Cristina Filip
Neonatal Intensive Care Unit
"M.S. Curie" Emergency Clinical Hospital for
    Children
and
Department of Pediatrics
Pediatric Cardiology
"Carol Davila" University of Medicine and
    Pharmacy
Bucharest, Romania

Florina Fringu
Cardiology Department
Rehabilitation Hospital
and
4th Department of Internal Medicine
"Iuliu Hatieganu" University of Medicine and
    Pharmacy
Cluj-Napoca, Romania

Delia Ghinga
Neonatology Department
Regina Maria Hospital
Cluj-Napoca, Romania

Ioana Golgot
Pediatric Cardiology
Pediatric Center
Cluj-Napoca, Romania

Alessandra Grison
Neonatal Intensive Care Unit
Pediatric Department
San Bortolo Hospital
Vicenza, Italy

Gabriel Gusetu
Cardiology Department
Rehabilitation Hospital
and
4th Department of Internal Medicine
"Iuliu Hatieganu" University of Medicine
    and Pharmacy
Cluj-Napoca, Romania

Raluca Hudrea
Neonatology Department
Regina Maria Hospital
Cluj-Napoca, Romania

Daniela Iacob
Pediatric Clinic No 3
Emergency Clinical Hospital for Children
and
Mother and Child Department
"Iuliu Hatieganu" University of Medicine
    and Pharmacy
Cluj-Napoca, Romania

Vasile Iliese
Laboratory of Interventional Cardiology
Carol Davila Central Military Universitary
Emergency Hospital
Bucharest, Romania

Maria Ilina
Department of Paediatric Cardiology
Royal Hospital for Children
Glasgow, United Kingdom

Diana Irimie
Cardiology Department
Rehabilitation Hospital
and
4th Department of Internal Medicine
"Iuliu Hatieganu" University of Medicine
    and Pharmacy
Cluj-Napoca, Romania

Sabina Istratoaie
Pharmacology Department
"Iuliu Hatieganu" University of Medicine
    and Pharmacy
and
Cardiology Department
Heart Institute
Cluj-Napoca, Romania

Diana Jecan Toader
Pediatric Clinic No 2
Cluj-Napoca Children's Emergency Clinical
    Hospital
Cluj-Napoca, Romania

Maria-Evelyn Kecskes
Department of Pediatric Cardiology
'Marie-Sklodowska Curie' Emergency
    Children's Hospital
Bucharest, Romania

Gabriela Kelemen
Pediatric Clinic No 1
Emergency Clinical Hospital for Children
Cluj-Napoca, Romania

Kristel Köbas
Children's Clinic
Tartu University Hospital
Tartu, Estonia

Rein Kolk
Department of Cardiology
Institute of Clinical Medicine, University
    of Tartu
Tartu, Estonia

Nikola Krmek
Department of Pediatrics
University Hospital Center "Sestre Milosrdnice"
Zagreb, Croatia

Stefan Kurath-Koller
Pediatric Cardiology Electrophysiology
Medical University of Graz
Austria

Alice Maltret
Department of Pediatric Cardiology
Hospital Necker, AP-HP
Paris, France

Andrei Mihordea
Cardiology Department
Spitalul Clinic Judeţean de Urgenţă
    "Sf. Spiridon"
University Hospital in Iaşi
Iaşi, Romania

Ioan Alexandru Minciuna
Cardiology Department
Rehabilitation Hospital
Cluj-Napoca, Romania

Nicoleta Motoc
Pneumology Department
"Leon Daniello" Clinical Hospital of
    Pneumophthisiology
and
"Iuliu Hatieganu" University of Medicine
    and Pharmacy
Cluj-Napoca, Romania

Lucian Muresan
Cardiology Department
"Emile Muller" Hospital
Mulhouse, France

Lavinia Oniga
Cardiology Outpatient Clinic
"Leon Daniello" Clinical Hospital of
    Pneumophthisiology
Cluj-Napoca, Romania

Emanuel Palade
Thoracic Surgery Department
"Leon Daniello" Clinical Hospital of
    Pneumophthisiology
and
"Iuliu Hatieganu" University of Medicine
    and Pharmacy
Cluj-Napoca, Romania

Dana Pop
Cardiology Department
Rehabilitation Hospital
and
4th Department of Internal Medicine
"Iuliu Hatieganu" University of Medicine
    and Pharmacy
Cluj-Napoca, Romania

Alexandra Popa
Pediatric Clinic No 1
Emergency Clinical Hospital for
    Children
and
Department 8 Mother and Child Pediatric
    Clinic No 1
"Iuliu Hatieganu" University of Medicine
    and Pharmacy
Cluj-Napoca, Romania

Boingiu Rares
Department of Cardiology
Carol Davila Central Military Universitary
    Emergency Hospital
Bucharest, Romania

Radu Rosu
Cardiology Department
Rehabilitation Hospital
and
4th Department of Internal Medicine
"Iuliu Hatieganu" University of Medicine
    and Pharmacy
Cluj-Napoca, Romania

Marta Rotella
Neonatal Intensive Care Unit, Pediatric
    Department
San Bortolo Hospital
Vicenza, Italy

Roxana Rusu
Pediatric Clinic No 2
Cluj-Napoca Children's Emergency Clinical
    Hospital
Cluj-Napoca, Romania

Massimo Spanghero
Cardiology Department
San Bortolo Hospital
Vicenza, Italy

Adrian Stef
Department of Surgery
Iuliu Hatieganu" University of Medicine
    and Pharmacy
and
Clinical Department of Anesthesia and
    Intensive Care
Heart Institute "Niculae Stancioiu"
Cluj-Napoca, Romania

Crina Sufana
Pediatric Clinic No 1
Emergency Clinical Hospital for Children
Cluj-Napoca, Romania

Ayse Sulu
Department of Pediatric Cardiology
Eskisehir Osmangazi University
Eskisehir, Turkey

Raluca Tomoaia
Cardiology Department
Rehabilitation Hospital
and
4th Department of Internal Medicine
"Iuliu Hatieganu" University of Medicine
    and Pharmacy Cluj-Napoca
Cluj-Napoca, Romania

Camelia Vidrea
Neonatology Department
Regina Maria Hospital
Cluj-Napoca, Romania

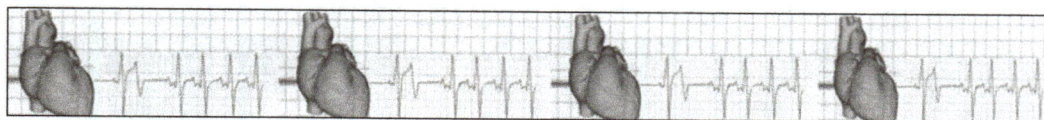

Case 1 Asymptomatic Outflow Tract Ventricular Tachycardia

Crina Sufana and Daniela Iacob

CLINICAL CASE

A 14-year-old asymptomatic girl who played baseball and football was evaluated for sport competitions. She had no complaints of palpitations or dyspnea. Frequent premature ventricular contractions (PVCs) were found in the electrocardiogram (ECG) in the form of ventricular bigeminy. Her heart rate was 80 bpm. Her blood pressure was normal: 100/60 mmHg. Echocardiography showed normal heart chambers with a normal left ventricular ejection fraction of 65%, and normal dimensions for the right ventricle and right ventricular outflow tract. A Holter ECG was performed by the pediatric cardiologist, which showed high burden PVCs. Her blood levels of vitamin D were low at 28 ng/ml 25-OH vitamin D; the rest of the biochemical values being normal. She had no treatment.

Info pacient		
Sex:	Feminin	
Greutatea:		
Inaltime:		
Fumător:		
Pacemaker:	prezent	

Info înregistrări		
DEMAREAZA:	20.12.2024, 11:50	
Finalizare:	21.12.2024, 11:43	
Durata:	23:52	
Iesiri:	12	
Calitate semnal:	100%	

Personalul de specialitate
Medic:
Tehnician:

Medicatie

Motiv admitere

Anamneza

Concluzie

Ritm cardiac			
Total bătăi		125 889	(0% paced)
HR max / min		154 / 49 bpm	
Media HR		Ø 88 bpm	
HR Max / Min Sinus		154 / 49 bpm	
Media HR (Treaz/Adormit)		94 / 77 bpm	
Index circadian		1,22	
Tahicardie / Bradicardie		18 % / < 1 %	

Pauze		
RR Max	1 578 ms	
Pauze (>2000ms)	0	

Fibrilație atrială / Flutter atrial		
Total AF	4	(< 1%)
AF HR Max	96 bpm	
Cel mai lung AF	Ø 69 bpm	00:03:03

Bradicardie		
Cea mai mică	Ø 51 bpm	12 sec
Cea mai mare	Ø 53 bpm	14 sec

ST		
St ridicare max	0,25 mV	II
ST depresurizare max	-0,20 mV	aVR

Ectopie ventriculară			
V Total		66247	(53%)
V / Ora Max		4 319	pe oră
Episoade Tahicardie V		1 075	Σ 01:12:16
Cea mai rapidă Tahicardie V		Ø 144 bpm	2 sec
V Cea mai lungă secvență		Ø 99 bpm	00:04:23
Triplete / Execută		2597	Σ 8553 bătăi
Cuplete		5500	Σ 11000 bătăi
Bigeminism		11722	Σ 38808 bătăi
Trigeminism		4855	Σ 14113 bătăi

Ectopie supraventriculară		
S Tot	0	(< 1%)
Episoade Tahicardie SV	-	
Cea mai rapidă Tahicardie SV	-	
S Cea mai lungă secvență	-	
Triplete / Execută	0	Σ 0 bătăi
Cuplete	0	Σ 0 bătăi

Figure 1.1 Summary table shows the highest and lowest rate during 24 hours monitoring (154/49 bpm); PVC burden is very high at 66247/24 hours.

DOI: 10.1201/9781003545040-1

7	Ectopii						Run-uri V sunt compuse din mai puţin de 5 bătăi. Run-uri S sunt compuse din mai puţin de 20 bătăi.																
Interval		TOTAL	act.	HR[bpm]			Bătăi V					Modele V			Bătăi S					Modele S			Pauza	Buton
De la	Dur.	Batai	[%]	Min	Media	Max	∑	Individu	Bi	Tri	Cvadr	Cupl	Tripl	Ruleaz	∑	Individu	Bi	Tri	Cvadr	Cupl	Tripl	Ruleaz		
(1) 11:50	00:09	960	21,00	84	106	136	577	0	68	55	3	32	15	3	0	0	0	0	0	0	0	0	0	0
(1) 12:00	01:00	6155	15,00	81	103	154	3262	0	792	352	6	430	105	67	0	0	0	0	0	0	0	0	0	0
(1) 13:00	01:00	6336	26,00	71	106	132	3227	0	871	476	7	474	71	41	0	0	0	0	0	0	0	0	0	0
(1) 14:00	01:00	6042	15,00	77	101	132	4285	0	786	143	6	376	107	84	0	0	0	0	0	0	0	0	0	0
(1) 15:00	01:00	6065	15,00	69	101	134	3502	0	514	119	24	231	129	42	0	0	0	0	0	0	0	0	0	0
(1) 16:00	01:00	6831	25,00	90	114	149	4319	5	904	347	20	570	58	77	0	0	0	0	0	0	0	0	0	0
(1) 17:00	01:00	6053	21,00	84	101	144	3907	4	974	232	4	580	91	84	0	0	0	0	0	0	0	0	0	0
(1) 18:00	01:00	6559	35,00	89	109	142	3820	7	969	278	29	621	106	73	0	0	0	0	0	0	0	0	0	0
(1) 19:00	01:00	5747	19,00	74	96	131	3160	3	651	173	20	402	73	62	0	0	0	0	0	0	0	0	0	0
(1) 20:00	01:00	5182	17,00	66	86	135	2744	13	407	156	31	117	105	35	0	0	0	0	0	0	0	0	0	0
(1) 21:00	01:00	4914	12,00	65	82	138	2524	1	261	92	21	64	51	16	0	0	0	0	0	0	0	0	0	0
(1) 22:00	01:00	4905	12,00	62	82	120	2447	0	289	126	24	69	85	11	0	0	0	0	0	0	0	0	0	0
(1) 23:00	01:00	5368	16,00	65	89	132	2450	1	443	265	14	175	52	22	0	0	0	0	0	0	0	0	0	0
(2) 00:00	01:00	4885	8,00	60	81	121	3160	2	454	158	28	121	113	26	0	0	0	0	0	0	0	0	0	0
(2) 01:00	01:00	4347	4,00	64	72	130	2820	1	429	42	30	36	269	8	0	0	0	0	0	0	0	0	0	0
(2) 02:00	01:00	4562	4,00	57	76	129	1962	1	199	150	7	28	0	2	0	0	0	0	0	0	0	0	0	0
(2) 03:00	01:00	4701	5,00	66	78	105	1847	0	489	447	2	88	4	1	0	0	0	0	0	0	0	0	0	0
(2) 04:00	01:00	4830	7,00	58	81	142	1892	7	273	230	26	100	21	2	0	0	0	0	0	0	0	0	0	0
(2) 05:00	01:00	4092	5,00	53	68	116	1278	88	84	56	77	26	8	0	0	0	0	0	0	0	0	0	0	0
(2) 06:00	01:00	4052	5,00	55	68	98	1259	85	23	220	88	289	0	0	0	0	0	0	0	0	0	0	0	0
(2) 07:00	01:00	3967	5,00	49	66	100	1240	31	161	115	128	53	17	5	0	0	0	0	0	0	0	0	0	0
(2) 08:00	01:00	4274	5,00	59	71	101	2003	35	398	207	97	204	195	23	0	0	0	0	0	0	0	0	0	0
(2) 09:00	01:00	4389	5,00	59	73	100	1601	16	357	117	240	29	21	0	0	0	0	0	0	0	0	0	0	0
(2) 10:00	01:00	6011	20,00	65	100	137	3481	10	522	178	15	184	106	54	0	0	0	0	0	0	0	0	0	0
(2) 11:00	00:43	4662	25,00	87	111	138	3480	1	404	121	4	201	33	24	0	0	0	0	0	0	0	0	0	0
Σ adormit	09:00	41742	7,00	53	77	142	19115	185	2683	1694	296	932	552	72	0	0	0	0	0	0	0	0	0	0
Σ treaz	14:52	84147	17,00	49	94	154	47132	122	9039	3161	655	4568	1283	690	0	0	0	0	0	0	0	0	0	0
TOTAL	23:52	125889	13,00	49	88	154	66247	307	11722	4855	951	5500	1835	762	0	0	0	0	0	0	0	0	0	0

Figure 1.2 Summary table shows the distribution of PVCs during daytime and nighttime. There is a high burden for each hour during the day and night.

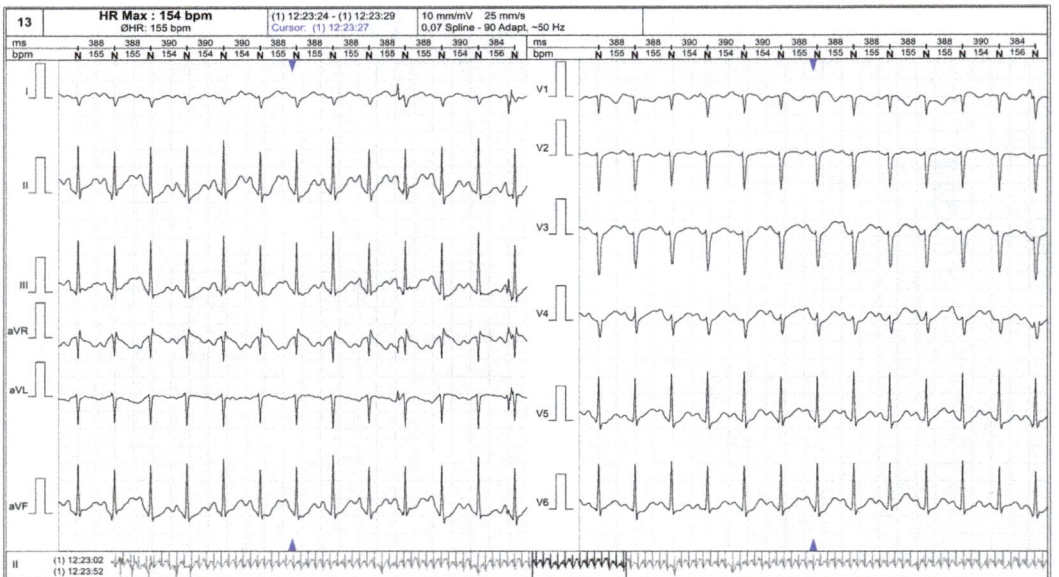

Figure 1.3 The image shows the highest rate during 24 hours monitoring; sinus rhythm is present with a rate of 154 bpm. No PVCs are present.

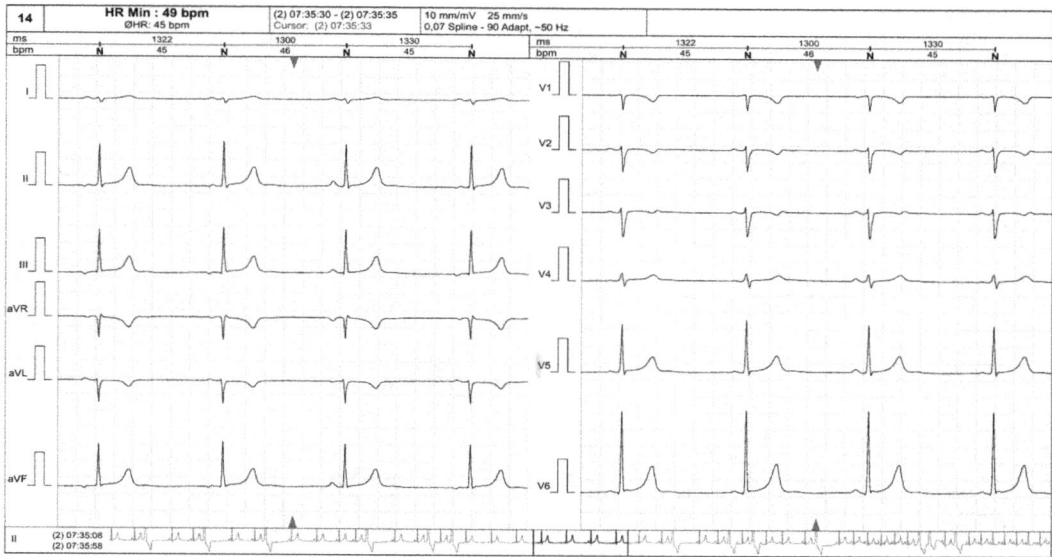

Figure 1.4 The tracing shows the lowest rate during monitoring; no PVC can be seen; sinus rhythm is present with a rate of 49 bpm.

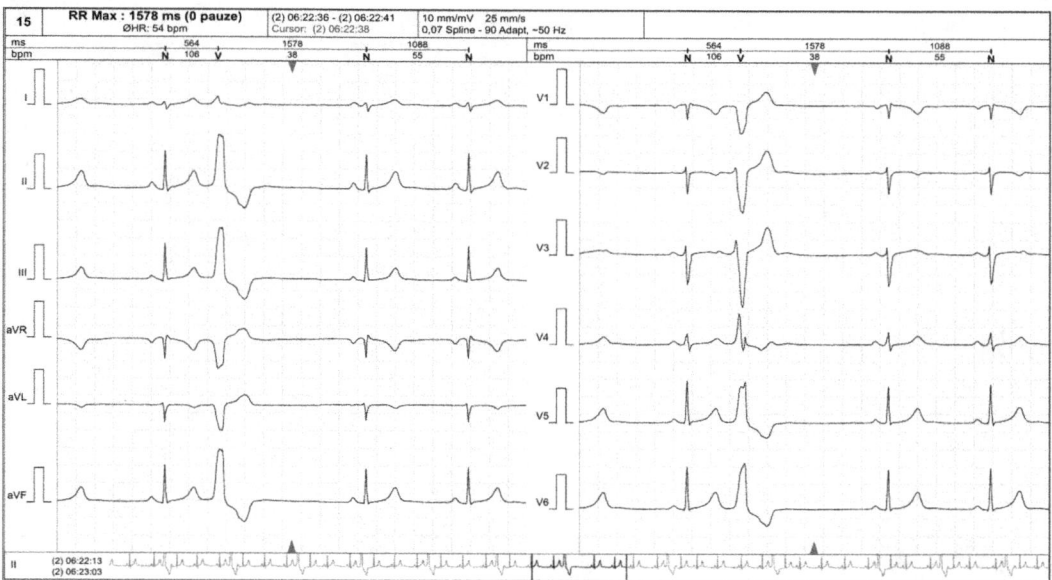

Figure 1.5 The tracing shows premature ventricular contractions. It has a left bundle branch block (LBBB) morphology with inferior axis (positive QRS in leads II, III and AVF), and precordial transition in lead V3. It is a mean PVC; compared to early PVCs and late PVCs it occurs after the T wave and before the next P wave.

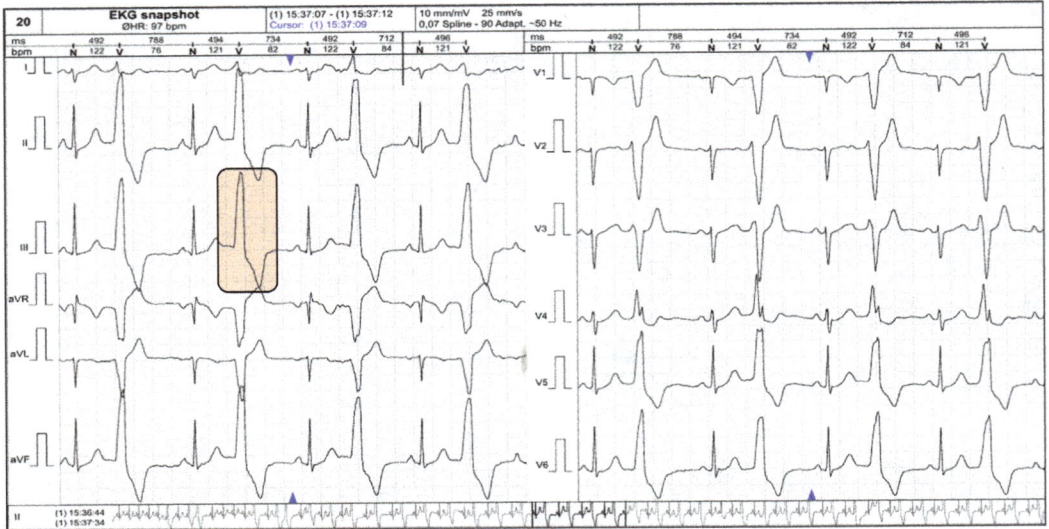

Figure 1.6 The tracing shows ventricular bigeminy. Every second beat is a ventricular premature contraction with an outflow tract morphology. The PVC is positive in the inferior leads: II, III and avF, suggesting a superior ventricular origin. However, in lead V2, the r wave in sinus rhythm is smaller than the r wave during PVC, suggesting an left ventricular outflow tract (LVOT) origin. An electrophysiological study could differentiate between a right ventricular outflow tract (RVOT) and an LVOT origin.

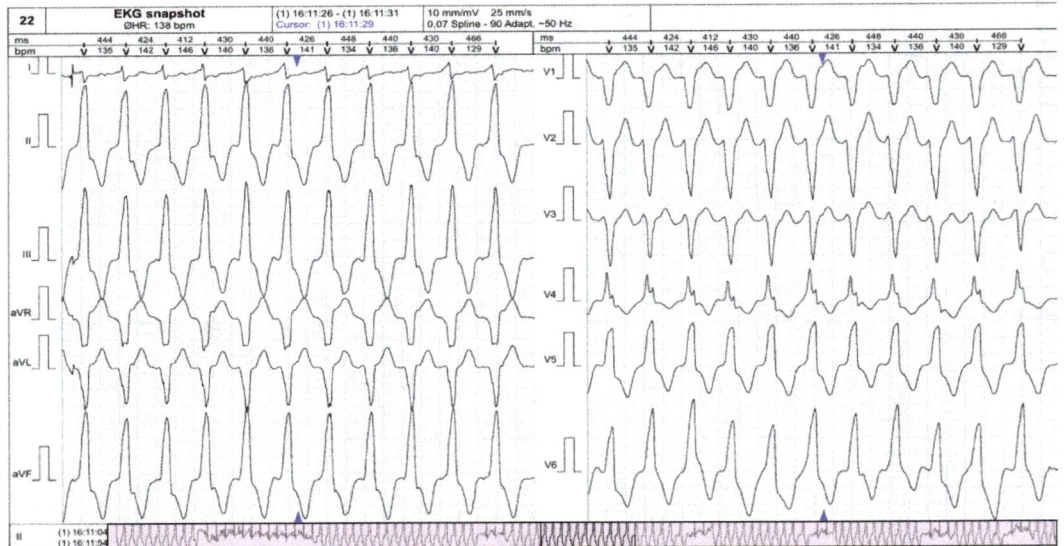

Figure 1.7 The tracing shows repeated episodes of nonsustained ventricular tachycardia (VT). The bottom line shows episodes of VT less than 30 seconds in duration, that resume with sinus rhythm. The RR interval during tachycardia is not regular.

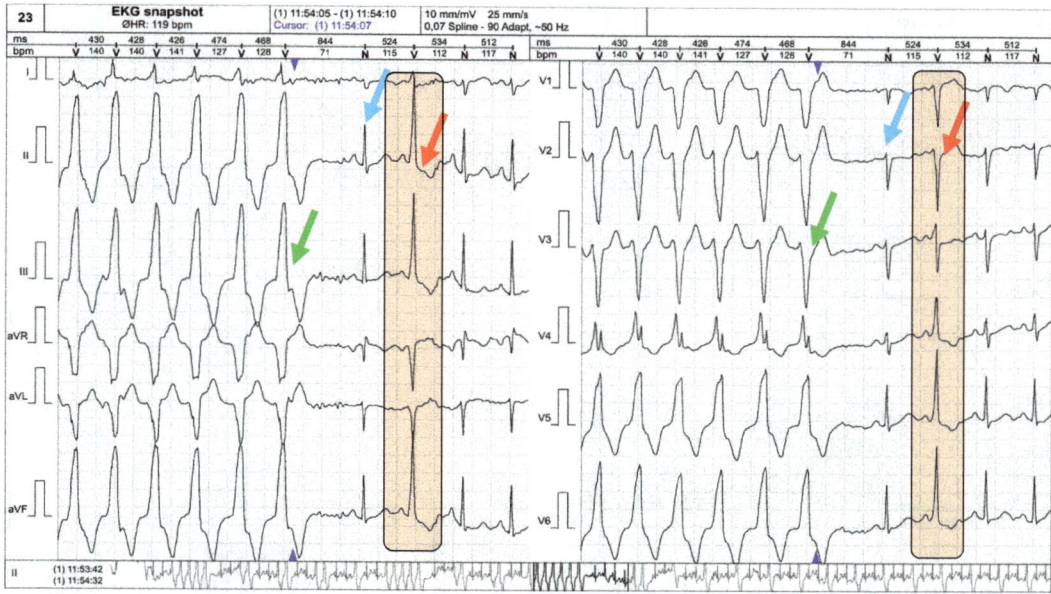

Figure 1.8 The tracing shows a fusion beat marked with a red arrow. It is a late PVC that occurs after the P wave. Ventricular activation through the normal conduction system fuses with ventricular activation determined by the abnormal outflow tract focus and produces an intermediate QRS. The T wave shows characteristics of both sinus beat and PVC beat: negative in leads V1, V2, positive in leads V3 to V6.

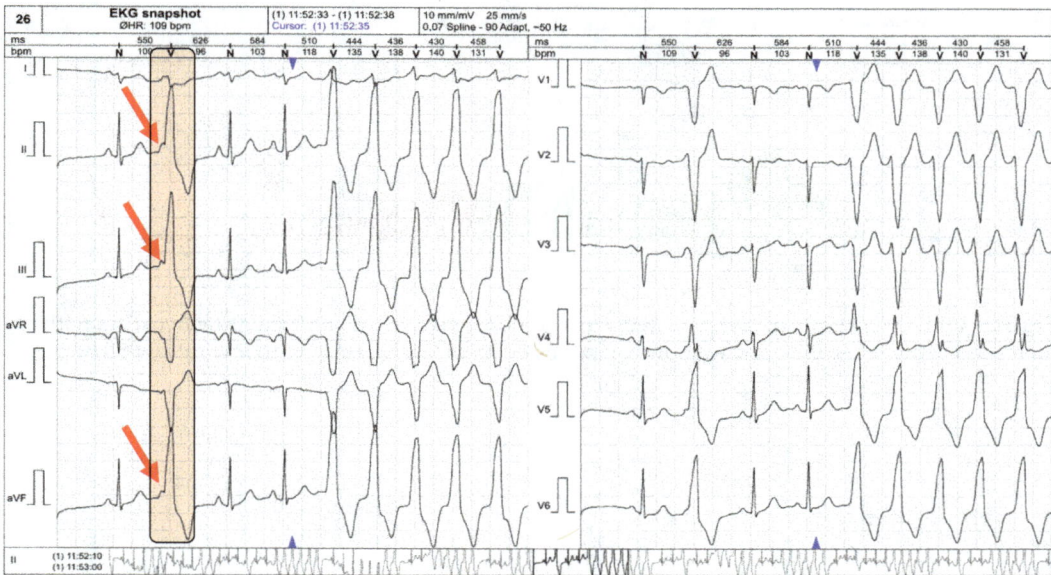

Figure 1.9 In this image late PVC occurs exactly on the P wave during the atrial activation, mimicking Wolff–Parkinson–White (WPW) pattern.

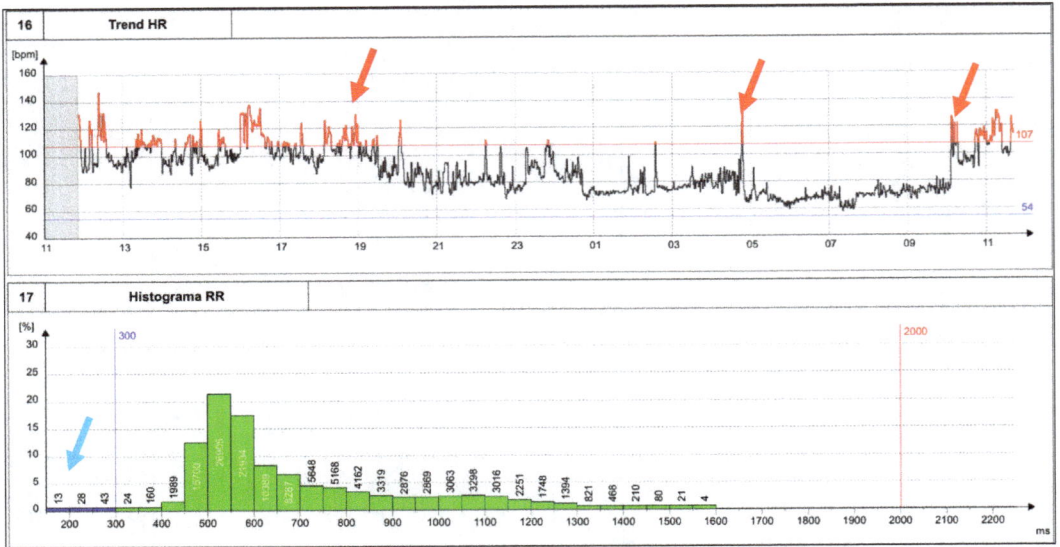

Figure 1.10 Heart rate trend and RR histogram. The red arrow marks episodes of ventricular tachycardia. Blue arrows mark short RR intervals, which also correspond to episodes of ventricular tachycardia.

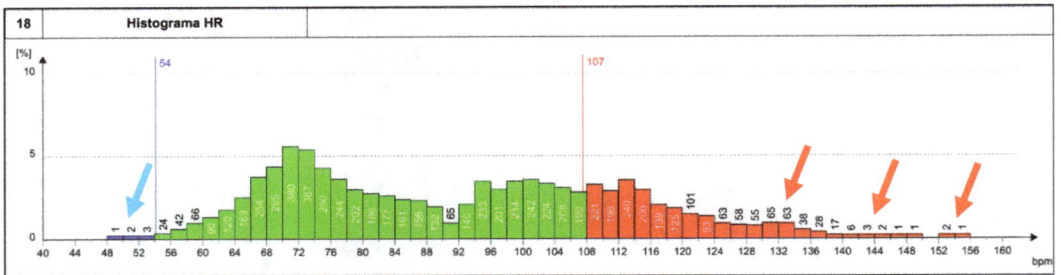

Figure 1.11 Heart rate histogram. Red arrows show episodes of ventricular tachycardia with increased heart rates. Blue arrow shows episodes of sinus bradycardia with low rates < 50 bpm.

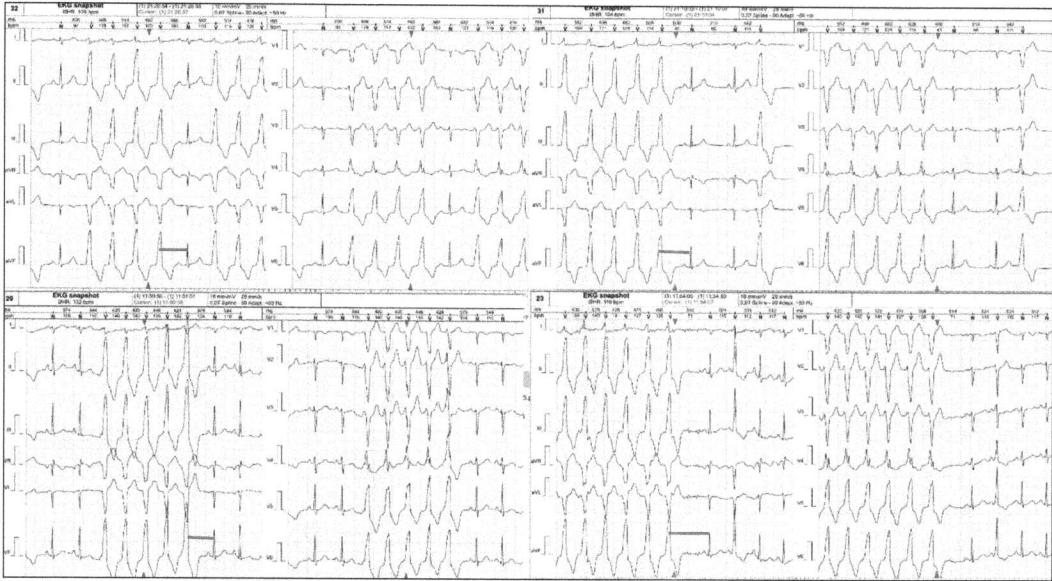

Figure 1.12 The image shows 4 instances when arrhythmia stops. The interval between the last VT beat and the first sinus beat is different, confirming the ventricular origin of the tachycardia.

HOLTER SUMMARY

The monitoring showed high burden PVCs 53% in an asymptomatic girl. PVCs were distributed equally throughout each 24-hour period. Bigeminy and repeated episodes of nonsustained ventricular tachycardia were also present. The patient continued to be asymptomatic during non-sustained ventricular tachycardias (NSVTs).

DISCUSSION

In structurally normal hearts, ventricular tachycardia typically originates from the outflow tracts. Outflow tract ectopy may present as frequent premature ventricular complexes, nonsustained ventricular tachycardia, and sustained ventricular tachycardia.

The outflow tracts are superior structures within the ventricles, and activation from these sites is oriented inferiorly, resulting in a QRS morphology that is positive in the inferior leads (II, III, and aVF) and negative in aVL and aVR. Typically, right ventricular origin results in left bundle branch block morphology, whereas left ventricular origin produces right bundle branch block morphology. However, lead V1 may improve the precision of ECG localization within the outflow and ventricles. Lead V1 is both a right-sided and an anterior lead. Given that the RVOT is positioned anteriorly and to the left within the human body, when the impulse initiates in the RVOT and propagates posteriorly and leftward, lead V1 is expected to have a QS morphology. In assessing outflow tract PVCs, the detection of a R wave in V1 should exclude anterior RVOT and prompt the examination of a more posterior origin, potentially generating an anteriorly directed vector toward lead V1. Consideration should be given to the posterior right ventricular outflow tract, the anterior left ventricular outflow tract, and the posterior left ventricular outflow tract. All these structures are posterior to the anterior RVOT and can lead to R waves in lead V1. A point of origin from the posterior right ventricular outflow tract may have a minimal r wave in lead V1. Given that the posterior right ventricular outflow tract is contiguous with the anterior left ventricular outflow tract, it is prudent to map the adjacent LVOT from the femoral artery to find an earlier activation location if the automated focus is localized towards the posterior RVOT. The aorta is a central structure inside the heart, with the left ventricular outflow tract positioned posterior to the right ventricular outflow tract. As a result, the left ventricular outflow tract is positioned distant from lead V1, allowing for the propagation of an LVOT origin toward V1, which generates a R wave in V1.

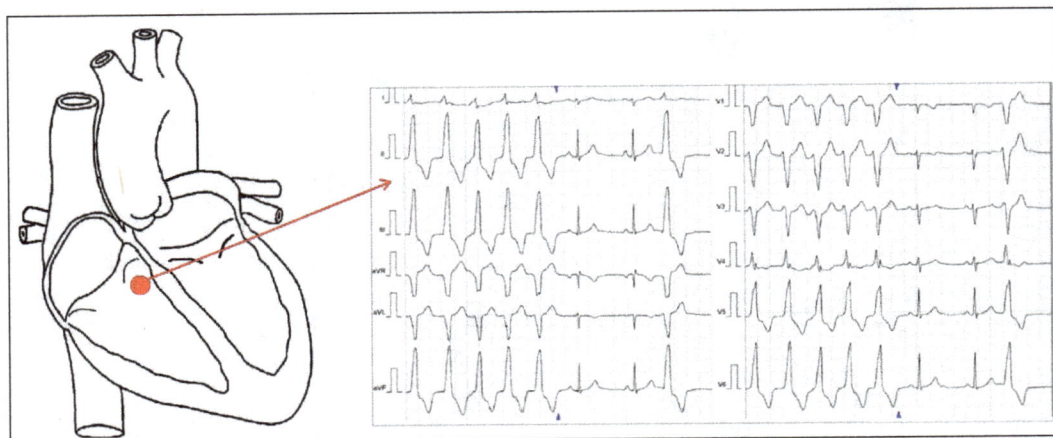

Figure 1.13 Schematic representation of RVOT ventricular arrhythmias. They have an LBBB morphology with inferior axis and ventricular transition after V3.

The prognosis for outflow tract ventricular arrhythmias is often favorable; nevertheless, there exists a risk of developing premature ventricular contraction-related cardiomyopathy if the PVCs burden exceeds 24% (some authors mention a burden of 10%).

Treatment for RVOT arrhythmias can include either disregarding any medication, offering antiarrhythmic drugs, or performing catheter ablation. The options are dependent on symptomatology, and the arrhythmia burden per 24 hours. Verapamil, which blocks calcium channels, can be an effective treatment by targeting calcium-dependent delayed after-depolarizations that may be the cause of an abnormal RVOT automatic focus. The automatic focus can also be treated with beta blockers. Class I C antiarrhythmic drugs like Propafenone or Flecainide can also be effective in reducing PVC burden. Catheter ablation of the autonomic focus is the most effective intervention for lowering ventricular arrhythmia burden. A comprehensive understanding of the anatomy of the RVOT improves the safety of right ventricular outflow tract VT ablation.

BIBLIOGRAPHY

1. Sehar N, Mears J, Bisco S, Patel S, Lachman N, Asirvatham SJ. Anatomic guidance for ablation: Atrial flutter, fibrillation, and outflow tract ventricular tachycardia. *Indian Pacing Electrophysiol J* 2010; 10(8):339–356.

2. Asirvatham SJ. Correlative anatomy for the invasive electrophysiologist: Outflow tract and supravalvar arrhythmia. *J Cardiovasc Electrophysiol* 2009; 20(8):955–968.

3. Srivathsan KS, Bunch TJ, Asirvatham SJ, Edwards WD, Friedman PA, Munger TM, et al. Mechanisms and utility of discrete great arterial potentials in the ablation of outflow tract ventricular arrhythmias. *Circ Arrhythm Electrophysiol* 2008; 1(1):30–38.

4. Tabatabaei N, Asirvatham SJ. Supravalvular arrhythmia: Identifying and ablating the substrate. *Circ Arrhythm Electrophysiol* 2009; 2(3):316–326.

5. Gard JJ, Asirvatham SJ. Outflow tract ventricular tachycardia. *Tex Heart Inst J* 2012; 39(4):526–528. PMID: 22949769; PMCID: PMC3423273.

6. Ward RC, van Zyl M, DeSimone CV. Idiopathic ventricular tachycardia. *J Clin Med* 25 January 2023; 12(3):930. doi: 10.3390/jcm12030930. PMID: 36769578; PMCID: PMC9918172.

7. Farzaneh-Far A, Lerman BB. Idiopathic ventricular outflow tract tachycardia. *Heart* 2005 February; 91(2):136–138. doi: 10.1136/hrt.2004.033795. PMID: 15657214; PMCID: PMC1768719.

8. Bera D, Saggu D, Yalagudri S, Kadel JK, Sarkar R, Devidutta S, Christopher J, Pavri B, Narasimhan C. Outflow-tract ventricular tachycardia: Can 12 lead ECG during sinus rhythm identify underlying cardiac sarcoidosis? *Indian Pacing Electrophysiol J.* 2020 May–June; 20(3):83–90. doi: 10.1016/j.ipej.2020.02.003. Epub 2020 Feb 29. PMID: 32119909; PMCID: PMC7244880.

9. Lu YY, Chen YC, Lin YK, Chen SA, Chen YJ. Electrical and structural insights into right ventricular outflow tract arrhythmogenesis. *Int J Mol Sci.* 2023 July 22; 24(14):11795. doi: 10.3390/ijms241411795. PMID: 37511554; PMCID: PMC10380666.

10. Fuenmayor AJ. Treatment or cure of right ventricular outflow tract tachycardia. *J Atr Fibrillation.* 2014 June 30; 7(1):1038. doi: 10.4022/jafib.1038. PMID: 27957079; PMCID: PMC5135148.

11. Kanei Y, Friedman M, Ogawa N, Hanon S, Lam P, Schweitzer P. Frequent premature ventricular complexes originating from the right ventricular outflow tract are associated with left ventricular dysfunction. *Ann Noninvasive Electrocardiol.* 2008 Jan.; 13(1):81–85. doi: 10.1111/j.1542-474X.2007.00204.x. PMID: 18234010; PMCID: PMC6932157.

12. Fonseca M, Parreira L, Farinha JM, Marinheiro R, Esteves A, Gonçalves S, Caria R. Premature ventricular contractions of the right ventricular outflow tract: is there an incipient underlying disease? New insights from a speckle tracking echocardiography study. *Indian Pacing Electrophysiol J.* 2021 May–Jun; 21(3):147–152. doi: 10.1016/j.ipej.2021.02.007. Epub 2021 Feb. 16. PMID: 33607220; PMCID: PMC8116808.

13. Clark BC, Ceresnak SR, Pass RH, Nappo L, Sumihara K, Dubin AM, Motonaga K, Moak JP. Can the 12-lead ECG distinguish RVOT from aortic cusp PVCs in pediatric patients? *Pacing Clin Electrophysiol.* 2020 Mar.; 43(3):308–313. doi: 10.1111/pace.13885. PMID: 32040211.

14. Fries B, Johnson V, Rutsatz W, Schmitt J, Bogossian H. Lokalisation ventrikulärer Extrasystolen im 12-Kanal-EKG [Localization of ventricular premature contractions by 12-lead ECG]. *Herzschrittmacherther Elektrophysiol.* 2021 Mar; 32(1):21–26. German. doi: 10.1007/s00399-021-00746-7. Epub 2021 Feb. 3. PMID: 33533995.

15. Yamada T. Twelve-lead electrocardiographic localization of idiopathic premature ventricular contraction origins. *J Cardiovasc Electrophysiol.* 2019 Nov.; 30(11):2603–2617. doi: 10.1111/jce.14152. Epub 2019 Sep 22. PMID: 31502322.

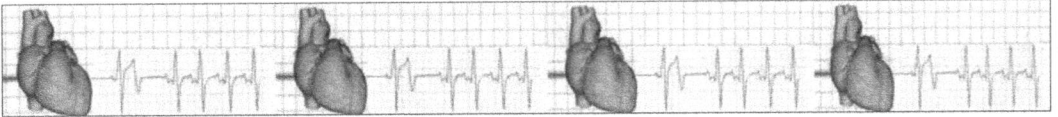

Case 2 Tuberous Sclerosis with Ventricular Arrhythmia

Cecilia Lazea, Crina Sufana, and Sabina Istratoaie

CLINICAL CASE

A 3-year-old girl was diagnosed with tuberous sclerosis and left ventricular tumors. She presented episodes of large QRS tachycardia detected during Holter ECG monitoring. A treatment with beta blockers was initiated following the confirmation of the arrhythmia, consisting of 2 × 10 mg Propranolol per day, resulting in the total remission of arrhythmic episodes.

Concluzie

Ritm cardiac		
Total bătăi	153 489	(0% paced)
HR max / min	**160 / 65 bpm**	
Media HR	**Ø 106 bpm**	
HR Max / Min Sinus	160 / 65 bpm	
Media HR (Treaz/Adormit)	114 / 94 bpm	
Index circadian	1,21	
Tahicardie / Bradicardie	13 % / < 1 %	

Pauze		
RR Max	**1 456 ms**	
Pauze (>2000ms)	**0**	

Fibrilaţie atrială / Flutter atrial		
Total AF	-	
AF HR Max	0 bpm	
Cel mai lung AF	-	

Bradicardie		
Cea mai mică	Ø 73 bpm	34 sec
Cea mai mare	Ø 73 bpm	34 sec

ST		
St ridicare max	6,68 mV	V1
ST depresurizare max	-2,24 mV	V1

Ectopie ventriculară		
V Total	0	(< 1%)
V / Ora Max	0	pe oră
Episoade Tahicardie V		-
Cea mai rapidă Tahicardie V		-
V Cea mai lungă secvenţă		-
Triplete / Execută	0 Σ 0 bătăi	
Cuplete	0 Σ 0 bătăi	
Bigeminism	0 Σ 0 bătăi	
Trigeminism	0 Σ 0 bătăi	

Ectopie supraventriculară		
S Tot	6	(< 1%)
Episoade Tahicardie SV		-
Cea mai rapidă Tahicardie SV		-
S Cea mai lungă secvenţă		-
Triplete / Execută	0 Σ 0 bătăi	
Cuplete	0 Σ 0 bătăi	

Figure 2.1 The summary page shows that the highest rate was 160 bpm and the lowest rate was 65 bpm. There was a low percentage of PACs < 1%/24 hours.

DOI: 10.1201/9781003545040-2

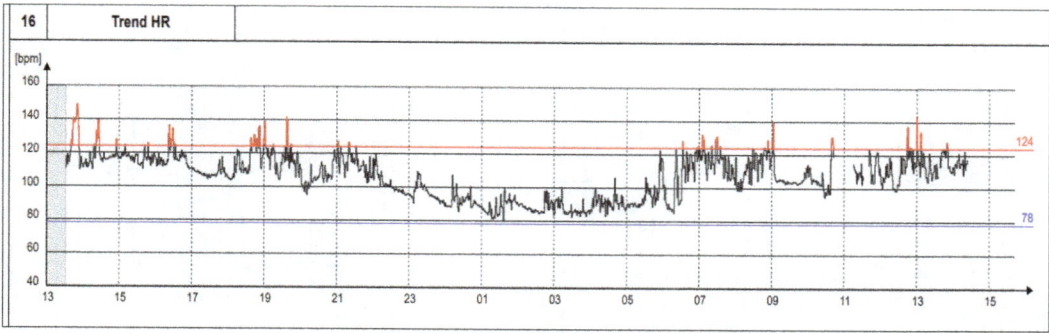

Figure 2.2 The heart rate trend shows the mean heart rate during the 24-hour period of monitoring. The red color marks rates above 124 bpm.

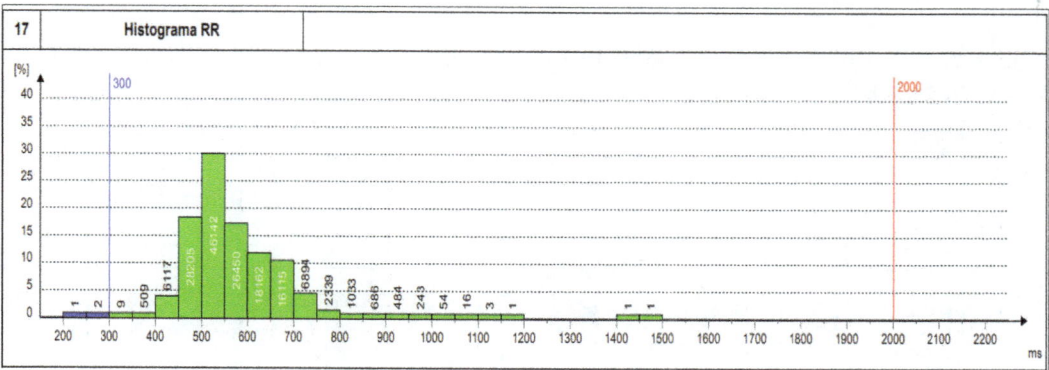

Figure 2.3 The RR histogram shows short RR intervals 200–300 ms corresponding to episodes of tachycardia and increased RR intervals 1400–1500 ms corresponding to pauses in the cardiac electrical activity.

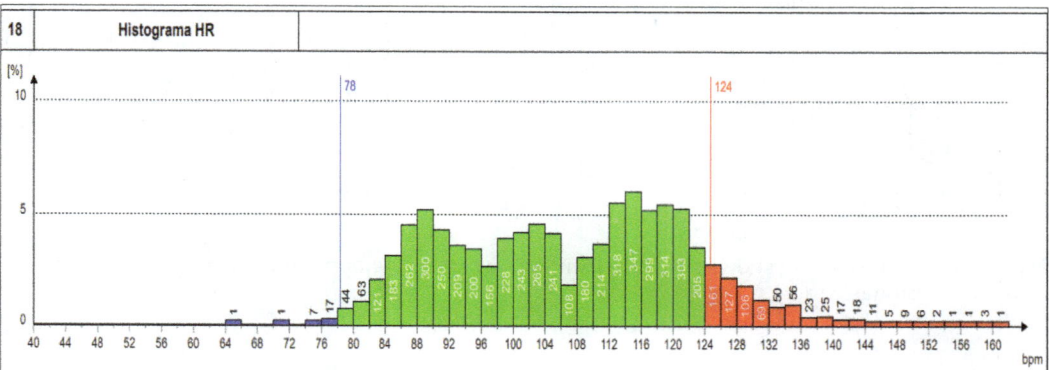

Figure 2.4 The HR histogram shows the heart rate tracing, including the heart rate distribution, with episodes of tachycardia of up to 160 bpm.

11

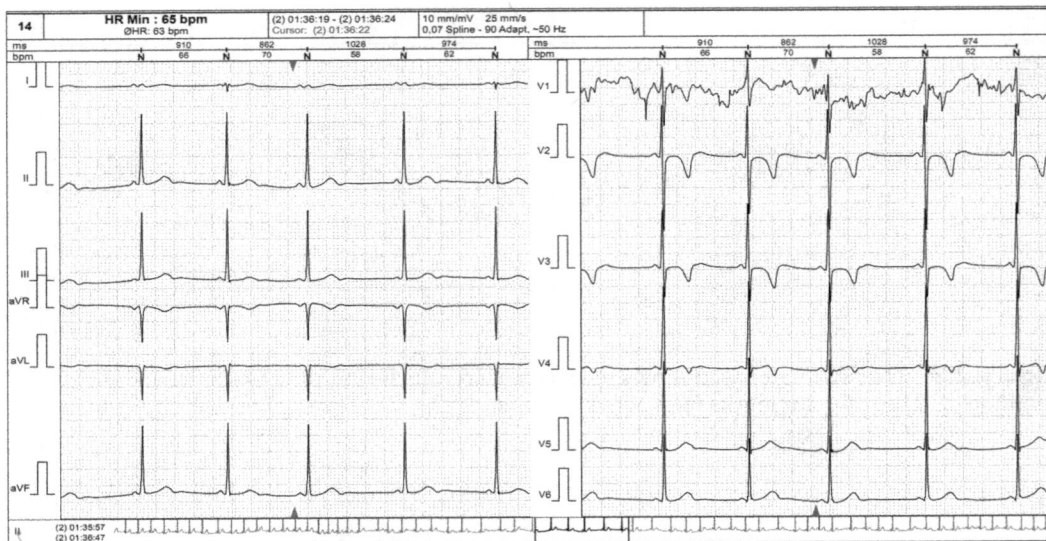

Figure 2.5 The tracing shows sinus rhythm with a rate of 65 bpm and negative T waves in lead V1–V3, biphasic in V4.

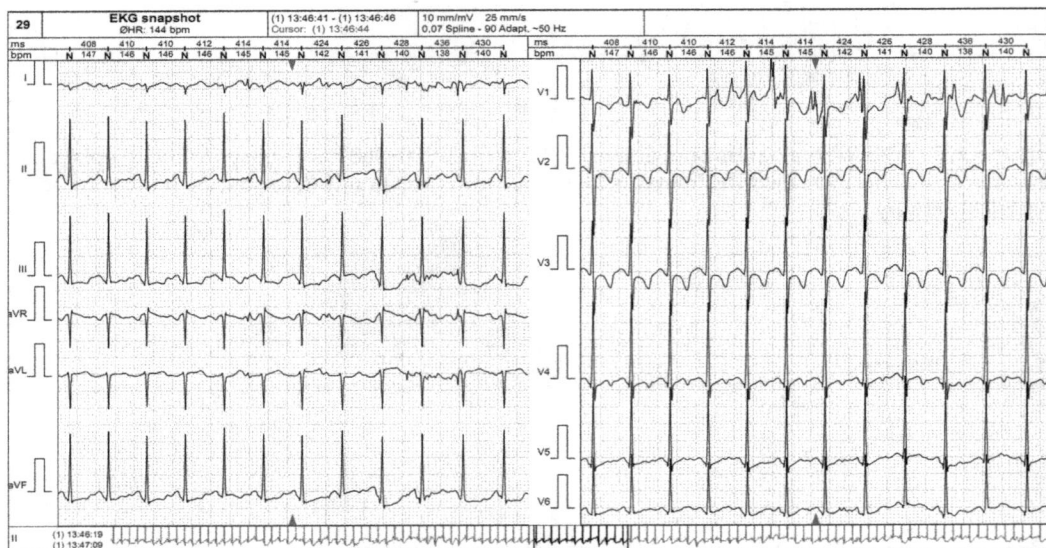

Figure 2.6 The tracing shows sinus rhythm with a rate of 144 bpm and negative T waves in lead V1–V3, biphasic in V4.

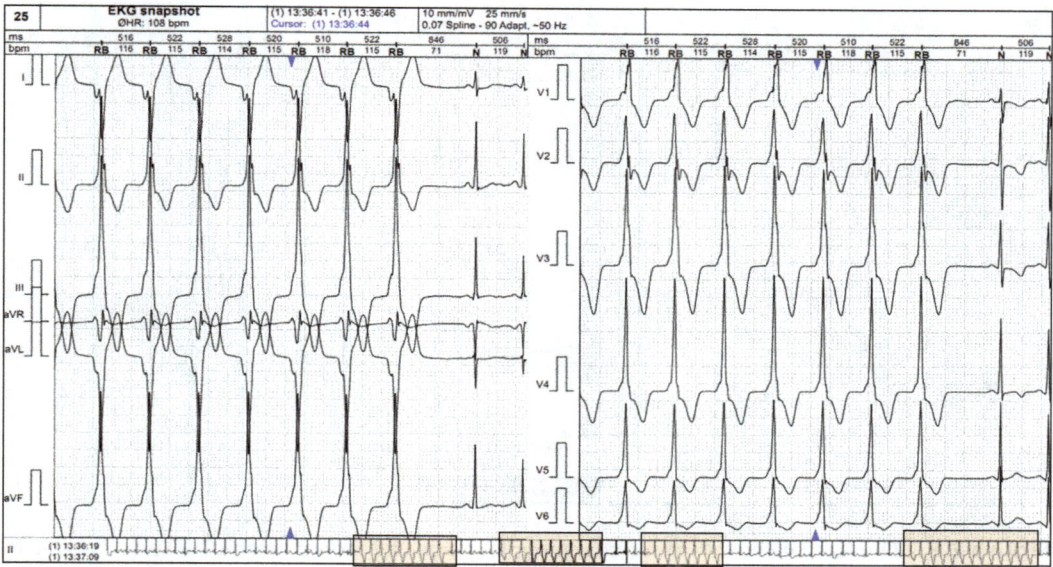

Figure 2.7 The tracing shows an episode of nonsustained large QRS tachycardia, followed by sinus rhythm and again episodes of tachycardia (bottom).

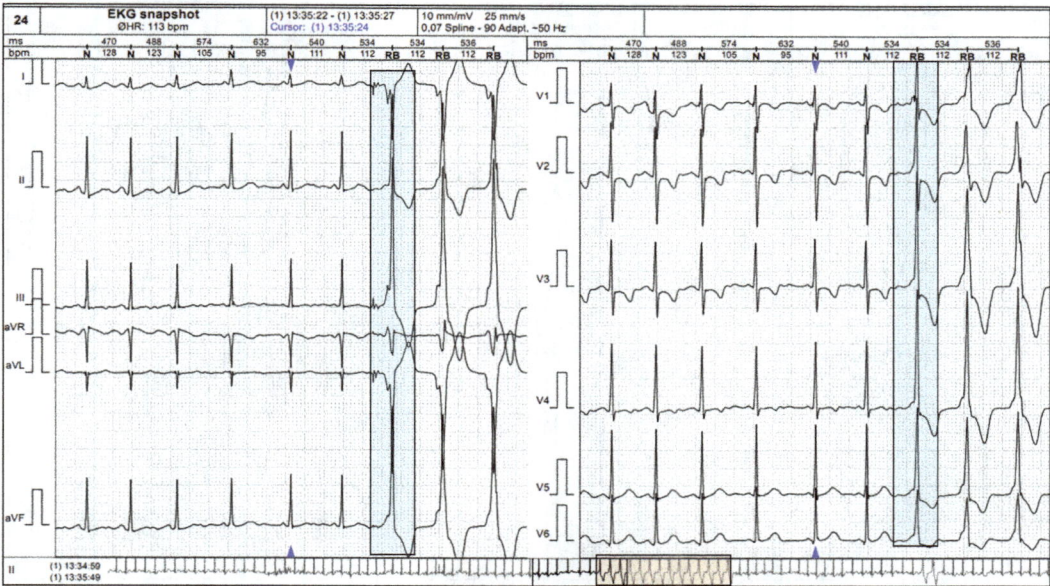

Figure 2.8 The tracing shows the first 3 beats of an episode of nonsustained ventricular tachycardia. The first beat marked with a blue square is a fusion beat between normal sinus rhythm and PVC, followed by 13 beats of monomorphic VT.

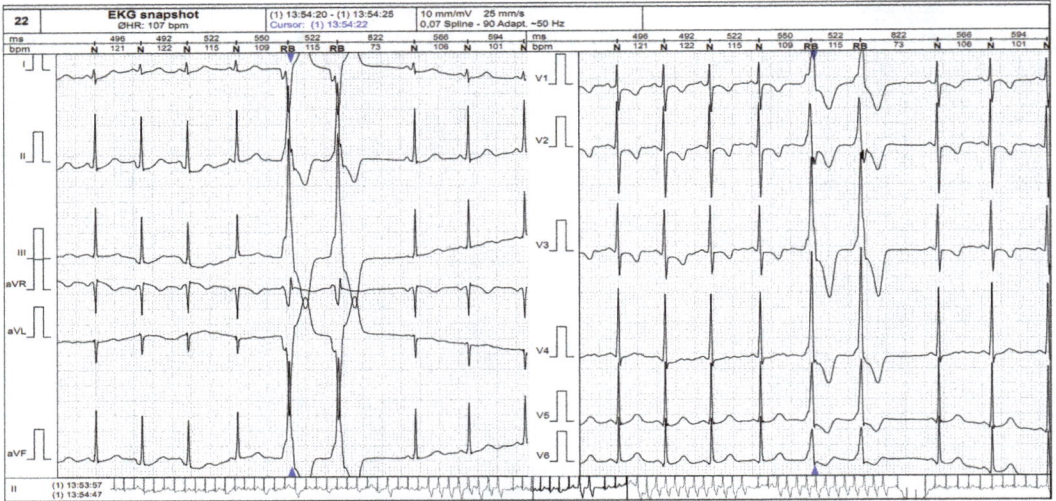

Figure 2.9   The tracing shows a ventricular couplet made of 2 monomorphic PVCs. No visible P wave is present inside the couplet.

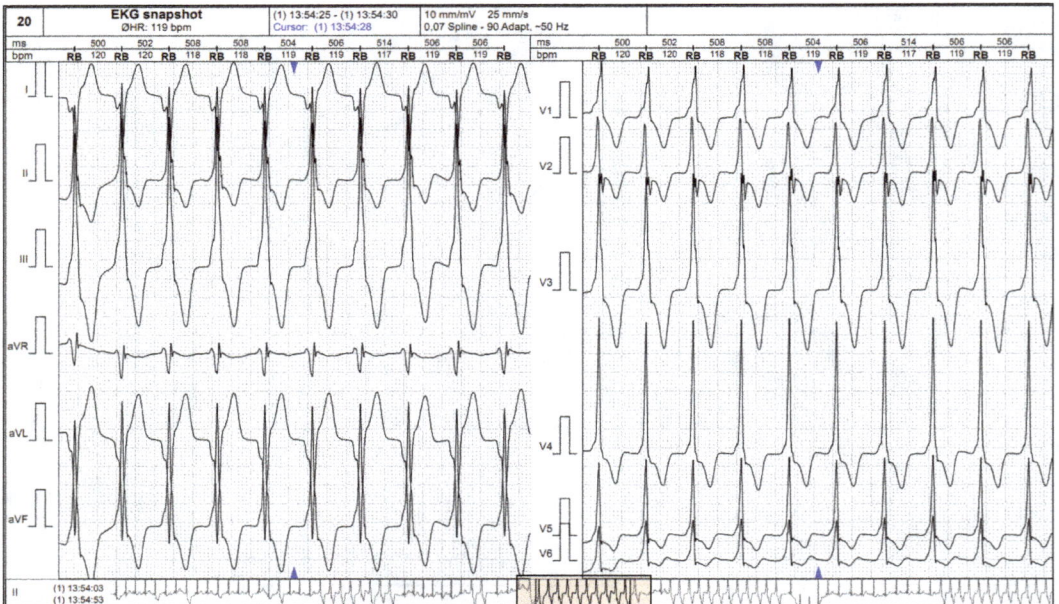

Figure 2.10   The tracing shows an episode of nonsustained ventricular tachycardia (12 consecutive beats). No visible P wave is present inside the VT episode. Positive concordance of QRS complexes is observed in the precordial leads, which can be present both in ventricular tachycardia and in the Wolff-Parkinson-White pattern.

HOLTER SUMMARY

The monitoring indicates the presence of a large QRS tachycardia, without visible P waves, suggesting ventricular tachycardia due to tuberous sclerosis lesions situated at the level of the lateral mitral valve. The QRS is large, with positive concordance in the precordial leads, positive QRS in the inferior lead and negative QRS in the lateral leads: I and avL. A differential diagnosis should be made with ventricular preexcitation.

DISCUSSION

Tuberous sclerosis is a hereditary disease characterized by a very diverse phenotype that can impact many organs. The central nervous system findings include the triad of cognitive impairment, facial angiofibromas, and seizures. Tuberous sclerosis is defined by the presence of extensive hamartomas, which are aberrant proliferations of normal tissues. Cardiac rhabdomyomas are hamartomatous lesions or benign tumors formed by cardiac myocytes, and they constitute the classic newborn presentation of cardiac abnormalities in tuberous sclerosis. Other heart manifestations include arrhythmias, which manifest later in life. The genes TSC1 and TSC2, which encode hamartin and tuberin, were identified as the primary cause of tuberous sclerosis.

Heart tumors are uncommon; nonetheless, rhabdomyomas represent the predominant primary heart tumor in pediatric patients. Cardiac rhabdomyomas often develop between 20 and 30 weeks of gestation. Tumors are identified more often in prenatal echocardiography than in postnatal echocardiography, leading to greater accuracy in the assessment of fetal echocardiograms. Fetal cardiac rhabdomyoma may manifest in utero as an abnormal mass on ultrasonography, cardiac arrhythmia, ericardial effusion, or hydrops fetalis. Cardiac rhabdomyomas can grow during the second part of gestation, a phenomenon attributable to maternal changes in hormones linked to pregnancy. Cardiac rhabdomyomas often do not produce symptoms or hemodynamic impairment during the gestational period, but may manifest symptoms shortly after birth of the baby or within the first year of life. Tumors may block inflow or outflow tracts, potentially resulting in ventricular dysfunction with low ejection fraction and heart failure.

Cardiac rhabdomyomas are often well-defined and non-encapsulated. Micropathology reveals aberrant myocyte architecture, with tumor sizes varying from a few millimeters to several centimeters. Tumors are generally situated in the ventricles, resulting in ventricular arrhythmias,

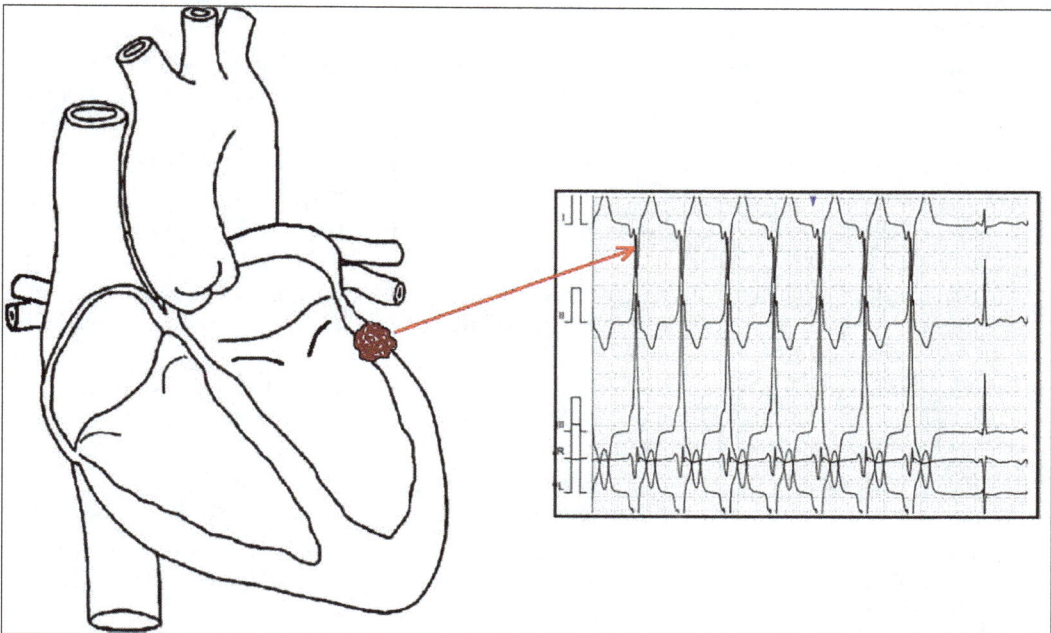

Figure 2.11   A cardiac tumor situated near the lateral mitral ring might lead to episodes of ventricular tachycardia with positive concordance in the precordial leads, negative QRS in lateral limb leads I and avL and also positive QRS in inferior leads.

or they may impair ventricular function by reducing the ejection fraction or disrupting the valve function, causing outflow obstruction (pseudo-mitral valve stenosis). Cardiac rhabdomyomas are generally observed as numerous, echogenic, nodular masses situated within the ventricular myocardium, occasionally extending into the ventricular chamber. Cardiac rhabdomyomas spontaneously regress in the majority of patients within the first year of life, leading to a decreased incidence in patients with tuberous sclerosis beyond the age of two years.

Ventricular tachycardia may result from tumors situated in the ventricles. Ventricular arrhythmias typically first appear either prenatally or within the initial months of life. The association of ventricular intramural rhabdomyomas with ventricular arrhythmias is uncommon in adolescents as those tumors regress with age. The literature review indicates cases where cardiac rhabdomyomas are associated with ventricular arrhythmia or sudden death. In the majority of patients, symptoms started at an early age or even prenatally. Due to the tendency of rhabdomyomas to regress, conservative treatment is typically adequate in most instances.

Two mechanisms have been identified for severe arrhythmias linked to rhabdomyoma: (1) a reentry circuit at the interface with normal myocardium may induce sustained monomorphic ventricular tachycardia; (2) a segment of the intracardiac tumor located on the mitral or tricuspid annulus can facilitate rapid conduction between the atria and ventricles, resulting in ventricular preexcitation. Consequently, radiofrequency ablation is feasible in certain patients with accessory pathways abnormally created by the intracardiac tumor.

Initial treatment with antiarrhythmic drugs such as Propranolol, Sotalol, and Amiodarone has demonstrated efficacy in managing ventricular tachycardia. ICD implantation is a viable option in the absence of response to antiarrhythmic medications. Resection of the tumor may totally reduce symptoms if surgically accessible.

BIBLIOGRAPHY

1. Nir A, Tajik AJ, Freeman WK, Seward JB, Offord KP, Edwards WD, Mair DD, Gomez MR. Tuberous sclerosis and cardiac rhabdomyoma. *Am J Cardiol.* 1995; 76:419–421.

2. Jacobs JP, Konstantakos AK, Holland FW, II, Herskowitz K, Ferrer PL, Perryman RA. Surgical treatment for cardiac rhabdomyomas in children. *Ann Thorac Surg.* 1994; 58:1552–1555.

3. Mlczoch E, Hanslik A, Luckner D, Kitzmüller E, Prayer D, Michel-Behnke I. Prenatal diagnosis of a gigantic cardiac rhabdomyoma in tuberous sclerosis complex – a new therapeutic option with everolimus. *Ultrasound Obstet Gynecol.* 2014; 45:618–621.

4. De Rosa G, De Carolis MP, Pardeo M, Bersani I, Tempera A, De Nisco A, Caforio L, Romagnoli C, Piastra M. Neonatal emergencies associated with cardiac rhabdomyomas: An 8-year experience. *Fetal Diagn Ther.* 2011; 29:169–177.

5. Foster ED, Spooner EW, Farina MA, Shaher RM, Alley RD. Cardiac rhabdomyoma in the neonate: Surgical management. *Ann Thorac Surg.* 1984; 37:249–253.

6. Shepherd CW, Gomez MR, Crowson CS. Causes of death in patients with tuberous sclerosis. *Mayo Clin Proc.* 1991; 66:792–796.

7. Enbergs A, Borggrefe M, Kurlemann G, Fahrenkamp A, Scheld HH, Jehle J, Breithardt G. Ventricular tachycardia caused by cardiac rhabdomyoma in a young adult with tuberous sclerosis. *Am Heart J.* 1996; 132:1263–1265.

8. Kathare PA, Muthuswamy KS, Sadasivan J, Calumbar N, Koneti NR. Incessant ventricular tachycardia due to multiple cardiac rhabdomyomas in an infant with tuberous sclerosis. *Indian Heart J.* 2013; 65:111–113.

9. Scurry J, Watkins A, Acton C, Drew J. Tachyarrhythmia, cardiac rhabdomyomata and fetal hydrops in a premature infant with tuberous sclerosis. *J Paediatr Child Health.* 1992; 28:260–262.

10. Hirakubo Y, Ichihashi K, Shiraishi H, Momoi MY. Ventricular tachycardia in a neonate with prenatally diagnosed cardiac tumors: A case with tuberous sclerosis. *Pediatr Cardiol.* 2005; 26:655–657.

11. Chao AS, Chao A, Wang TH, Chang YC, Chang YL, Hsieh CC, Lien R, Su WJ. Outcome of antenatally diagnosed cardiac rhabdomyoma: Case series and a meta-analysis. *Ultrasound Obstet Gynecol.* 2008; 31:289–295.

12. Degueldre SC, Chockalingam P, Mivelaz Y, Di Bernardo S, Pfammatter JP, Barrea C, Sekarski N, Jeannet PY, Fouron JC, Vial Y, Meijboom EJ. Considerations for prenatal counselling of patients with cardiac rhabdomyomas based on their cardiac and neurologic outcomes. *Cardiol Young.* 2010; 20:18–24.

13. Black MD, Kadletz M, Smallhorn JF, Freedom RM. Cardiac rhabdomyomas and obstructive left heart disease: Histologically but not functionally benign. *Ann Thorac Surg.* 1998; 65:1388–1390.

14. Tworetzky W, McElhinney DB, Margossian R, Moon-Grady AJ, Sallee D, Goldmuntz E, van der Velde ME, Silverman NH, Allan LD. Association between cardiac tumors and tuberous sclerosis in the fetus and neonate. *Am J Cardiol.* 2003; 92:487–489.

15. Shen Q, Shen J, Qiao Z, Yao Q, Huang G, Hu X. Cardiac rhabdomyomas associated with tuberous sclerosis complex in children. *From presentation to outcome. Herz.* 2015 Jun; 40(4):675–678. doi: 10.1007/s00059-014-4078-1. Epub 2014 Mar 9. PMID: 24609800.

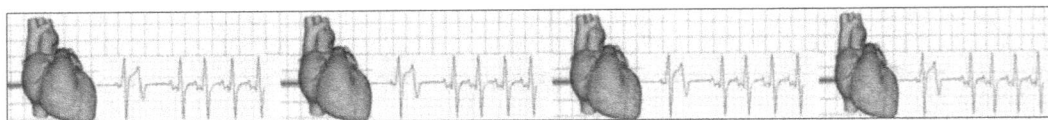

Case 3 Salvos of Atrial Tachycardia with Heart Failure

Vasile Iliese, Radu Andrei Dan, Boingiu Rares, Corina Diaconescu, and Iulia Ciobotariu

CLINICAL CASE

A male patient experienced recurring episodes of tachycardia that were refractory to antiar-rhythmic medications. The episode durations ranged from 10 seconds to 30 minutes. He exhib-ited significant symptoms of dyspnea and palpitations, ultimately resulting in left heart failure. The BNP level was 1200 pg/ml. He presented arrhythmia 80% of his daily activity. An electro-physiological study using three-dimensional mapping identified focal activity within the left atrium at the junction between the left superior pulmonary vein and the left atrial appendage. Radiofrequency ablation rendered the arrhythmia uninducible. A 30-day follow-up revealed no additional occurrences of arrhythmia, no dyspnea, and a BNP reduction to 30 ng/ml.

Clinic		Holter ECG
Cardiology		

Start of recording: 12.03.2024 09:55, Duration 23:58 h

SUMMARY

QRS Complexes	129438	Noise	26
VENTRICULAR EVENTS		SUPRAVENTRICULAR EVENTS	
Ventricular escapes:	1147	SVE (Prematurity <80%):	18247
PVC (Prematurity < 90%):	1046	SVE Tachycardia (>120 1/min):	3323
Bigeminy:	16	-longest: 7,5 s at 15:38	
Couplets:	950	-fastest: 210 bpm at 11:42	
Triplets:	536	ARRHYTHMIA	
VE Runs:	243	Arrhythmias:	13727
-fastest: 212 bpm at 13:06		-longest: 2,00 s at 03:16	
VE Tachycardia (>4):	66	Bradycardias (< 50 1/min):	427
-longest: 2,3 s at 20:56		-slowest: 40 bpm at 4:53	
-fastest: 205 bpm at 16:13		Pauses (>2000 ms):	22
		-longest: 2,13 s at 04:47	

HEART RATE		ST LEVEL	
Minimum	64 bpm at 07:57	mV at	
Mean	118 bpm	mV	
Maximum	151 bpm at 21:59	mV at	

Duration of atrial fibrillation: 1427, 63 min, 99.22% of recording duration
QRS Criteria: Normal, Sensitivity Ch 1: Mean, CH2: Mean

Figure 3.1 The summary page shows the high number of PACs: 18247/24 hours and frequent episodes of supraventricular tachycardias: 3323/24 hours. The longest episode had 7.5 seconds and the fastest rate was 210 bpm.

   DOI: 10.1201/9781003545040-3

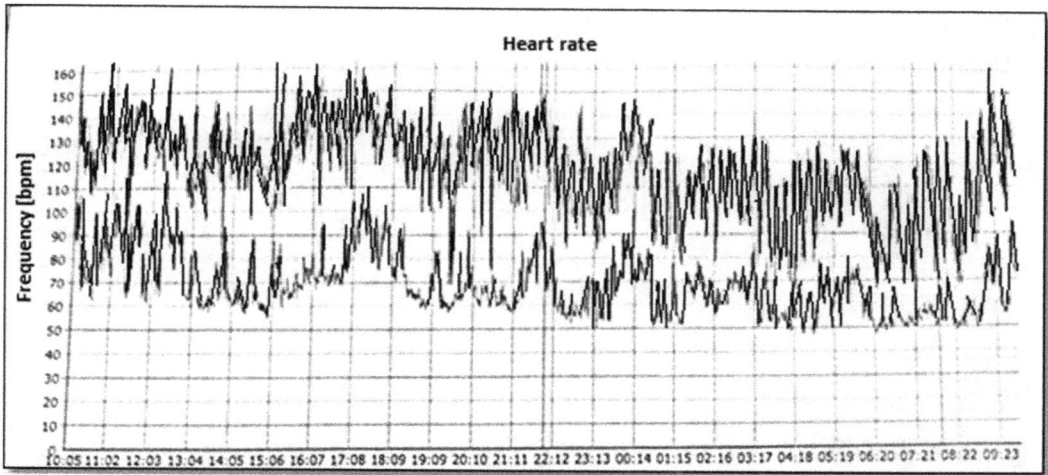

Figure 3.2 The heart rate trend shows high variability due to frequent episodes of supraventricular tachycardia.

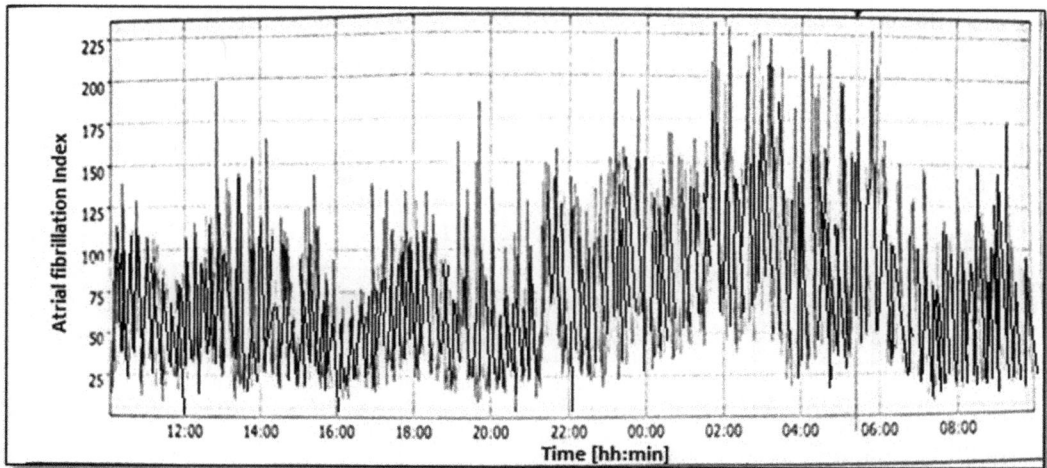

Figure 3.3 The graph illustrates multiple episodes of supraventricular tachycardia alternating with periods of normal heart rhythm, resulting in a spike-shaped pattern.

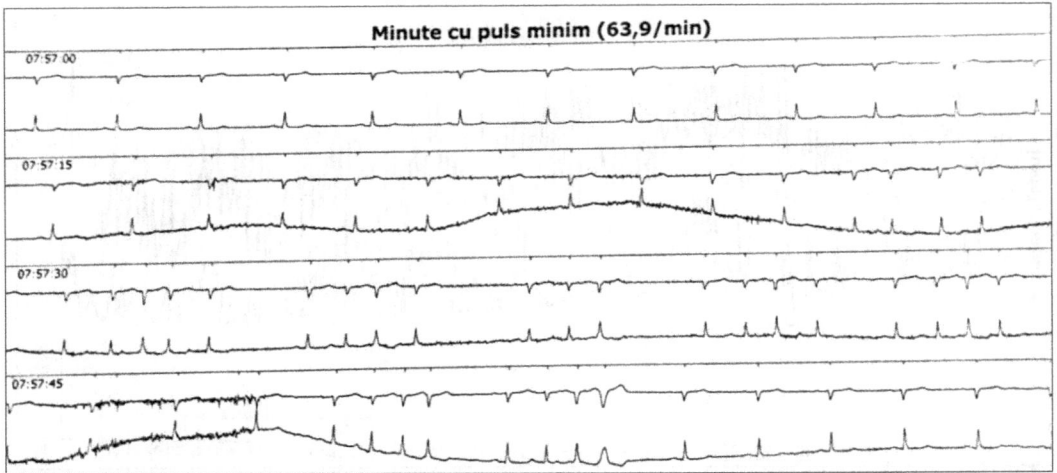

Figure 3.4 The graph depicts episodes of bradycardia. The first line contains 12 beats over a duration of 15 seconds, resulting in a rhythm of 48 beats per minute. The overall heart rate across the four lines is 63.9 bpm.

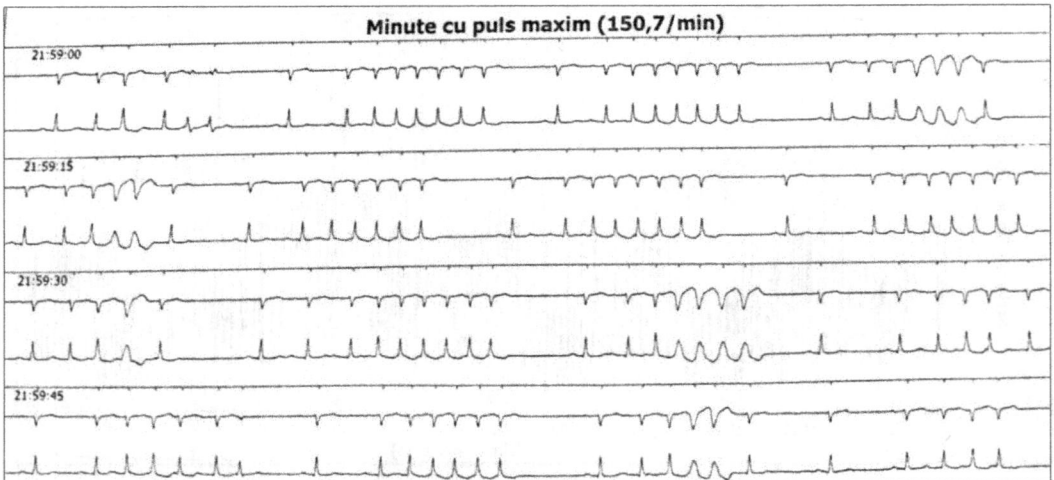

Figure 3.5 The graph depicts episodes of tachycardia. The overall heart rate across the four lines is 150.7 bpm.

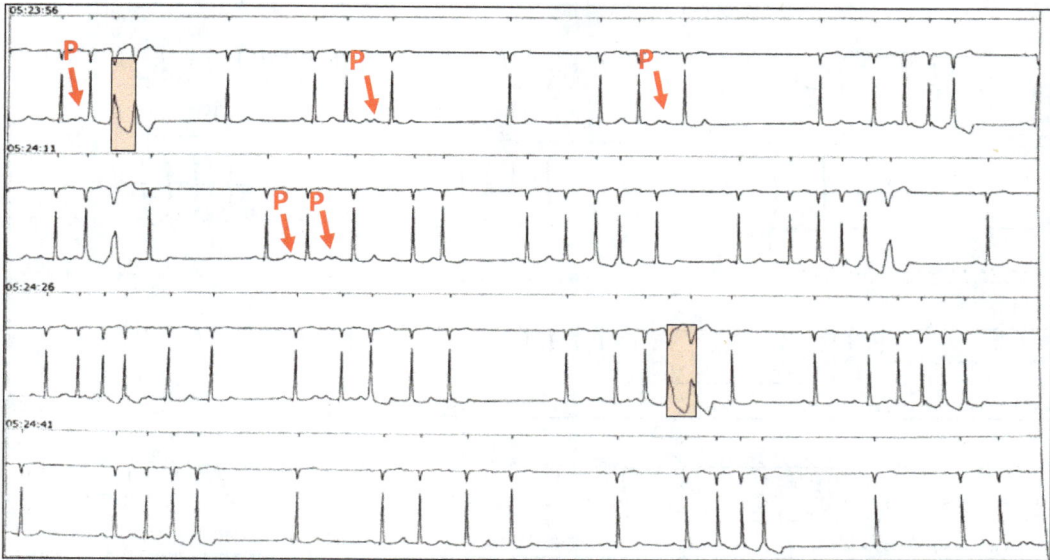

Figure 3.6 The strip shows salvos of PACs. Red arrow shows the P wave which has different morphology and PR interval compared to sinus P wave. Some episodes present intermittent bundle branch block, the RR interval being shorter than the rest of RRs within the salvos (red square).

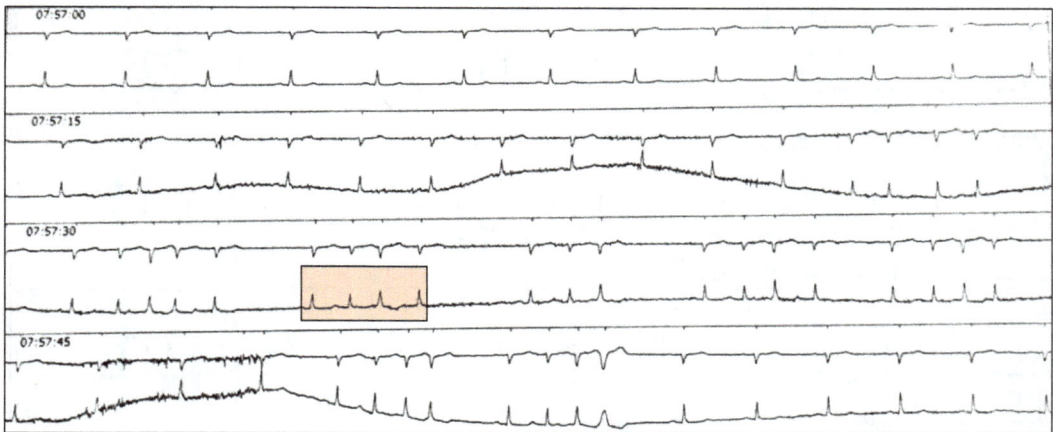

Figure 3.7 The strip shows salvos of PACs.

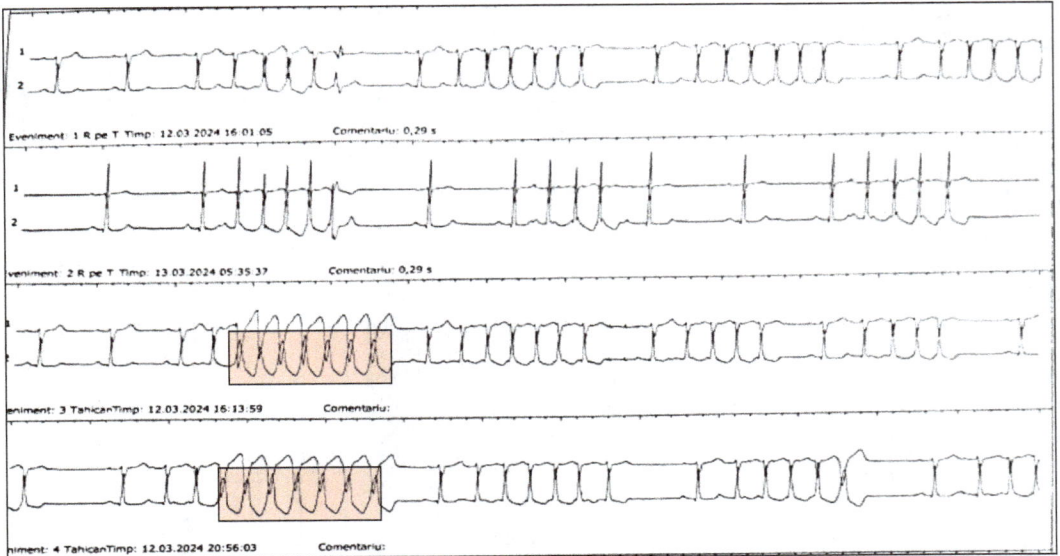

Figure 3.8 The strip shows salvos of PACs. Some episodes present intermittent bundle branch block, the RR interval being shorter than the rest of RRs within the salvos (red square).

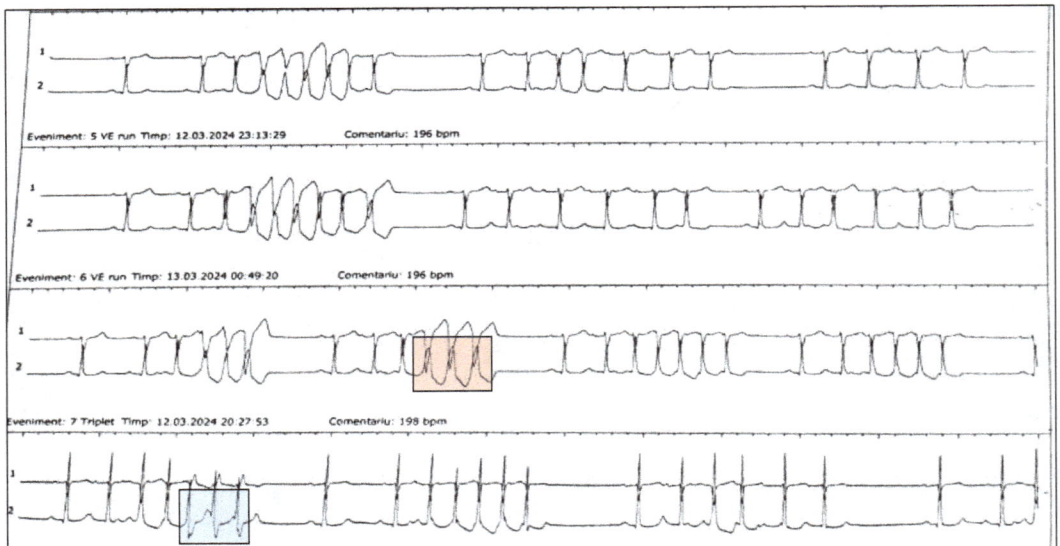

Figure 3.9 The strip shows salvos of PACs. Some episodes present intermittent bundle branch block, with other morphology compared to previous images (it may indicate RBBB in the blue squares and LBBB in the red squares).

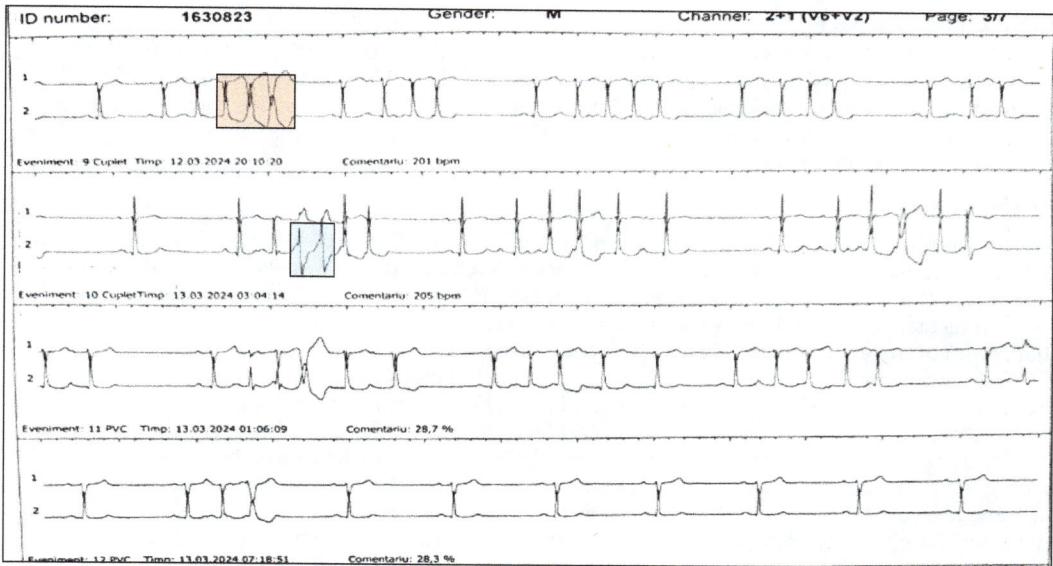

Figure 3.10 Salvos of PACs. Intermittent bundle branch block, with 2 morphologies, indicative of RBBB and LBBB aberrancy.

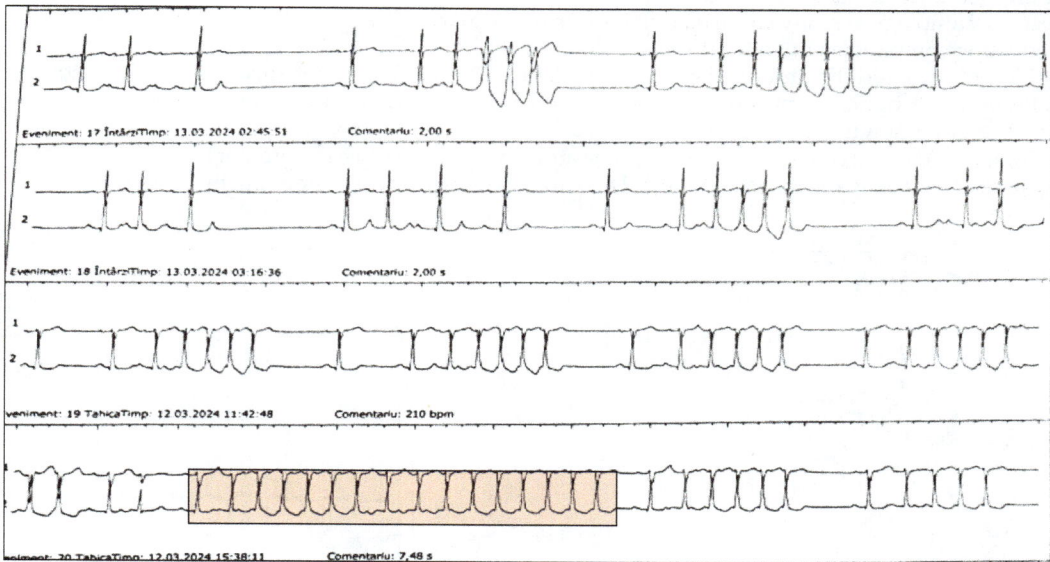

Figure 3.11 Longest episode of atrial tachycardia 7.48 seconds.

HOLTER SUMMARY

The 24-hour monitoring period indicated repeated episodes of atrial tachycardia lasting 3–12 beats, with durations of up to 7.5 seconds and a rate reaching 210 bpm. Some episodes showed large QRS complexes attributable to rate-dependent bundle branch block. The monitoring was conducted during therapy with antiarrhythmic medications, revealing the limited efficacy of these drugs on arrhythmia burden.

DISCUSSION

Atrial automatic tachycardia is a rare arrhythmia in children that typically persists for months or years. In a 12-lead electrocardiogram it is characterized by distinct P waves accompanied by an abnormal PR interval. Irregularities in the atrial rate, P-wave axis, or morphology differentiate it from sinus tachycardia, whereas the occurrence of second-degree atrioventricular block without disruption of the arrhythmia rules out all types of reentrant tachycardias.

Previous research on dogs with sustained atrial pacing clearly indicated that persistent atrial tachycardia causes a reduction in left ventricular ejection fraction, apparent as early as one week post-tachycardia onset, and reaching its lowest level at four weeks after the onset. Damiano et al. also investigated the reversibility of these hemodynamic anomalies induced by atrial tachy-pacing. After the cessation of tachycardia, the left ventricular ejection fraction normalized to baseline levels within 2 weeks, but left ventricular end-diastolic left ventricular volumes remained increased for up to 3 months post-pacing termination. In humans, the proof of atrial tachycardia-related cardiomyopathy mostly consists of case reports describing the improvement or resolution of congestive heart failure after catheter ablation or pharmacological termination of persistent atrial tachycardia. In our patient the BNP levels decreased significantly, from 1200 to 30 ng/ml. Automatic atrial tachycardia is challenging to manage with antiarrhythmic medications and may lead to dilated cardiomyopathy or heart failure, as shown in our case.

The diagnosis of automatic ectopic focal atrial tachycardia may be deduced from the surface electrocardiogram. However, the diagnosis of an ectopic focal tachycardia is confirmed by electrophysiological study. In our patient we had a suspicion of ectopic atrial tachycardia due to the appearance of the P wave and PR interval which were different to those of sinus rhythm. The electrophysiological study confirmed the origin of the arrhythmia inside the left atrium and the activation compatible with a focal source.

"Salvo" was initially described by Lown et al. in 1973 describing brief episodes of PVCs with rates up to 188 bpm. The phrase was also adopted for atrial arrhythmias, meaning short episodes of PACs also known as non-sustained atrial tachycardia.

Infants and children with automatic ectopic atrial tachycardia typically present a significant therapeutic challenge as medication with Digoxin proves ineffective in stopping the arrhythmia.

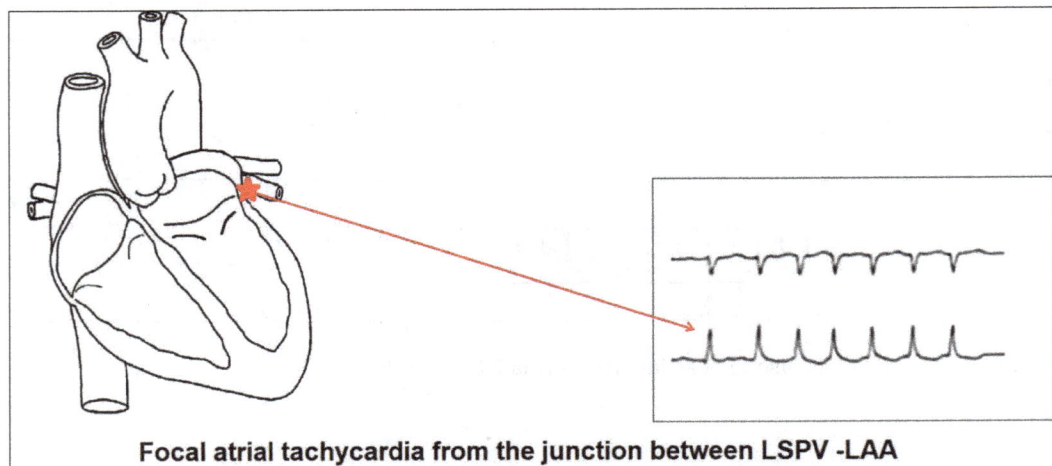

Focal atrial tachycardia from the junction between LSPV -LAA

Figure 3.12   Focal atrial tachycardia has a narrow QRS complex. However, sometimes it may be conducted to the ventricles with LBBB or RBBB aberrancy.

Electrical cardioversion and overdrive pacing are also unsuccessful as they merely inhibit the focal activation for a maximum of a few seconds. Furthermore, our patient had short episodes of atrial tachycardia of 2–5 seconds, and in such cases electrical cardioversion and overdrive pacing are useless. Digoxin is the most commonly used drug for blocking re-entry circuits; it is, however, rarely successful in ectopic foci such as focal atrial tachycardia. It is still used in children as it prevents congestive heart failure and can decrease the ventricular rate resulting from A to V block. Propranolol is a beta blocker that can be used to lower the rate of atrial tachycardia and sometimes inhibit the atrial focus. However, case reports with Propranolol and Sotalol showed disappointing results.

Accurate localization of the atrial focus can be difficult. Traditional mapping with two-dimensional fluoroscopy has been used to identify the ectopic site. However, this method sometimes proves challenging and involves prolonged fluoroscopy exposure. The variability in success rates for X-ray-guided RF ablation is mostly attributable to difficulties in localizing the foci. The electromagnetic three-dimensional mapping technology facilitates identification of ectopic foci without the use of X-ray exposure, and enables effective radiofrequency ablation.

BIBLIOGRAPHY

1. Rabbani LE, Wang PJ, Couper GL, Friedman PL. Time course of improvement in ventricular function after ablation of incessant automatic atrial tachycardia. *Am Heart J.* 1991 March; 121(3 Pt 1): 816–819. doi: 10.1016/0002-8703(91)90193-l. PMID: 2000748.

2. Paul T, Janousek J. New antiarrhythmic drugs in pediatric use: Propafenone. *Pediatr Cardiol.* 1994 July–August; 15(4): 190–197. doi: 10.1007/BF00800674. PMID: 7991437.

3. Kang KT, Etheridge SP, Kantoch MJ, et al. Current management of focal atrial tachycardia in children: A multicenter experience. *Circ Arrhythm Electrophysiol.* 2014; 7: 664–670.

4. Walsh EP, Saul JP, Hulse JE, et al. Transcatheter ablation of ectopic atrial tachycardia in young patients using radiofrequency current. *Circulation.* 1992; 86: 1138–1146.

5. Kugler JD, Danford DA, Deal BJ, et al. Radiofrequency catheter ablation for tachyarrhythmias in children and adolescents. *N Engl J Med.* 1994; 330: 1481–1487.

6. Dhala AA, Case CL, Gillette PC. Evolving treatment strategies for managing atrial ectopic tachycardia in children. *Am J Cardiol.* 1994; 74: 283–286.

7. Cummings RM, Mahle WT, Strieper MJ, et al. Outcomes following electroanatomic mapping and ablation for the treatment of ectopic atrial tachycardia in the pediatric population. *Pediatr Cardiol.* 2008; 29: 393–397.

8. Koike K, Hesslein PS, Finlay CD, Williams WG, Izukawa T, Freedom RM. Atrial automatic tachycardia in children. *Am J Cardiol.* 1988; 61: 1127–1130.

9. Keane JF, Plauth WH, Nadas AS. Chronic ectopic tachycardia of infancy and childhood. *Am Heart J.* 1972; 84: 748–757.

10. Gillette PC, Garson A. Electrophysiologic and pharmacologic characteristics of automatic ectopic atrial tachycardia. *Circulation.* 1977; 56(4 Pt 1): 571–575.

11. Damiano RJ Jr, Tripp HF Jr, Asano T, Small KW, Jones RH, Lowe JE. Left ventricular dysfunction and dilatation resulting from chronic supraventricular tachycardia. *J Thorac Cardiovasc Surg.* 1987 July; 94(1): 135–143. PMID: 3599999.

12. Burchell SA, Spinale FG, Crawford FA, Tanaka R, Zile MR. Effects of chronic tachycardia-induced cardiomyopathy on the beta-adrenergic receptor system. *J Thorac Cardiovasc Surg.* 1992 October; 104(4): 1006–1012. PMID: 1328769.

13. Crawford FA Jr, Gillette PC, Case CL, Zeigler V. Surgical management of dysrhythmias in infants and small children. *Ann Surg.* 1992 September; 216(3): 318–326. doi: 10.1097/00000658-199209000-00011. PMID: 1417181; PMCID: PMC1242616.

14. Tomita M, Spinale FG, Crawford FA, Zile MR. Changes in left ventricular volume, mass, and function during the development and regression of supraventricular tachycardia-induced cardiomyopathy: Disparity between recovery of systolic versus diastolic function. *Circulation.* 1991 February; 83(2): 635–644. doi: 10.1161/01.cir.83.2.635. PMID: 1991381.

15. Cohen J, Scherf D. Consideration on impulse formation in the left atrium and its diagnosis by electrocardiogram. *Am J Cardiol.* 1973; 31: 799.

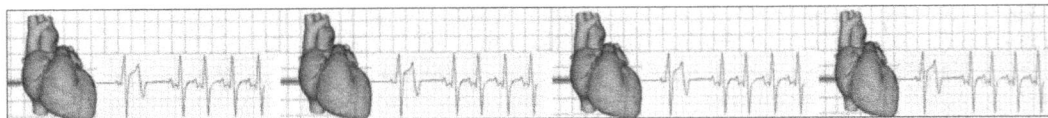

Case 4 Multifocal Atrial Tachycardia in a Newborn

Gabriela Abrudan, Cismaru Gabriel, and Cecilia Lazea

CLINICAL CASE

A 5 day-old female neonate had episodes of tachycardia 200 bpm. The ECG was normal, echocardiography showed nonobstructive hypertrophic cardiomyopathy with 2 atrial septal defects and aneurysm of the interatrial septum. Lab tests were normal, except for low levels of 25-OH vitamin D (24.1ng/ml). No lung disease was detected.

Ritm cardiac		
Total bătăi	169 235	(0% paced)
HR max / min	**212 / 59 bpm**	
Media HR	**Ø 124 bpm**	
HR Max / Min Sinus	211 / 59 bpm	
Media HR (Treaz/Adormit)	127 / 119 bpm	
Index circadian	1,07	
Tahicardie / Bradicardie	7 % / 35 %	

Pauze		
RR Max	**1 134 ms**	
Pauze (>2000ms)	0	

Fibrilaţie atrială / Flutter atrial		
Total AF	-	
AF HR Max	0 bpm	
Cel mai lung AF	-	

Bradicardie		
Cea mai mică	Ø 78 bpm	28 sec
Cea mai mare	Ø 100 bpm	00:15:38

ST		
St ridicare max	0,38 mV	V5
ST depresurizare max	-0,21 mV	III

Ectopie ventriculară		
V Total	5563	(3%)
V / Ora Max	472	pe oră
Episoade Tahicardie V		-
Cea mai rapidă Tahicardie V		-
V Cea mai lungă secvenţă	Ø 204 bpm	0 sec
Triplete / Executã		21 Σ 65 bătăi
Cuplete		101 Σ 202 bătăi
Bigeminism		476 Σ 1127 bătăi
Trigeminism		121 Σ 248 bătăi

Ectopie supraventriculară		
S Tot	25116	(15%)
Episoade Tahicardie SV		78 Σ 00:11:24
Cea mai rapidă Tahicardie SV	Ø 212 bpm	5 sec
S Cea mai lungă secvenţă	Ø 126 bpm	33 sec
Triplete / Executã		1809 Σ 15225 bătăi
Cuplete		282 Σ 564 bătăi

Figure 4.1 The summary page shows a maximum heart rate of 212 and a minimum rate of 59 bpm. The mean heart rate was 124 bpm. There were 25116 PACs, with 76 episodes of atrial tachycardia; the longest had a duration of 33 seconds and the fastest heart rate was 212 bpm.

DOI: 10.1201/9781003545040-4

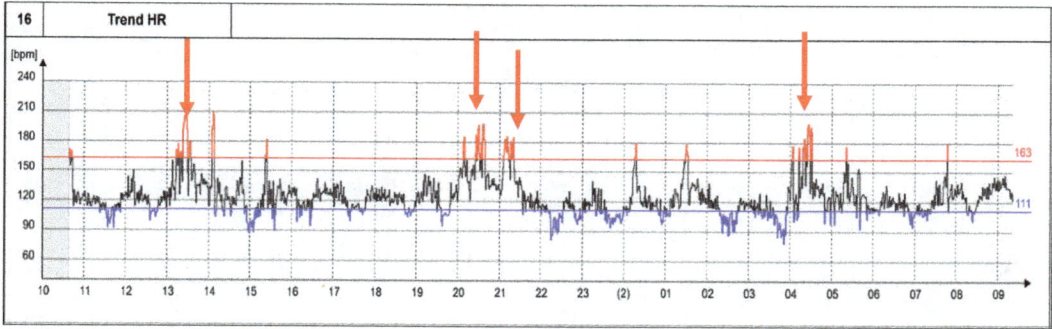

Figure 4.2 The heart rate trend shows repeated episodes of tachycardia up to 210 bpm.

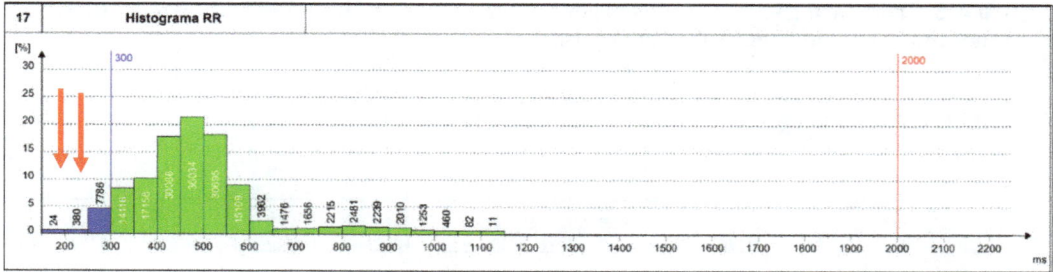

Figure 4.3 The RR histogram shows short RR intervals of 200–300 ms, corresponding to fast atrial rates during tachycardia.

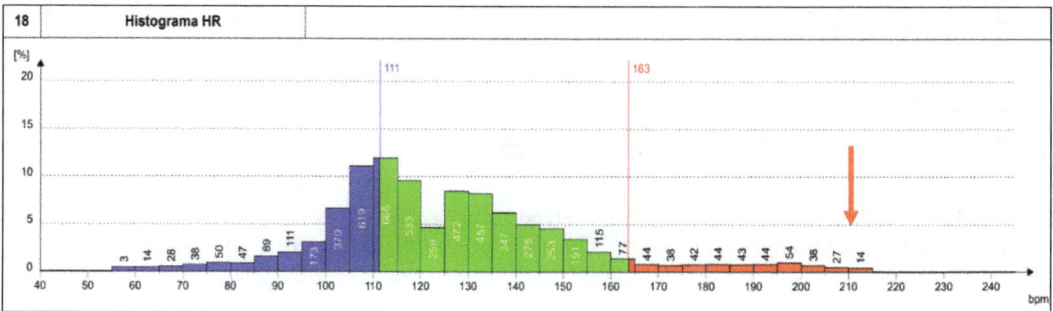

Figure 4.4 The HR histogram shows fast rates during tachycardia up to 210 bpm.

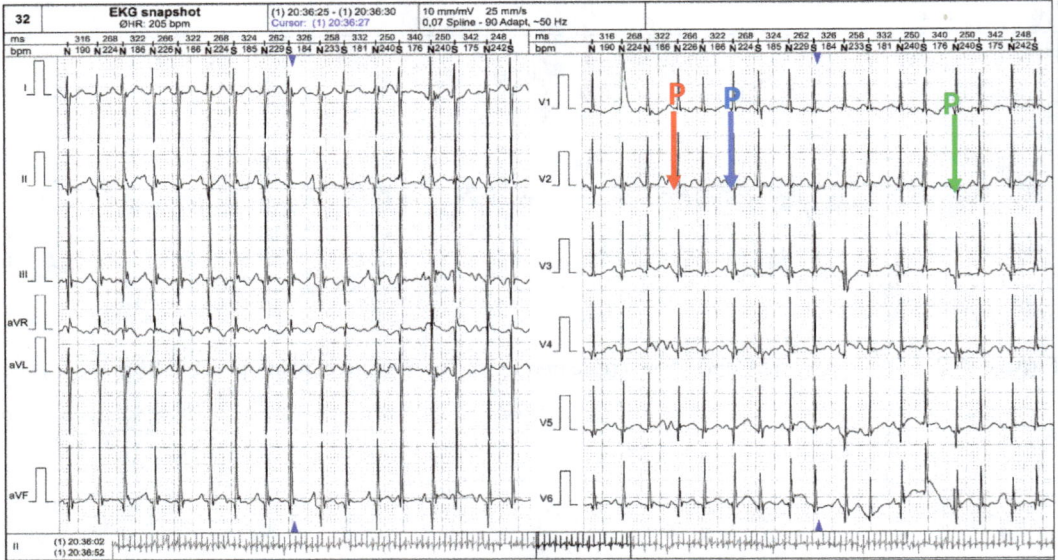

Figure 4.5 The tracing shows an episode of multifocal atrial tachycardia with more than 3 P wave morphologies and irregular PP intervals.

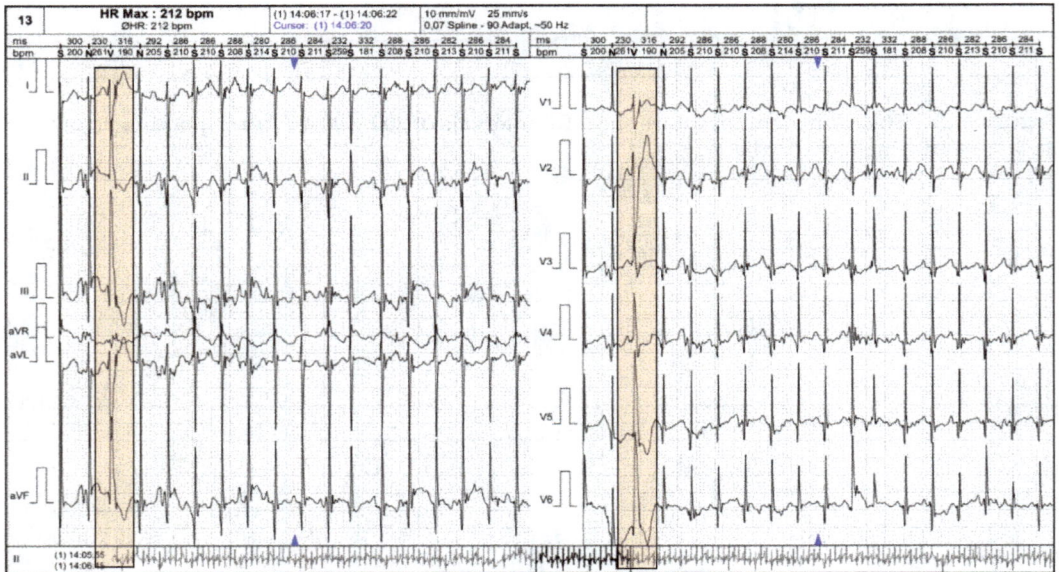

Figure 4.6 The tracing shows a multifocal atrial tachycardia with a rate of 212 bpm and multiple P wave morphologies. The marked beat is a premature ventricular contraction.

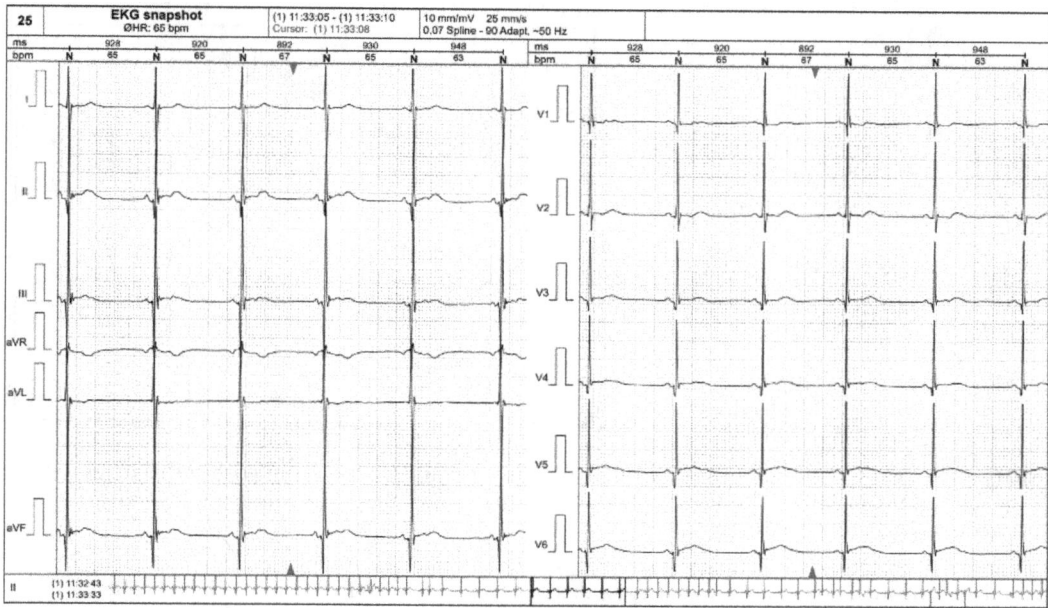

Figure 4.7 The lowest recorded rate during sinus rhythm.

HOLTER SUMMARY

The monitoring reveals episodes of multifocal atrial tachycardia with a rate of up to 212 bpm. During the episodes, there are more than 3 morphologies of the P wave, with irregular PP intervals. The longest episode of MAT had a duration of 33 seconds. The fastest episode of MAT had a rate of 212 bpm and a duration of 5 seconds. Approximately 3% of the beats were premature ventricular contractions.

DISCUSSION

Multifocal atrial tachycardia is characterized by fast atrial rhythm (> 100 bpm) with a minimum of three morphologically distinct P waves. It is additionally characterized by irregular P–P, R–R, and P–R intervals. Between the P waves there is an isoelectric baseline and the atrial rate is around 400/min. The duration of multifocal tachycardia is minutes to hours, followed by a return to sinus rhythm before another arrhythmic recurrence.

The mechanism of MAT is given by impulses from numerous automatic foci activating the atrium at a rapid pace > 400/minutes. Similar to focal atrial tachycardia, MAT does not respond to electrical cardioversion. Another hypothesis suggests that the diverse morphologies of P waves in MAP are the result of the varied propagation of impulses that originate from a single focus. This hypothesis is sustained by the work of Bevilacqua et al. who ablated MAP at a single site in the right atrium located on the interatrial septum, at the posterior rim of the fossa ovalis. Despite the multifocal pattern, the ablation was carried out at a single focus. The incomplete development of the atrium may also contribute to the age distribution of MAT being predominantly infantile (< 1 year of age). Pickoff et al. have reported that neonatal puppies exhibit atrial vulnerability, with low atrial effective refractory periods, and increasing atrial refractory period as the dog grows.

In children, multifocal atrial tachycardia occurs especially in infants younger than one year of age. The incidence in neonates is 0.02%. It manifests with poor feeding, irritability, respiratory distress and lethargy. Southall et al. conducted a prospective evaluation of ECGs in 3383 healthy infants. Individuals with anomalies underwent multiple 24-hour Holter monitoring for 3 consecutive years. Out of 3,383 infants, two exhibited MAT, both of whom were asymptomatic at 3 years old.

Numerous investigations indicated an association between the RyR2 mutation and MAT. Broendberg et al. documented five cases of MAT among 51 individuals with identified RyR2 mutations. Lin et al. examined the cardiovascular abnormalities associated with RASopathy in a cohort of 61 patients diagnosed with Costello syndrome. In their study, 15 out of 61 patients with

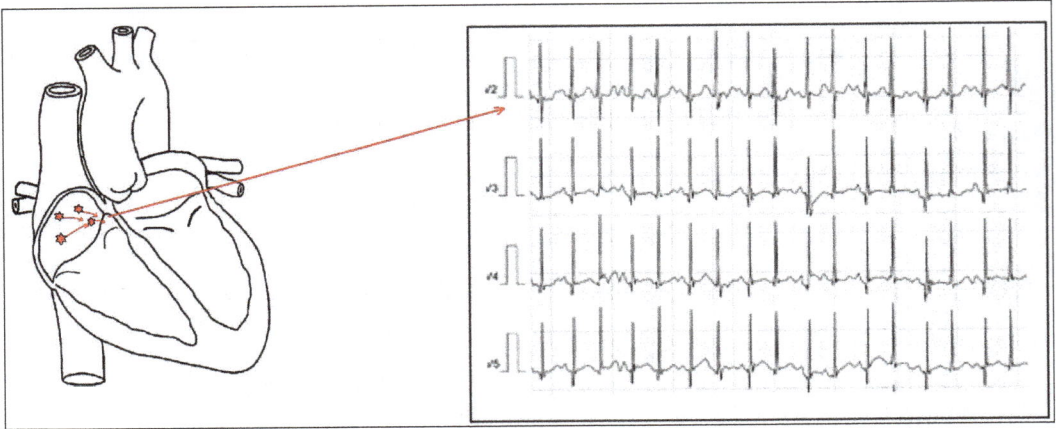

Figure 4.8 Multifocal atrial tachycardia originates in multiple foci from within the atrium, it is characterized by fast atrial rhythm (> 100 bpm) with a minimum of three morphologically distinct P waves and irregular P–P intervals.

Costello syndrome, or 25%, presented episodes of MAT. Most MAT data in pediatric patients indicate that over 20% had concurrent pulmonary disease; however the prevalence is significantly lower compared to adults, where it reaches 60%. In the study by Wu et al., 17 out of 22 (77%) individuals with MAT exhibited respiratory disorders.

Digoxin, the most commonly used medication in neonates, is frequently used for MAT. It slows the ventricular response, but cannot stop the arrhythmia. Encainide was used by Strasburger et al, without effective response in arrhythmia control. Houyel used Flecainide with success, and Fish had a response to Propafenone in 5 of 6 patients. Amiodarone was also used with high success rates.

The majority of pediatric MAT patients are infants, who typically have a favorable prognosis, particularly in the absence of other comorbidities. Nevertheless, the clinical course of MAT in patients with other underlying comorbidities may vary, and up to 12% develop sudden cardiac death. Yeager et al. documented four infants diagnosed with MAT, three of whom died two to five months post-diagnosis.

BIBLIOGRAPHY

1. Bevilacqua LM, Rhee EK, Epstein MR, Triedman JK. Focal ablation of chaotic atrial rhythm in an infant with cardiomyopathy. *J Cardiovasc Electrophysiol*. 2000; 11: 577–581.

2. Hsieh MY, Lee PC, Hwang B, Meng CC. Multifocal atrial tachycardia in 2 children. *J Chin Med Assoc*. 2006; 69: 439–443. doi: 10.1016/S1726-4901(09)70288-6

3. Lipson MJ, Naimi S. Multifocal atrial tachycardia (chaotic atrial tachycardia): Clinical associations and significance. *Circulation*. 1970; 42: 397–407. doi: 10.1161/01.cir.42.3.397

4. Bradley DJ, Fischbach PS, Law IH, Serwer GA, Dick M 2nd. The clinical course of multifocal atrial tachycardia in infants and children. *J Am Coll Cardiol*. 2001; 38: 401–408. doi: 10.1016/s0735-1097(01)01390-0

5. Kastor JA. Multifocal atrial tachycardia. *N Engl J Med*. 1990; 322: 1713–1717. doi: 10.1056/NEJM199006143222405

6. Fish FA, Mehta AV, Johns JA. Characteristics and management of chaotic atrial tachycardia of infancy. *Am J Cardiol*. 1996; 78: 1052–1055. doi: 10.1016/s0002-9149(96)00536-x

7. Liberthson RR, Colan SD. Multifocal or chaotic atrial rhythm: Report of nine infants, delineation of clinical course and management, and review of the literature. *Pediatr Cardiol*. 1982; 2: 179–184. doi: 10.1007/BF02332108

8. Dodo H, Gow RM, Hamilton RM, Freedom RM. Chaotic atrial rhythm in children. *Am Heart J*. 1995; 129: 990–995. doi: 10.1016/0002-8703(95)90121-3

9.   Salim MA, Case CL, Gillette PC. Chaotic atrial tachycardia in children. *Am Heart J.* 1995; 129: 831–833. doi: 10.1016/0002-8703(95)90339-9

10. Beitzke A. Multifocal (chaotic) atrial tachycardia in infancy. *Helv Paediatr Acta.* 1979; 34: 319–327.

11. Zeevi B, Berant M, Sclarovsky S, Blieden LC. Treatment of multifocal atrial tachycardia with amiodarone in a child with congenital heart disease. *Am J Cardiol.* 1986; 57: 344–345. doi: 10.1016/0002-9149(86)90920-3

12. Houyel L, Fournier A, Davignon A. Successful treatment of chaotic atrial tachycardia with oral flecainide. *Int J Cardiol.* 1990; 27: 27–29. doi: 10.1016/0167-5273(90)90187-a

13. Bouziri A, Khaldi A, Hamdi A, et al. Multifocal atrial tachycardia: An unusual cause of cardiogenic shock in a newborn. *Tunis Med.* 2011; 89: 59–61.

14. Chen H, Ma Y, Wang Y, Luo H, Xiao Z, Chen Z, Liu Q, Xiao Y. Progress of Pathogenesis in Pediatric Multifocal Atrial Tachycardia. *Front Pediatr.* 2022 Jun. 22;10:922464. doi: 10.3389/fped.2022.922464. PMID: 35813391; PMCID: PMC9256911

15. Huh J. Clinical Implication of Multifocal Atrial Tachycardia in Children for Pediatric Cardiologist. *Korean Circ J.* 2018 Feb.; 48(2):173–175. doi: 10.4070/kcj.2018.0037. PMID: 29441751; PMCID: PMC5861009.

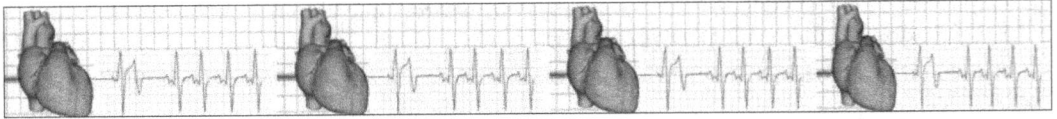

Case 5 Junctional Rhythm Mimicking WPW Pattern

Andrei Mihordea, Ioana Golgot, and Cismaru Gabriel

CLINICAL CASE

A 12-year-old girl exhibited repeated episodes of paroxysmal tachycardia at 160 bpm, lasting from 3 to 50 minutes. Treatment with Propranolol was ineffective; hence, it was substituted with Flecainide. An electrophysiological investigation was conducted due to repeated recurrences while on Flecainide. A dual nodal pathway was identified, with inducible typical slow-fast atrioventricular nodal tachycardia. The slow pathway was ablated. No evidence of an accessory pathway was found. Intermittently she had an asymptomatic junctional rhythm at a rate of 90–110 bpm.

Ritm cardiac		
Total bătăi	116 628	(0% paced)
HR max / min	176 / 48 bpm	
Media HR	Ø 81 bpm	
HR Max / Min Sinus	176 / 48 bpm	
Media HR (Treaz/Adormit)	92 / 61 bpm	
Index circadian	1,51	
Tahicardie / Bradicardie	16 % / 11 %	

Pauze	
RR Max	4 832 ms
Pauze (>2000ms)	5

Fibrilație atrială / Flutter atrial	
Total AF	-
AF HR Max	0 bpm
Cel mai lung AF	-

Bradicardie		
Cea mai mică	Ø 50 bpm	12 sec
Cea mai mare	Ø 52 bpm	00:09:08

ST		
St ridicare max	-	
ST depresurizare max	-0,38 mV	II

Ectopie ventriculară		
V Total	0	(< 1%)
V / Ora Max	0	pe oră
Episoade Tahicardie V	-	
Cea mai rapidă Tahicardie V	-	
V Cea mai lungă secvență	-	
Triplete / Execută	0 Σ 0 bătăi	
Cuplete	0 Σ 0 bătăi	
Bigeminism	0 Σ 0 bătăi	
Trigeminism	0 Σ 0 bătăi	

Ectopie supraventriculară		
S Tot	1057	(< 1%)
Episoade Tahicardie SV	7 Σ 00:05:41	
Cea mai rapidă Tahicardie SV	Ø 166 bpm	11 sec
S Cea mai lungă secvență	Ø 153 bpm	00:03:39
Triplete / Execută	4 Σ 31 bătăi	
Cuplete	2 Σ 4 bătăi	

Figure 5.1 The summary page shows a maximum rate of 176 bpm, a lowest rate of 48 bpm, and an episode of supraventricular tachycardia with a rate of 166 bpm and a duration of 11 seconds.

DOI: 10.1201/9781003545040-5

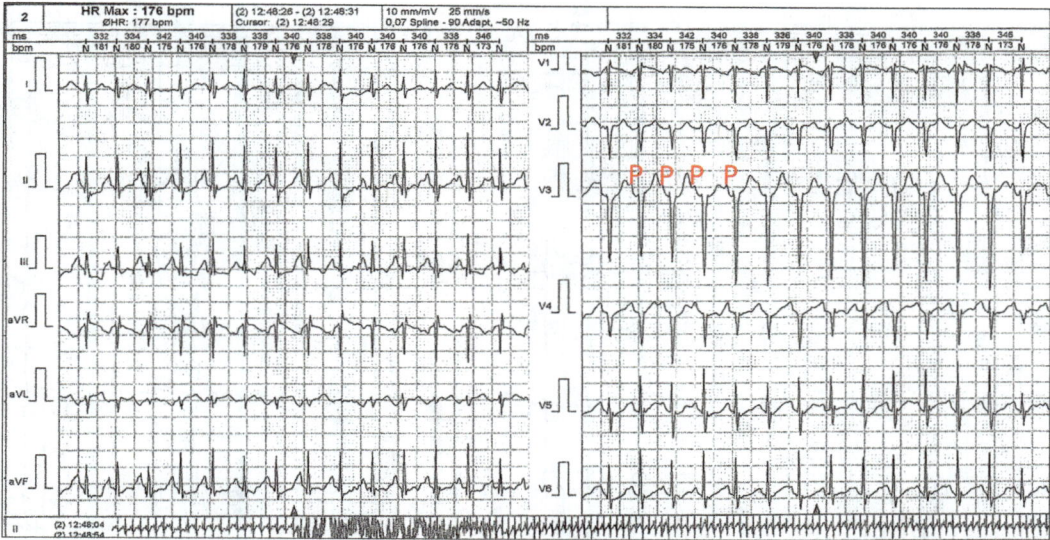

Figure 5.2 The tracing shows the highest rate detected, which is sinus rhythm during physical activity. The QRS complexes are narrow, preceded by P waves.

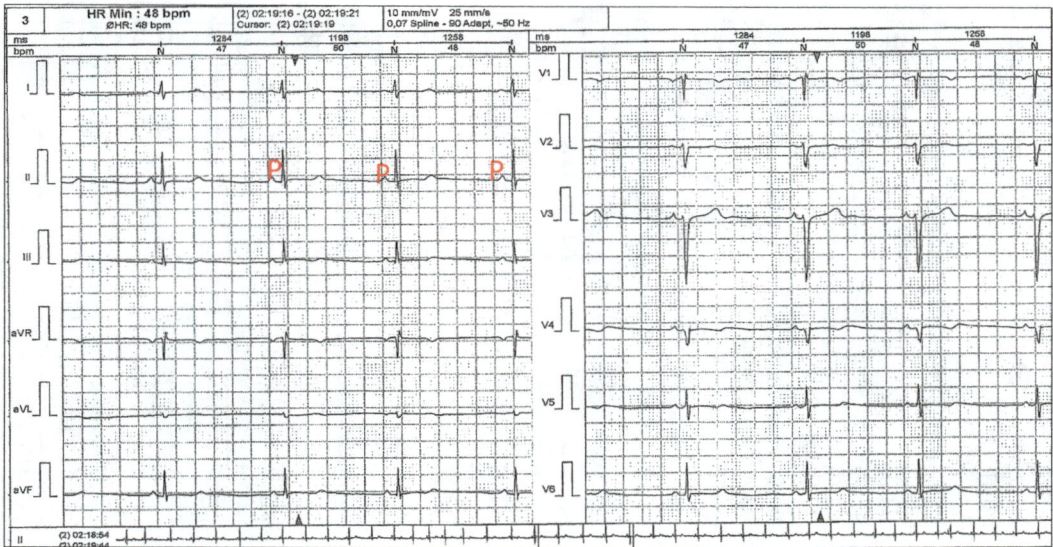

Figure 5.3 The tracing shows the lowest rate detected during Holter monitoring, which is a sinus rhythm, every QRS complex being preceded by a normal P wave.

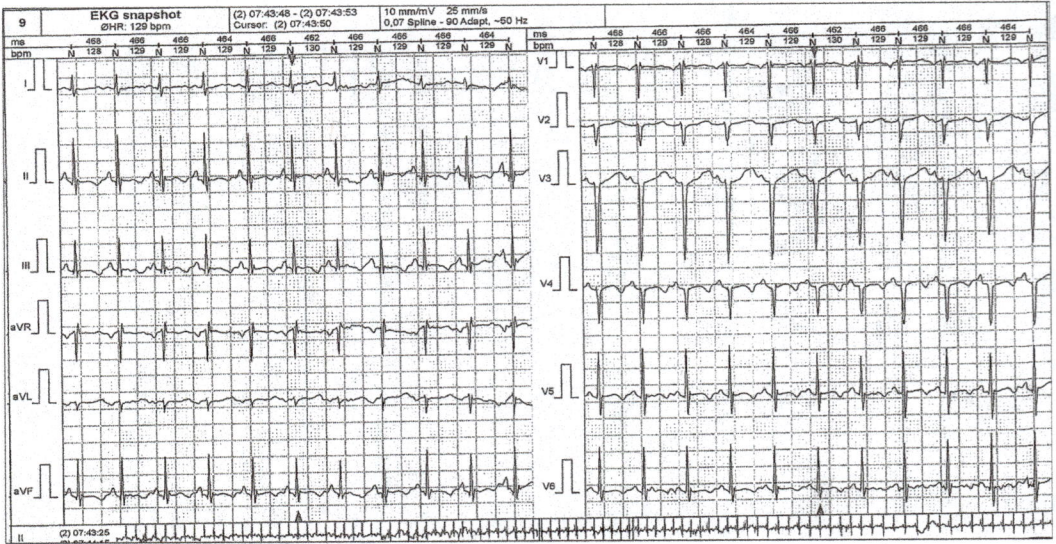

Figure 5.4 The tracing shows sinus rhythm 129 bpm, every QRS complex being preceded by a normal P wave.

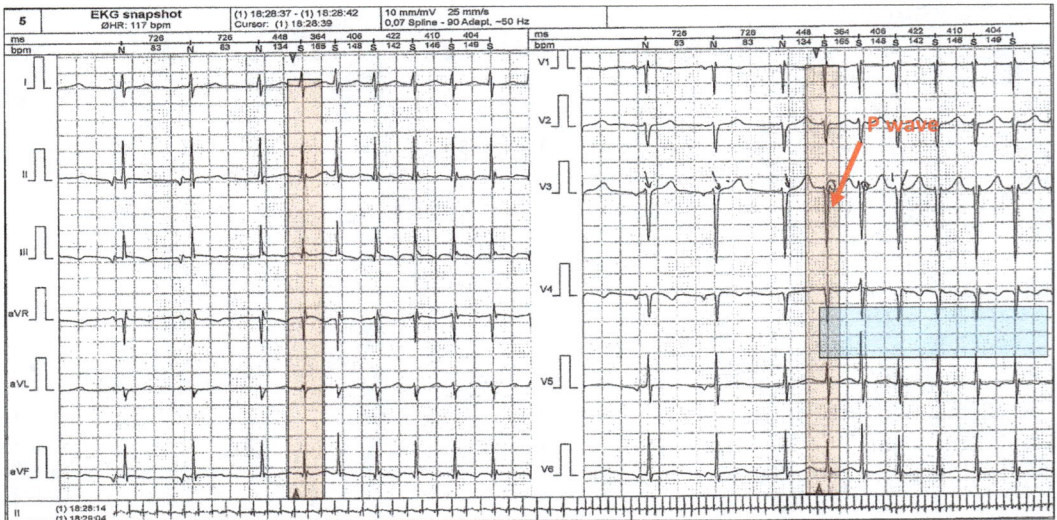

Figure 5.5 The image shows the onset of a paroxysmal supraventricular tachycardia (blue box), after the occurrence of a premature contraction (red box). The premature contraction is followed by a retrograde P wave, most likely conducted retrogradely through the fast nodal pathway (red arrow).

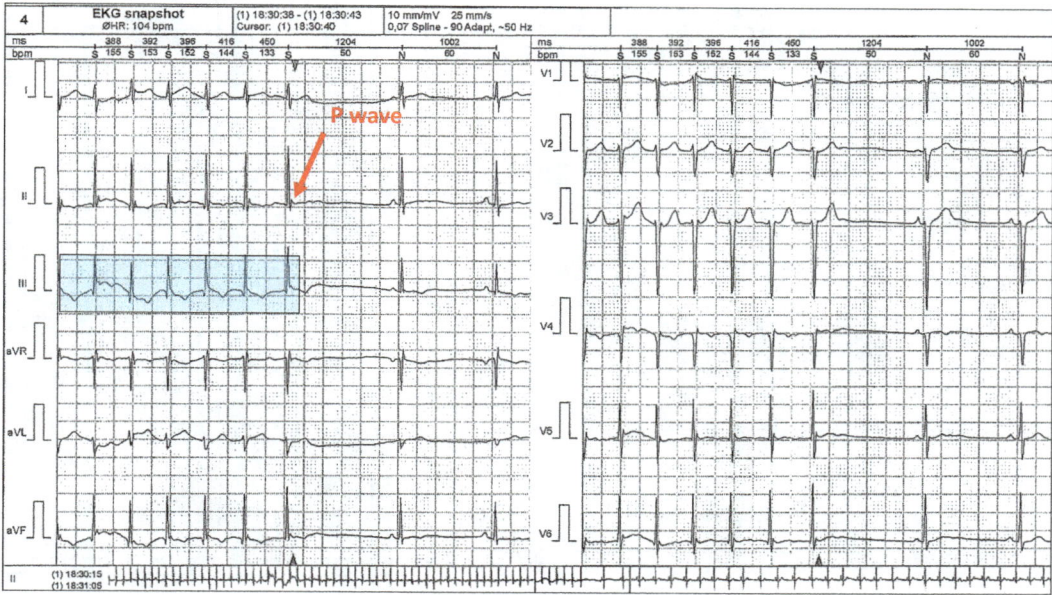

Figure 5.6 The tracing shows the termination of the supraventricular tachycardia with a P wave (atrial activation-red arrow). Afterwards, sinus rhythm resumes.

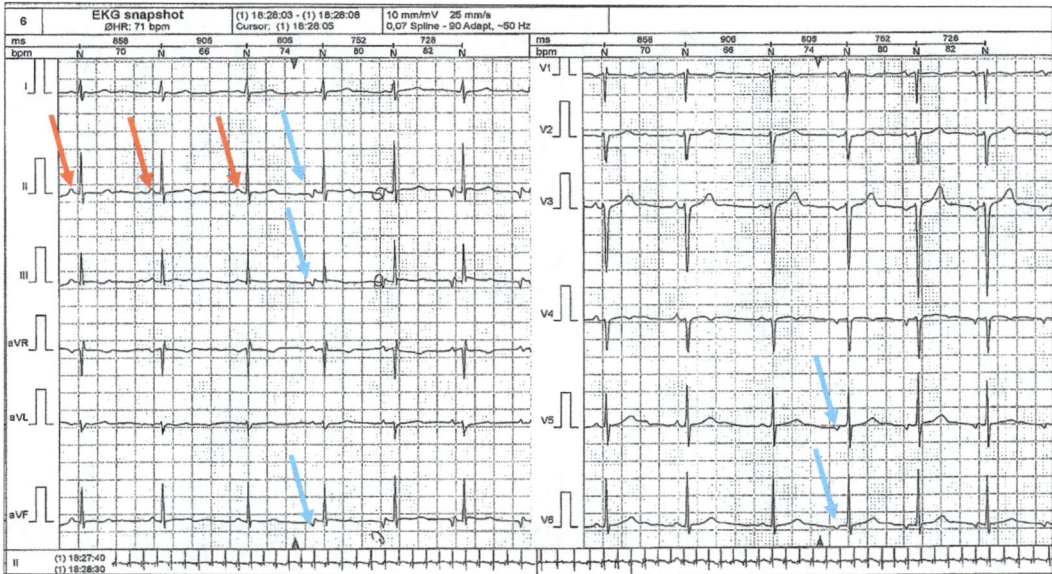

Figure 5.7 The tracing shows sinus rhythm (red arrows) alternating with low left atrial rhythm (the P wave is negative in inferior leads II, III, avF as well as in left lateral leads V5–V6).

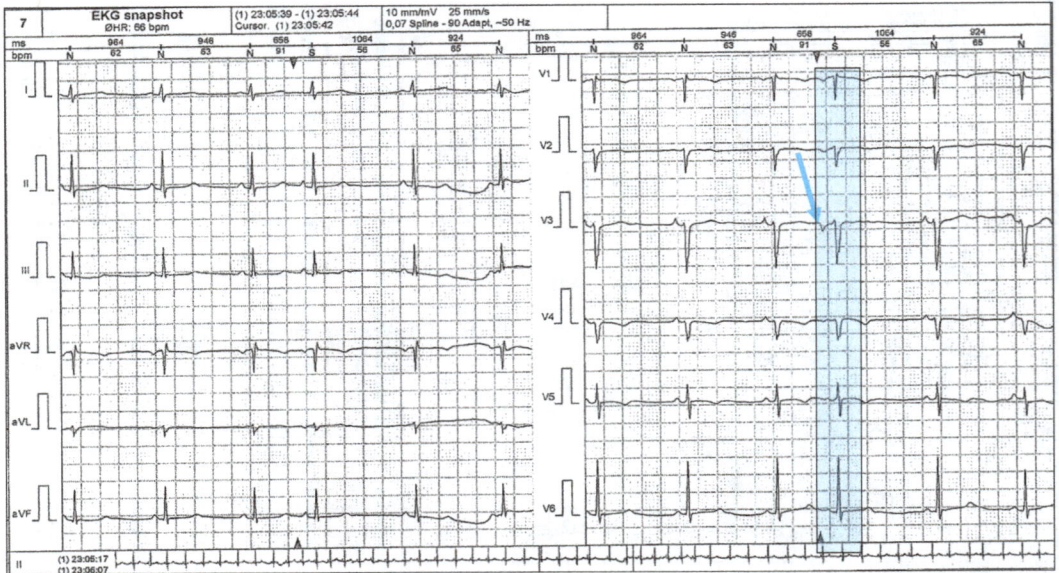

Figure 5.8 The tracing shows an atrial premature contraction. The P wave preceding the beat has a modified P wave of different morphology.

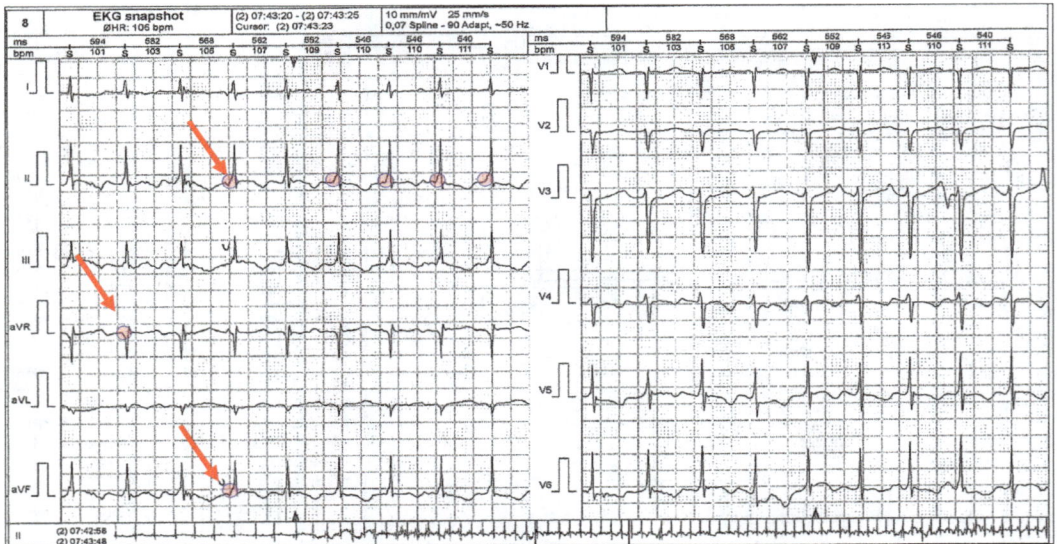

Figure 5.9 The tracing shows a regular heart rate of 106 bpm. The QRS complexes are narrow, similar to those of sinus rhythm; however, the initial portion of the QRS has an upstroke that looks like a delta wave. Although, there is no P wave preceding the delta wave. In fact this was confirmed as junctional rhythm during electrophysiological testing.

HOLTER SUMMARY

Upon a quick review of Holter tracings, there were complexes that had an upstroke slur which resembled a delta wave. However, there was no P wave before the delta wave. The electrophysiological study demonstrated that this was a junctional rhythm with P waves overlapping QRS complexes, mimicking delta waves. Sometimes "Fusion causes Confusion". The described phenomenon can be named a pseudo-WPW pattern.

Additionally, we detected a supraventricular tachycardia, triggered by a premature contraction, PSVT that terminates with an atrial activation (P wave). This excludes atrial tachycardia. The retrograde P wave observed at the end of the QRS complex, associated with an RP interval of less than 80 ms, supports the diagnosis of AVNRT (atrioventricular node reentrant tachycardia). The electrophysiological examination confirmed the presence of both slow and fast pathways at the level of the AV node, with inducible typical slow-fast reentrant tachycardia. The PSVT arrhythmia pattern resembled that observed during Holter ECG.

The premature contraction that induced PSVT (Figure 5.5) can be either a PAC or a PVC. Arguments for PAC are the narrow QRS complex with a T wave identical to the other sinus beats. However, the argument for PVC is the different morphology of the beat with a different amplitude of the QRS complex. This can be a PVC near the His bundle which explains the narrow QRS and the identical T wave.

DISCUSSION

The pseudo-WPW pattern is an ECG that mimics preexcitation, in the absence of an accessory pathway. Causes of pseudo-WPW may include late premature ventricular contractions that arrive after the P wave, left ventricular hypertrophy, idioventricular rhythm, tricuspid atresia, hypoplastic left heart syndrome and atrioventricular canal defect. More than 90% of patients with HCM have abnormal ECG. A small percentage have pseudo-delta wave, mimicking a WPW syndrome; however, in those cases electrophysiological study is normal with the exclusion of an accessory pathway.

In the study by Zellers et al. on 183 patients with tricuspid atresia, the authors looked for a short PR interval with a slurring of the QRS onset called a delta wave. The patient's ages ranged from 4 months to 21 years, with 55% being males. The authors found during electrophysiological testing that only 20% of patients had an accessory pathway. The other 80% had a pseudo-WPW pattern, with an absence of an accessory pathway during EP study.

Eduardo Sternick et al. reported 20 patients of 107 individuals from 2 families, with a unique mutation of PRKAG2 gene manifested by ECG modifications of sinus bradycardia, short PR interval, right bundle branch block and the presence of a slurring of the initial portion of the QRS complex, compatible with a delta wave. During an electrophysiological study, all of the patients had a short AH interval (< 60 ms), a normal HV interval and infranodal conduction disorders without any sign of an accessory pathway. They called the modification pseudo-Wolff–Parkinson–White Syndrome.

Accelerated junctional rhythm occurs when the rate of an AV junction surpasses that of the sinus node. This condition occurs when there is increased automaticity in the AV node associated with decreased automaticity in the sinus node. Junctional rhythm is characterized by a narrow complex rhythm; QRS duration is always 120ms (if there is no pre-existing bundle branch block or rate-related aberrant conduction); the ventricular rate is usually 60–110 bpm and P waves may be present and can appear before, during or after the QRS complex. In our case the P waves appeared just before the beginning of the QRS mimicking a delta wave.

AVNRT is generally paroxysmal and may arise spontaneously in patients or be triggered by effort or mental stress. It is more prevalent in women than in men, with around 75% of cases occurring in females, and it can manifest in young, healthy individuals. AVNRT is caused by a reentrant circuit inside the AV node. The circuit is formed between two pathways forming the re-entrant limbs of the circuit: the slow and fast pathways with different electrophysiological properties. The ECG reveals a retrograde P wave accompanied by a short RP interval of less than 80 ms. Retrograde conduction occurs via the fast pathway, resulting in a short RP interval. The retrograde P wave may be recognized by the pseudo S wave in inferior leads II, III, and aVF, or by the existence of a pseudo r' in leads aVR and V1. That is the P wave located within the terminal segment of the QRS complex.

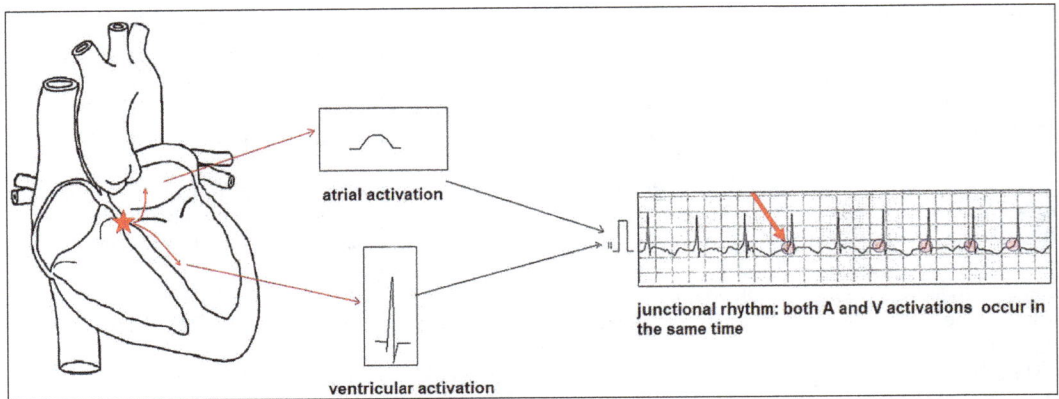

Figure 5.10   The pseudo-WPW pattern during junctional rhythm.

BIBLIOGRAPHY

1. Zellers TM, Porter CJ, Driscoll DJ. Pseudo-preexcitation in tricuspid atresia. *Tex Heart Inst J.* 1991; 18: 124–126.

2. Carlson AM, Turek JW, Law IH, Von Bergen NH. Pseudo-preexcitation is prevalent among patients with repaired complex congenital heart disease. *Pediatr Cardiol.* 2015; 36: 8–13.

3. Cohen M et al. PACES/HRS expert consensus statement on the management of the asymptomatic young patient with a Wolff–Parkinson–White (WPW, ventricular preexcitation) electrocardiographic pattern. *Heart Rhythm.* 2012; 9: 1006–1024.

4. Sternick EB, Antonio O, Magalhães LP, Gerken LM, Hong K, Santana O, Brugada P, Brugada J, Brugada R. Familial pseudo Wolff–Parkinson–White syndrome. *J Cardiovasc Electrophysiol.* 2006; 17: 724–732.

5. Scheinman MM. Familial preexcitation and pseudo-preexcitation syndromes. *J Cardiovasc Electrophysiol.* 2006 July; 17(7): 733–734. doi: 10.1111/j.1540-8167.2006.00474.x. PMID: 16836668.

6. Berkman NL, Lamb LE. The Wolff–Parkinson–White electrocardiogram. A follow-up study of five to twenty-eight years. *N Engl J Med.* 1968; 278(9): 492–494. doi: 10.1056/NEJM196802292780906

7. Hindman MC, Last JH, Rosen KM. Wolff–Parkinson–White syndrome observed by portable monitoring. *Ann Intern Med.* 1973; 79(5): 654–663. doi: 10.7326/0003-4819-79-5-654

8. Charron P, Genest M, Richard P, Komajda M, Pochmalicki G. A familial form of conduction defect related to a mutation in the PRKAG2 gene. *Europace.* 2007; 9(8): 597–600. doi: 10.1093/europace/eum071

9. Green M, Gollob M. Comment on "Familial pseudo-Wolff–Parkinson–White syndrome". *J Cardiovasc Electrophysiol.* 2006 December; 17(12): E9; author reply E10. doi: 10.1111/j.1540-8167.2006.00650.x. Epub 2006 November 10. PMID: 17096658.

10. Marrakchi S, Kammoun I, Kachboura S. Wolff–Parkinson–White syndrome mimics a conduction disease. *Case Rep Med.* 2014; 2014: 789537. doi: 10.1155/2014/789537. Epub 2014 July 9. PMID: 25114686; PMCID: PMC4119906.

11. Hafeez Y, Grossman SA. Junctional Rhythm. 2023 Feb 5. In: *StatPearls* [Internet]. Treasure Island (FL): StatPearls Publishing; 2025 Jan. PMID: 29939537.

12. Kerr CR, Mason MA. Incidence and clinical significance of accelerated junctional rhythm following open heart surgery. *Am Heart J.* 1985 Nov.; 110(5):966–969. doi: 10.1016/0002-8703(85)90193-0. PMID: 3877447.

13. Benezet-Mazuecos J, Lozano Rosado Á, Crosa J. Incessant accelerated idioventricular rhythm mimicking preexcitation. *J Electrocardiol.* 2020 Jul.–Aug; 61:137–140. doi: 10.1016/j.jelectrocard.2020.06.015. Epub 2020 Jun. 11. PMID: 32599292.

14. Kiger ME, McCanta AC, Tong S, Schaffer M, Runciman M, Collins KK. Intermittent versus Persistent Wolff-Parkinson-White Syndrome in Children: Electrophysiologic Properties and Clinical Outcomes. *Pacing Clin Electrophysiol.* 2016 Jan.; 39(1):14–20. doi: 10.1111/pace.12732. Epub 2015 Sep 11. PMID: 26256551.

15. Miyama H, Takatsuki S, Kimura T, Mitamura H, Ogawa S. Unusual Permanent Form of Junctional Reciprocating Tachycardia Associated With an Accessory Pathway With Bidirectional Conduction. *JACC Case Rep.* 2020 Feb. 19; 2(2):245–246. doi: 10.1016/j.jaccas. 2019.12.015. PMID: 34317213; PMCID: PMC8298563.

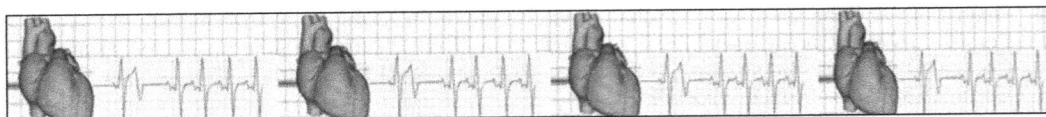

Case 6 Nonsustained Ventricular Tachycardia in a Patient with Dilated Cardiomyopathy

Simona Cainap, Cismaru Gabriel, and Adrian Stef

CLINICAL CASE

A 16-year-old male patient with muscular dystrophy and dilated cardiomyopathy, presenting a low ejection fraction of 20%, developed cardiac failure, necessitating high doses of inject-able Furosemide, sacubitril-valsartan SGLT2 inhibitor, and spironolactone as treatment. The Holter ECG demonstrated PVCs with multiple morphologies and episodes of nonsustained ventricular tachycardia. Due to the persistently poor ejection fraction for over two years, the decision was made to implant an internal defibrillator for the primary prevention of sudden cardiac death.

Concluzie

Ritm cardiac		
Total bătăi	114 862	(< 1% paced)
HR max / min	**125 / 89 bpm**	
Media HR	**Ø 110 bpm**	
HR Max / Min Sinus	125 / 89 bpm	
Media HR (Treaz/Adormit)	114 / 106 bpm	
Index circadian	1,08	
Tahicardie / Bradicardie	94 % / - %	

Pauze		
RR Max	**1 020 ms**	
Pauze (>2000ms)	0	

Fibrilaţie atrială / Flutter atrial		
Total AF	-	
AF HR Max	0 bpm	
Cel mai lung AF	-	

Bradicardie		
Cea mai mică	-	
Cea mai mare	-	

ST		
St ridicare max	-	
ST depresurizare max	-0,11 mV	aVF

Ectopie ventriculară		
V Total	3343	(3%)
V / Ora Max	260	pe oră
Episoade Tahicardie V	1 Σ 2 sec	
Cea mai rapidă Tahicardie V	Ø 123 bpm	2 sec
V Cea mai lungă secvenţă	Ø 123 bpm	2 sec
Triplete / Execută	17 Σ 52 bătăi	
Cuplete	331 Σ 662 bătăi	
Bigeminism	87 Σ 179 bătăi	
Trigeminism	105 Σ 218 bătăi	

Ectopie supraventriculară		
S Tot	7	(< 1%)
Episoade Tahicardie SV	-	
Cea mai rapidă Tahicardie SV	-	
S Cea mai lungă secvenţă	-	
Triplete / Execută	0 Σ 0 bătăi	
Cuplete	0 Σ 0 bătăi	

Figure 6.1 The summary page shows a maximum heart rate of 125 bpm and a minimum rate of 88 bpm. The PVC burden is moderate: 3% on 24 hours with episodes of bigeminy, trigeminy, couplets and triplets. The longest VT episode had 2 seconds duration.

DOI: 10.1201/9781003545040-6

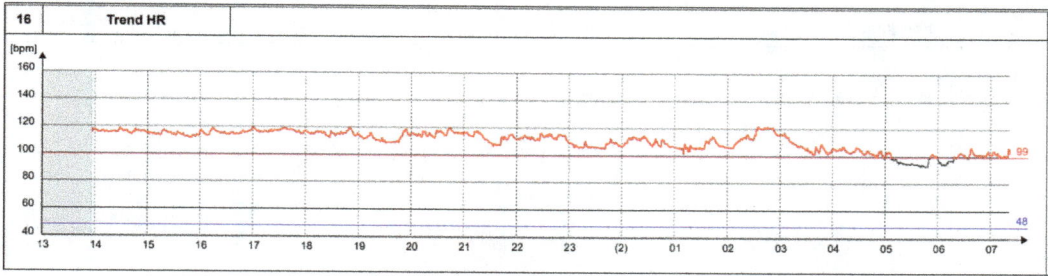

Figure 6.2 The heart rate histogram shows the mean rate over 24 hours of monitoring.

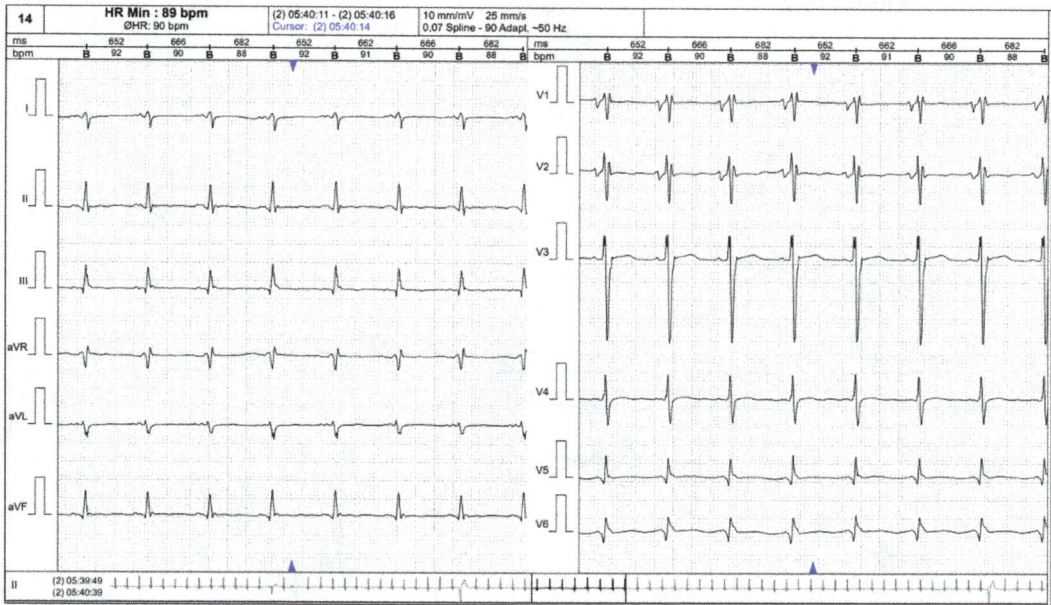

Figure 6.3 The minimum recorded rate was 89 bpm during normal sinus rhythm.

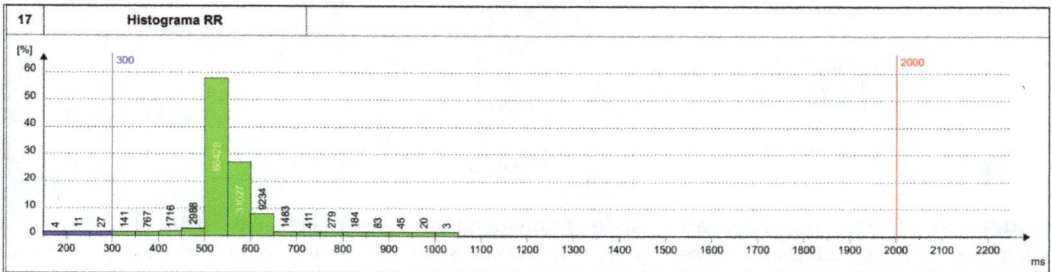

Figure 6.4 The RR histogram shows cycle length between 500 and 600 ms, corresponding to normal sinus rhythm 100–120 bpm. It rarely falls below 300 ms for several beats (blue color), indicative of episodes of nonsustained ventricular tachycardia.

41

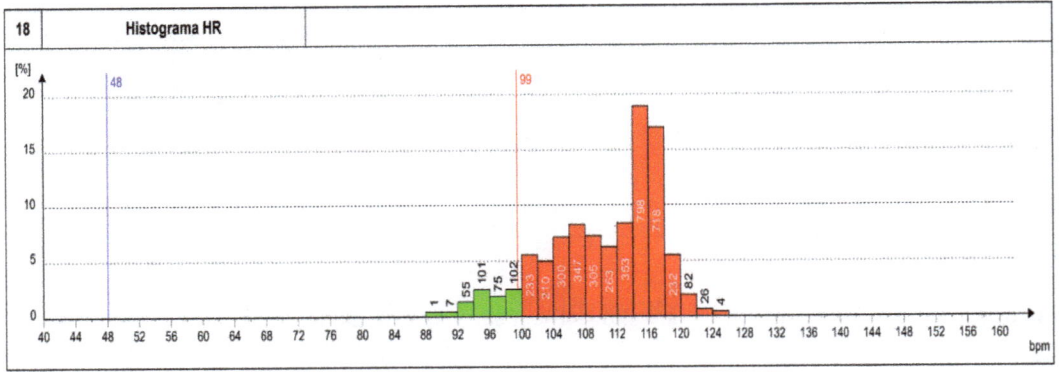

Figure 6.5 The HR histogram shows heart rates during 24 hours period of monitoring. The rate ranges from 89 to 125 bpm.

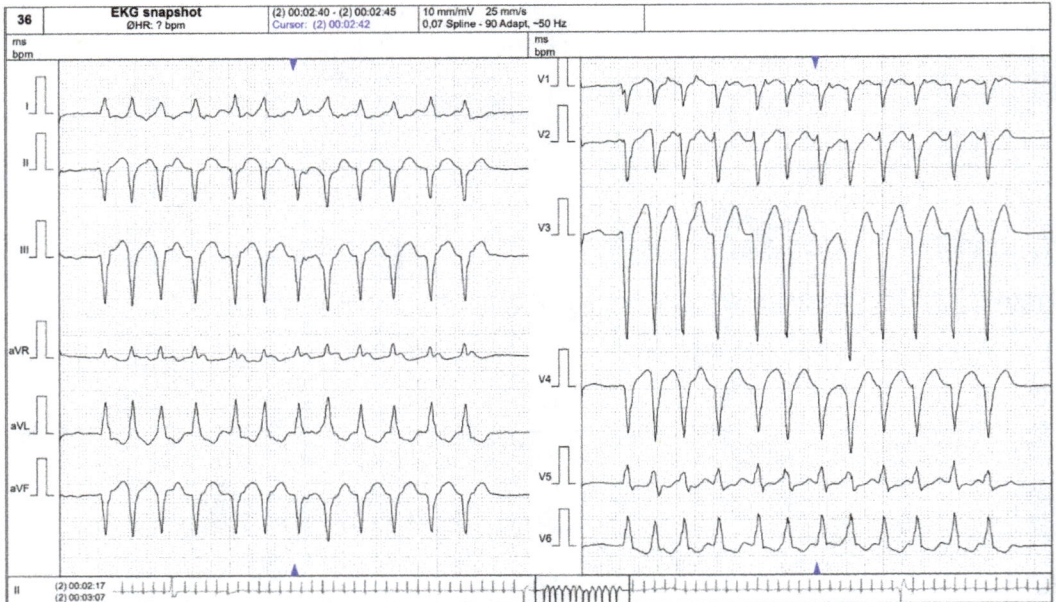

Figure 6.6 The tracing shows an episode of nonsustained ventricular tachycardia of 12 complexes. It is preceded and succeeded by regular sinus rhythm, as depicted in the lower section of the figure.

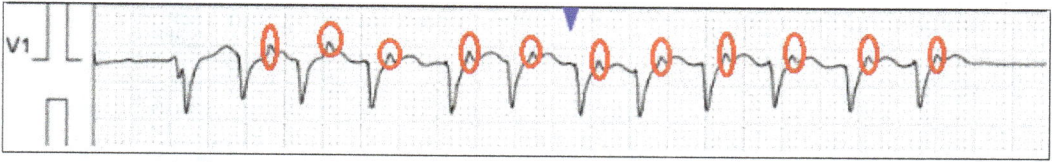

Figure 6.7 A magnified lead V1 reveals dissociated P waves confirming ventricular tachycardia.

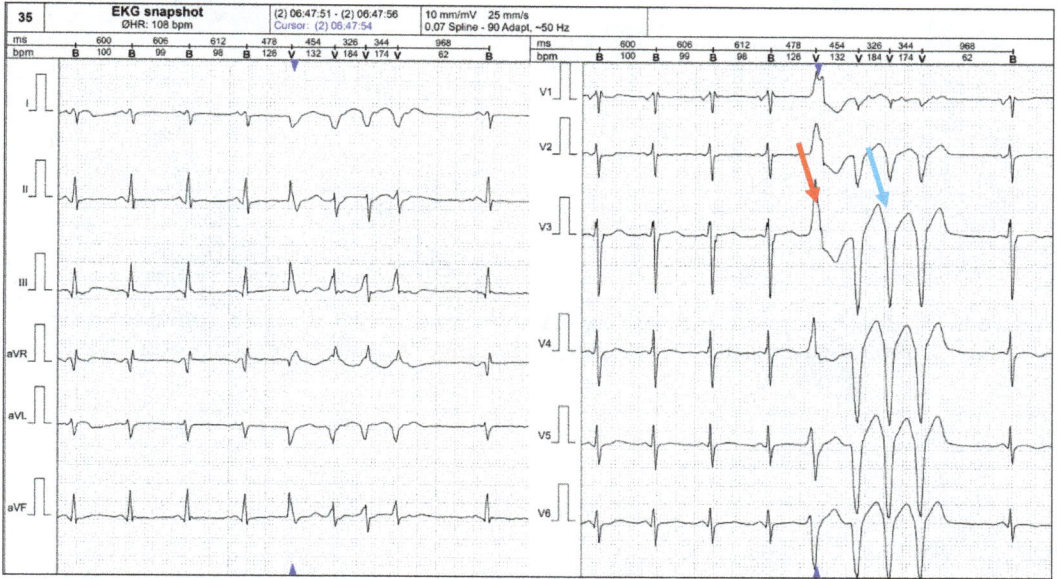

Figure 6.8 The tracing shows an episode of nonsustained ventricular tachycardia. The first ventricular beat marked with red arrow is different from the subsequent ventricular beats which look monomorphic (blue arrow).

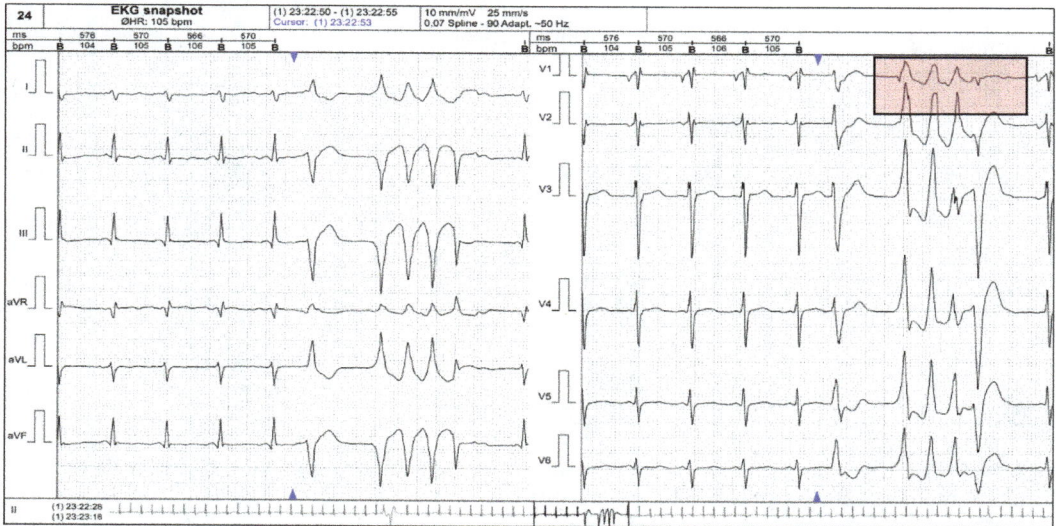

Figure 6.9 The tracing shows an episode of nonsustained ventricular tachycardia. In contrast to the episode depicted in Figure 6.6, it exhibits an RBBB pattern in lead V1, suggestive of a left ventricular origin.

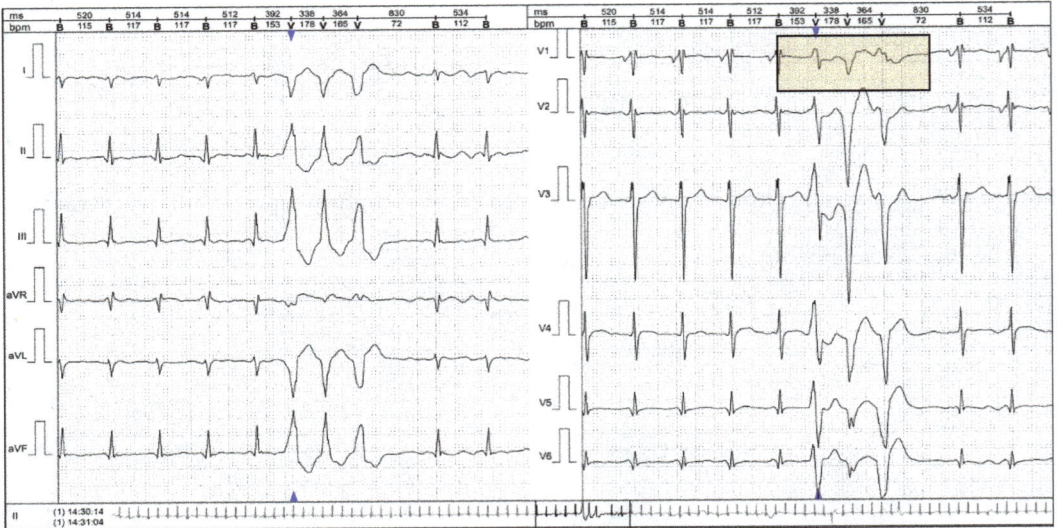

Figure 6.10 The tracing shows an episode of nonsustained ventricular tachycardia consisting of 3 premature ventricular beats. It may be referred to as NSVT, ventricular salvo, or triplet.

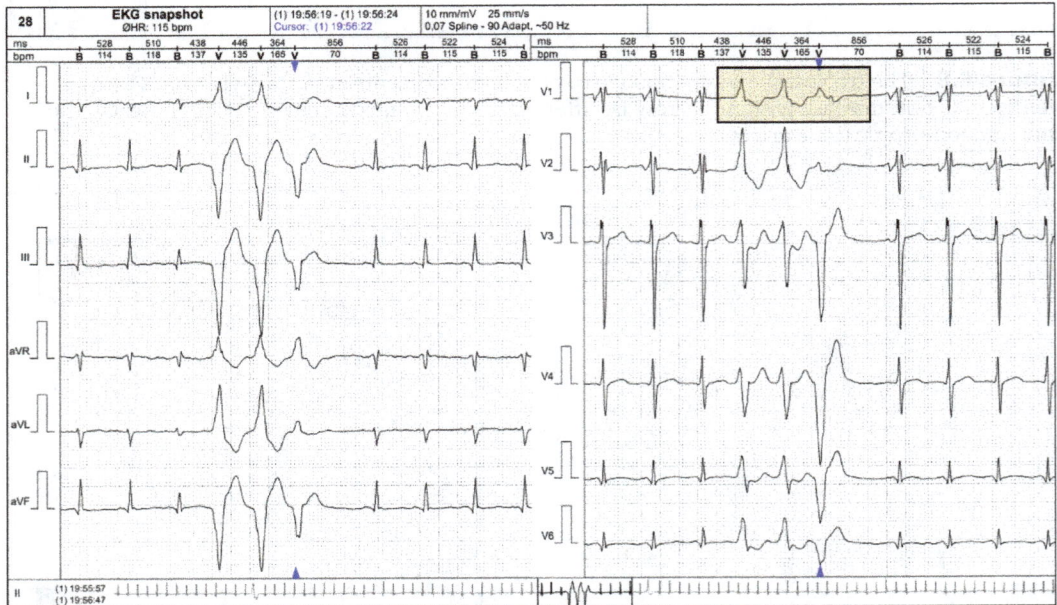

Figure 6.11 The tracing shows another episode of nonsustained ventricular tachycardia of different morphology compared to the prior events.

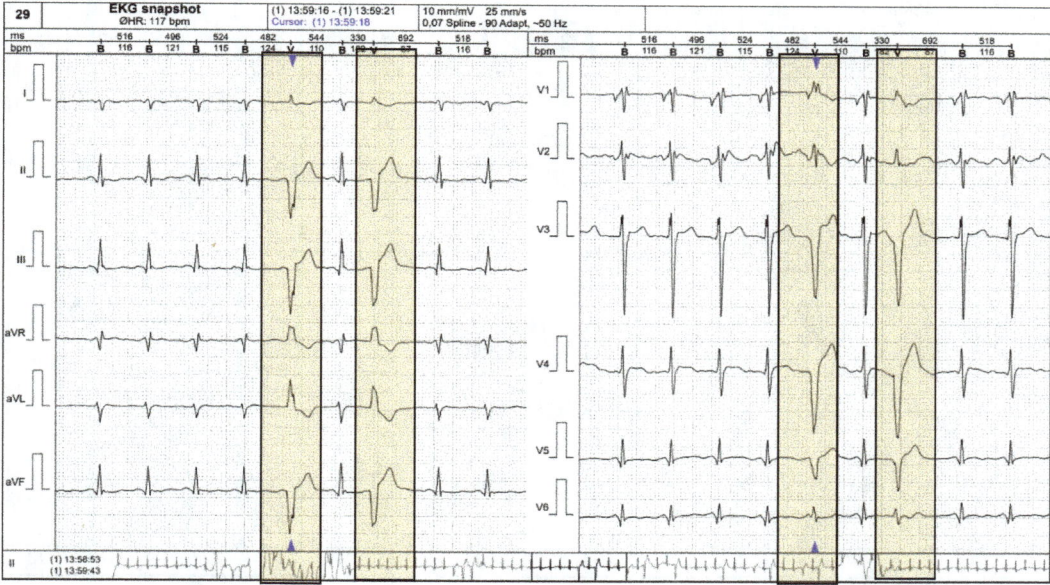

Figure 6.12 Premature ventricular contractions with an RBBB morphology.

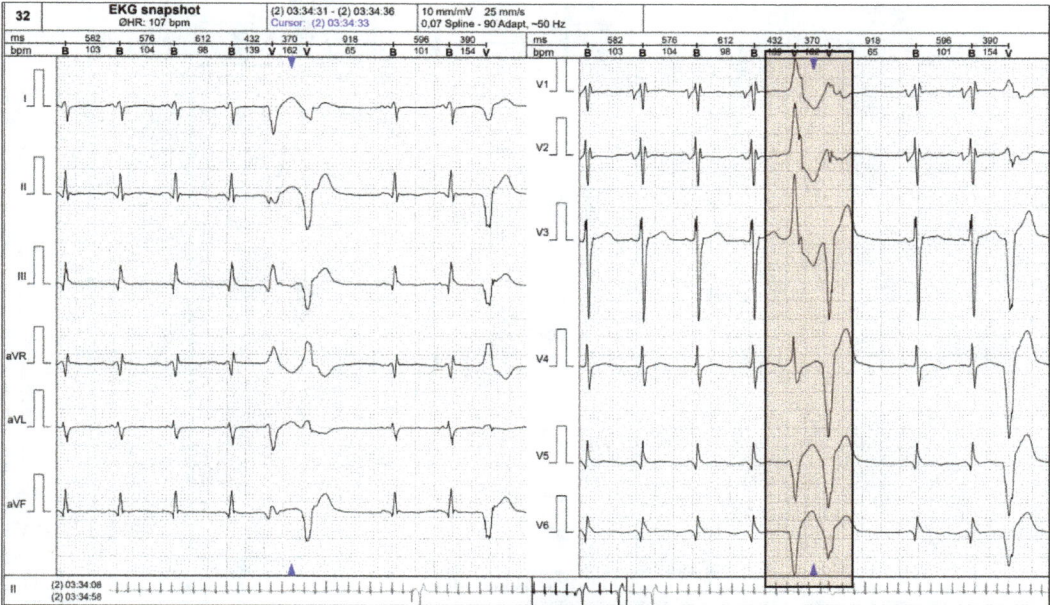

Figure 6.13 The tracing shows a ventricular couplet (2 consecutive PVCs).

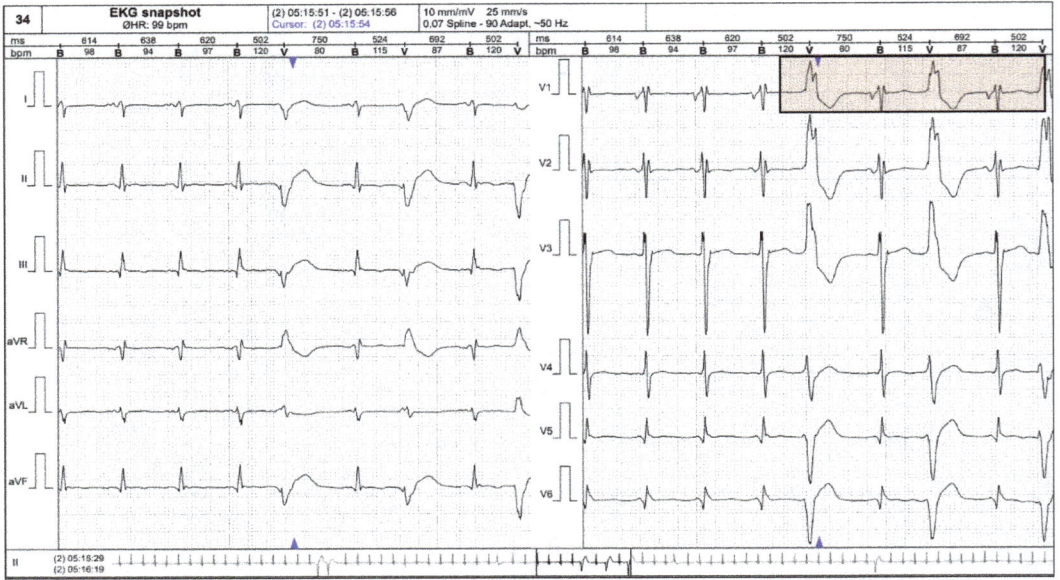

Figure 6.14 The tracing shows another pattern of PVCs with RBBB morphology.

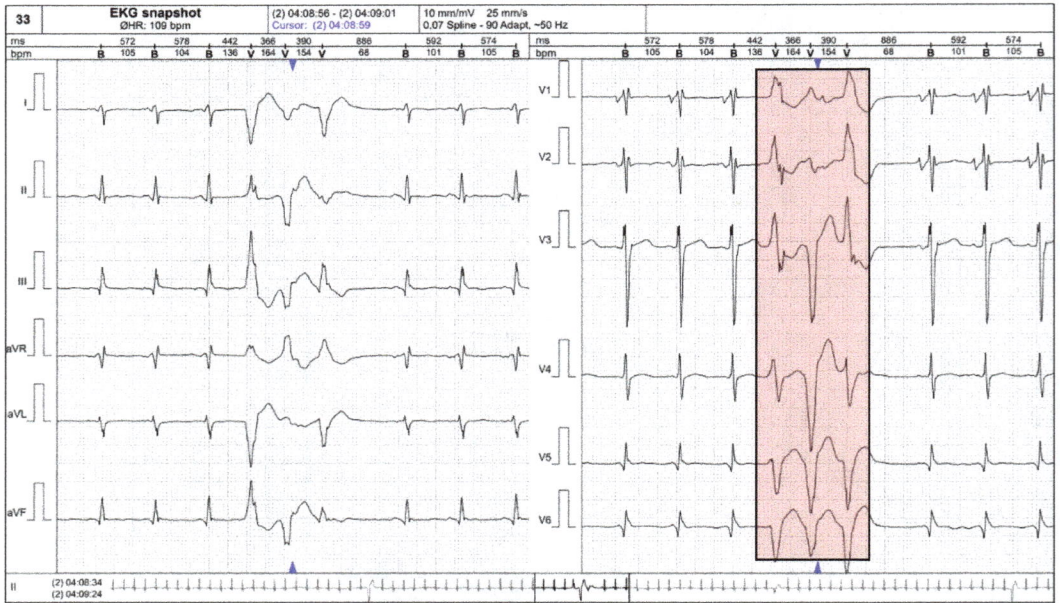

Figure 6.15 The tracing shows a ventricular triplet consisting of 3 different PVCs.

HOLTER SUMMARY

During 24 hours of Holter monitoring, 3372 PVCs were detected. We could identify at least 6 different morphologies suggesting origin in the left ventricle. There were also episodes of nonsustained ventricular tachycardia from 3 to 12 ventricular complexes, of different morphologies suggesting different localizations inside the left ventricle. The longest VT episode had a duration of 4.3 seconds with a heart rate of 177 bpm. There was no episode of sustained ventricular tachycardia of > 30 seconds.

DISCUSSION

Children with dilated cardiomyopathy (DCM) may experience various bradyarrhythmias and tachyarrhythmias.

The ventricular arrhythmogenic substrate for PVCs is characterized by several "irritable foci" caused by myocardial fibrosis, elevated catecholamine levels, or the distension of myocardial fibers. Ventricular arrhythmias can be classified in premature ventricular contractions, ventricular tachycardia and ventricular fibrillation.

Premature ventricular contractions may occur in repeating patterns: bigeminy- when every other second beat is a PVC, trigeminy- when every third beat is a PVC, couplet-in case of 2 consecutive beats, triplet-in case of three consecutive beats.

Ventricular tachycardia is defined by 3 or more consecutive ventricular beats at a rate of > 120 bpm (compared to 100 bpm in adults).

ECG characteristics of VT are:

- ventricular rate above 120 bpm

- 3 or more ventricular beats

- QRS wider than the normal QRS in sinus rhythm

- Ventriculo-atrial dissociation (as in Figure 6.7).

Ventricular tachycardia can be classified in terms of function of duration and morphology: Sustained VT > 30 seconds duration; Nonsustained VT less than 30 seconds duration but > 3 consecutive beats; Monomorphic VT = constant QRS morphology and axis; Polymorphic VT = more QRS morphologies and axis.

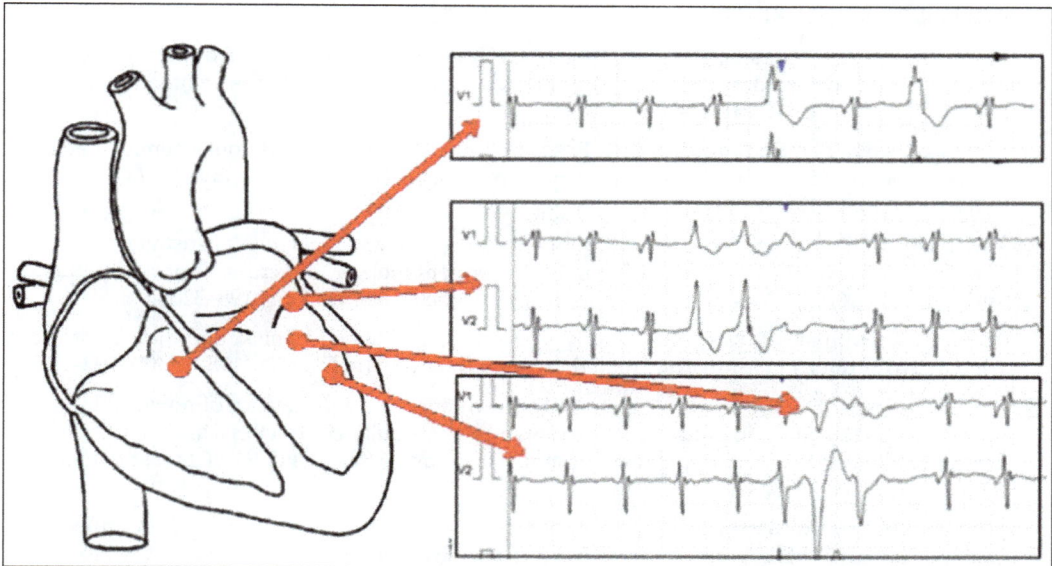

Figure 6.16 In dilated cardiomyopathy, several arrhythmogenic foci may exist within the ventricle, potentially giving rise to PVCs or VT. Therefore, the PVC morphologies are different due to the presence of several arrhythmogenic regions within the ventricle.

Ventricular tachycardia in children with dilated cardiomyopathy should be differentiated from supraventricular tachycardias with an RBBB aberrancy, or SVT with a preexisting RBBB or antidromic AV reentrant tachycardia using a left accessory pathway. If a wide QRS tachycardia is detected during ambulatory monitoring and the mechanism is unknown, an electrophysiological study can be performed to clarify the diagnosis.

The acute treatment of VT in children with dilated cardiomyopathy depends on the clinical situation. In case of hemodynamic compromise, a synchronized electrical shock is indicated using 1–2 J/kg energy for cardioversion. In case of hemodynamic stability, intravenous lidocaine is indicated 0.5–0.1 mg/kg that can be repeated up to 3 mg/kg/h. in continuous infusion. Ventricular tachycardia in dilated cardiomyopathy may also respond to intravenous beta blockers. In cases of significantly LV systolic dysfunction where beta blockers and Verapamil are contraindicated, Amiodarone may be administered with monitoring of blood pressure and ejection fraction.

Certain investigations indicated a poorer prognosis and an elevated risk of sudden cardiac death in patients with NSVT. In the GESICA trial, 516 patients (33.4% with NSVT) were examined using 24-hour Holter monitoring and followed for two years. Over this period, 87 out of 173 patients (50.3%) with nonsustained ventricular tachycardia (NSVT) and 106 out of 343 patients (30.9%) without NSVT died. The study demonstrated that NSVT is an independent indicator of increased overall mortality and sudden death risk. The lack of NSVT and ventricular repeated beats in a 24-hour Holter monitor suggests a reduced likelihood of sudden death.

However, in other cases, nonsustained ventricular tachycardia served as a predictor of sudden cardiac death only in univariate analysis, but not in multivariable analysis, or were not predictive of SCD, possibly due to the elevated incidence of nonsustained VT in patients with dilated cardiomyopathy.

BIBLIOGRAPHY

1. Hershberger RE, Hedges DJ, Morales A. Dilated cardiomyopathy: The complexity of a diverse genetic architecture. *Nat Rev Cardiol.* 2013; 10(9): 531–547.

2. Brembilla-Perrot B, Alla F, Suty-Selton C, Huttin O, Blangy H, Sadoul N, et al. Nonischemic dilated cardiomyopathy: Results of noninvasive and invasive evaluation in 310 patients and clinical significance of bundle branch block. *Pacing Clin Electrophysiol.* 2008; 31(11): 1383–1390.

3. Sekiguchi M, Hasegawa A, Hiroe M, Morimoto S, Nishikawa T. Inclusion of electric disturbance type cardiomyopathy in the classification of cardiomyopathy: EA current review. *J Cardiol.* 2008; 51(2): 81–88.

4. Spezzacatene A, Sinagra G, Merlo M, Barbati G, Graw SL, Brun F, et al. Arrhythmogenic phenotype in dilated cardiomyopathy: Natural history and predictors of life-threatening arrhythmias. *J Am Heart Assoc.* 2015; 4(10): e002149.

5. Holmes J, Kubo SH, Cody RJ, Kligfield P. Arrhythmias in ischemic and nonischemic dilated cardiomyopathy: Prediction of mortality by ambulatory electrocardiography. *Am J Cardiol.* 1985; 55(1): 146–151.

6. Doval HC, Nul DR, Grancelli HO, Varini SD, Soifer S, Corrado G, et al. Nonsustained ventricular tachycardia in severe heart failure. Independent marker of increased mortality due to sudden death: GESICA-GEMA Investigators. *Circulation.* 1996; 94(12): 3198–3203.

7. Meinertz T, Hofmann T, Kasper W, Treese N, Bechtold H, Stienen U, et al. Significance of ventricular arrhythmias in idiopathic dilated cardiomyopathy. *Am J Cardiol.* 1984; 53(7): 902–907.

8. Singh SN, Fisher SG, Carson PE, Fletcher RD. Prevalence and significance of nonsustained ventricular tachycardia in patients with premature ventricular contractions and heart failure treated with vasodilator therapy: Department of Veterans Affairs CHF STAT Investigators. *J Am Coll Cardiol.* 1998; 32(4): 942–947.

9. Grimm W, Christ M, Bach J, Müller HH, Maisch B. Noninvasive arrhythmia risk stratification in idiopathic dilated cardiomyopathy: Results of the Marburg Cardiomyopathy Study. *Circulation.* 2003; 108(23): 2883–2891.

10. Zecchin M, Di Lenarda A, Gregori D, Merlo M, Pivetta A, Vitrella G, et al. Are nonsustained ventricular tachycardias predictive of major arrhythmias in patients with dilated cardiomyopathy on optimal medical treatment? *Pacing Clin Electrophysiol.* 2008; 31(3): 290–299.

11. Pogwizd SM, McKenzie JP, Cain ME. Mechanisms underlying spontaneous and induced ventricular arrhythmias in patients with idiopathic dilated cardiomyopathy. *Circulation.* 1998; 98(22): 2404–2414.

12. Soejima K, Stevenson WG, Sapp JL, Selwyn AP, Couper G, Epstein LM. Endocardial and epicardial radiofrequency ablation of ventricular tachycardia associated with dilated cardiomyopathy: The importance of low-voltage scars. *J Am Coll Cardiol.* 2004; 43(10): 1834–1842.

13. Streitner F, Kuschyk J, Dietrich C, Mahl E, Streitner I, Doesch C, et al. Comparison of ventricular tachyarrhythmia characteristics in patients with idiopathic dilated or ischemic cardiomyopathy and defibrillators implanted for primary prevention. *Clin Cardiol.* 2011; 34(10): 604–609.

14. Merlo M, Pivetta A, Pinamonti B, Stolfo D, Zecchin M, Barbati G, et al. Long-term prognostic impact of therapeutic strategies in patients with idiopathic dilated cardiomyopathy: Changing mortality over the last 30 years. *Eur J Heart Fail.* 2014; 16(3): 317–324.

15. Towbin JA, Lorts A. Arrhythmias and dilated cardiomyopathy common pathogenetic pathways? *J Am Coll Cardiol.* 2011; 57(21): 2169–2171.

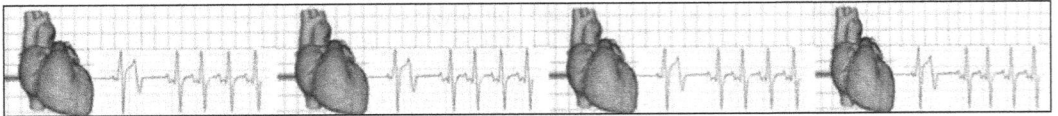

Case 7 Vagal Nerve Stimulation-Induced AV Block in an 11-Year-Old with Epilepsy

Stefan Kurath-Koller

CLINICAL CASE

An 11-year-old patient with a known history of epilepsy, refractory to medical treatment, was implanted with a vagal nerve stimulator (VNS) to control seizures. The patient presented to the pediatric emergency department due to recurrent episodes of apnea, predominantly occurring during sleep. The mother reported irregular breathing and multiple episodes of apnea, with no other associated symptoms. She attempted to use the VNS to alleviate the apnea, suspecting it might be related to seizures.

On examination. On examination, the patient's echocardiography was unremarkable. However, continuous monitoring ECG revealed several episodes of pauses in the cardiac electrical activity. Subsequent 24-hour ECG recording demonstrated recurrent episodes of AV block, characterized by the loss of conduction over multiple P waves and a maximum pause duration of up to 7 seconds. Notably, underlying sinus rhythm slowed down before phases of AV block, with slight PR prolongation and intermittent phases of 2:1 AV block.

During these pauses, the patient was largely asymptomatic but occasionally appeared absent. Assessing mental status and level of consciousness was challenging due to underlying developmental delay.

Considering the possibility of vagally mediated pauses, the VNS settings were reviewed by pediatric neurologists. It was found that the VNS was set to very high stimulation levels and prolonged action time. This led to the hypothesis that the VNS might be inducing AV block episodes. Despite reducing the VNS therapy to appropriate levels for seizure control, the pauses continued.

Given the persistence of the pauses, the decision was made to implant a cardiac pacemaker to ensure adequate heart rates. Post-implantation, the patient has been doing well, requiring approximately 1% ventricular pacing to prevent pauses.

This case highlights the potential for vagal nerve stimulation to induce significant AV block in pediatric patients with epilepsy. Careful monitoring and adjustment of VNS settings are crucial in some cases, however, additional interventions such as pacemaker implantation may be necessary to manage cardiac complications.

Herzfrequenzen (1-Min.-Durchschnitt)		Bradykardie	1	Tachykardie	0
Max. HF	138 1/min. am Mi. 03, 17:09	Summe	12 Sek., 0,0%	Summe	
Mittl. HF	119 1/min.	Längste	7 Schläge am Do. 04, 00:02	Längste	
Min. HF	71 1/min. am Mi. 03, 12:15	Min. Frequenz	27 1/min. am Do. 04, 00:02	Max. Frequenz	
Pause	39 , längste 6,62 Sek. um Mi. 03, 23:35				

Figure 7.1 Heart rate and bradycardia overview (HF = heart rate).

DOI: 10.1201/9781003545040-7

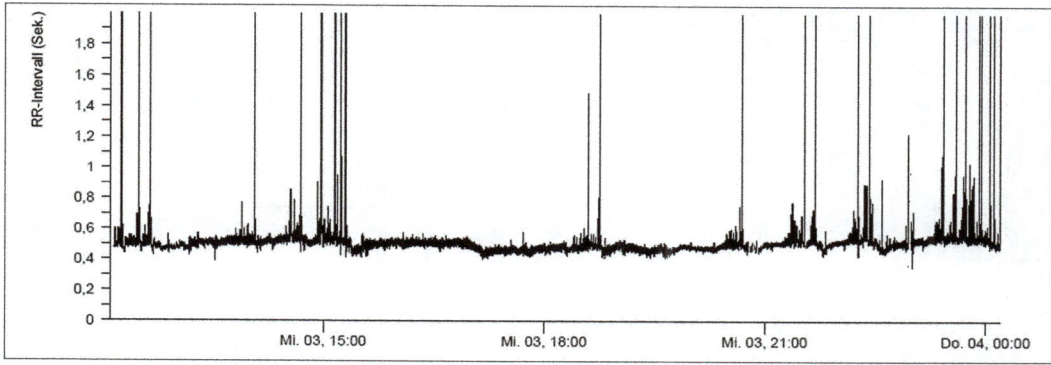

Figure 7.2 RR interval histogram in seconds over time.

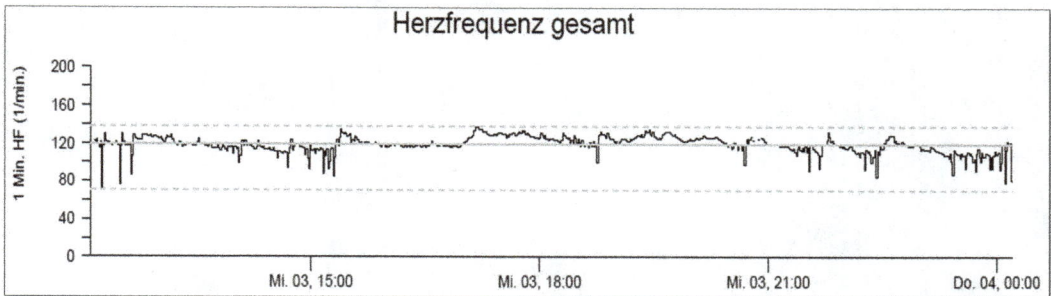

Figure 7.3 Heart rate histogram in beats per minute over time.

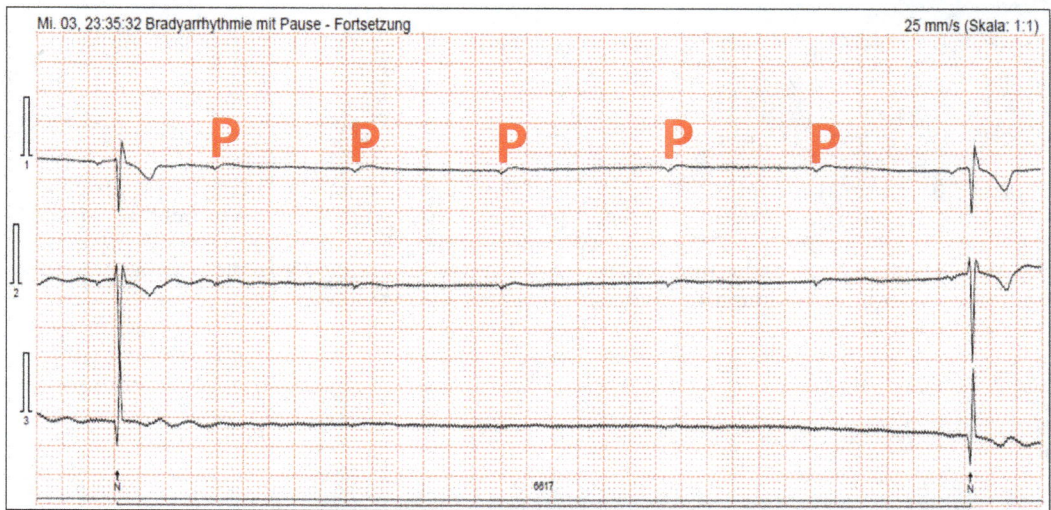

Figure 7.4 Longest pause (6.617 seconds) due to high degree AV block. Five unconducted P waves visible.

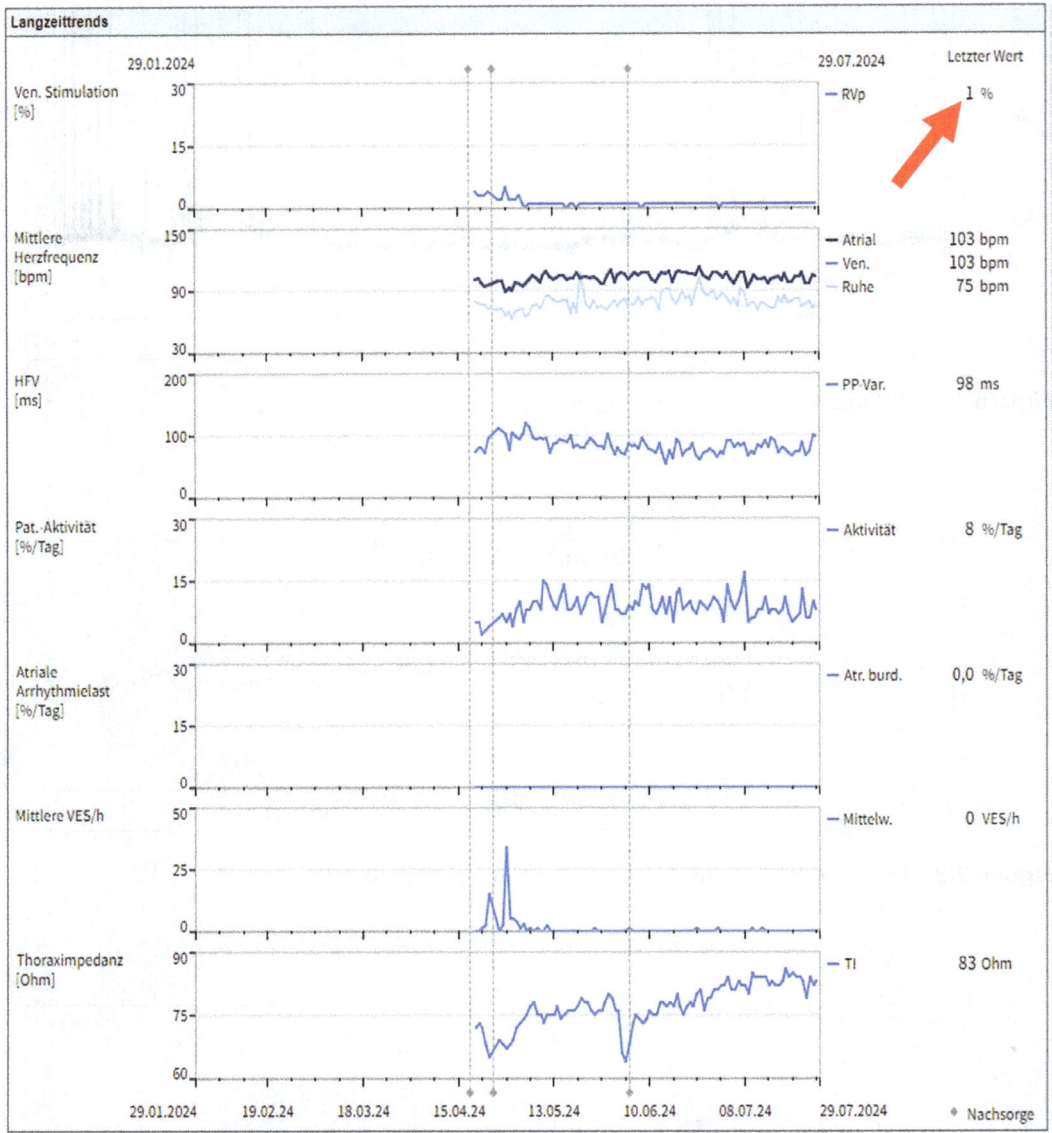

Figure 7.5 Pacemaker read out over 3 months following implantation. Top line: % ventricular stimulation (1% ventricular pacing). Second line: mean heart rate in beats per minute. Third line: Heart rate variability given as P-P variability in milliseconds. Fourth line: Patient activity in % per day. Fifth line: Atrial arrhythmia burden in % per day. Sixth line: Mean premature ventricular contractions per hour. Bottom line: Thoracic impedance in Ohm.

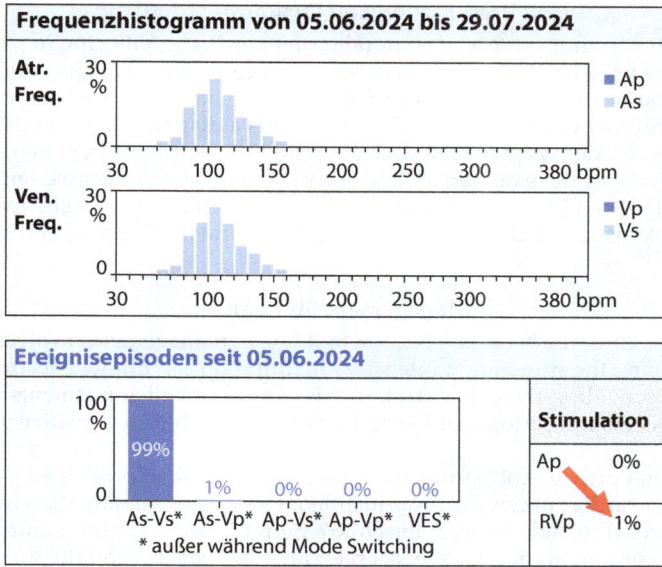

Figure 7.6 Pacemaker readout depicting atrial and ventricular rate histogram and pacing burden (1% RV pacing).

HOLTER SUMMARY

- Recurrent AV block: Multiple episodes of AV block with maximum pause duration of up to 7 seconds.

- Sinus rhythm: Slowed down prior to AV block phases.

- PR prolongation: Slight, intermittent 2:1 AV block.

- Frequency of pauses: Up to 20 pauses per hour, each lasting 4 to 6 seconds.

DISCUSSION

Vagal Nerve Stimulation and Cardiac Effects

Vagal nerve stimulation (VNS) is an established therapeutic option for patients with epilepsy refractory to medical treatment. By delivering electrical impulses to the vagus nerve, VNS can help reduce the frequency and severity of seizures. However, the vagus nerve also plays a critical role in autonomic control of the heart, and its stimulation can lead to significant cardiac effects. The most notable among these are bradyarrhythmias, including sinus bradycardia and AV block. These cardiac side effects are particularly relevant in pediatric patients, whose autonomic nervous systems may respond more sensitively to external stimulation.

Mechanisms of VNS-Induced Cardiac Arrhythmias

The vagus nerve influences heart rate and conduction primarily through its parasympathetic (cholinergic) effects. When VNS is activated, it can increase parasympathetic tone, leading to decreased heart rate and conduction velocity. This can manifest as sinus bradycardia or various degrees of AV block. In the case presented, the patient experienced recurrent episodes of AV block with significant pauses, suggesting that the VNS was indeed affecting cardiac conduction pathways.

The observed slowing of the sinus rhythm prior to the AV block episodes, along with PR prolongation and intermittent 2:1 AV block, is consistent with enhanced vagal tone. These findings indicate that the VNS was likely set to a level where its effects on the heart were pronounced, overshadowing its intended therapeutic action on seizure activity.

Clinical Presentation and Diagnostic Challenges

This case underscores the importance of comprehensive cardiac monitoring in patients with VNS, especially when they present with symptoms such as apnea or syncope. The patient's recurrent apnea episodes, initially attributed to seizure activity by the mother, were later found to be associated with significant cardiac pauses. This highlights a diagnostic challenge, as symptoms of cardiac arrhythmias can mimic or coexist with neurological symptoms in patients with epilepsy.

The patient's underlying developmental delay further complicated the assessment of symptoms and mental status. This complexity necessitates a multidisciplinary approach, involving pediatric cardiologists, neurologists, and electrophysiologists, to accurately diagnose and manage such cases.

Management Strategies

Upon identifying the cardiac effects of VNS, the first line of management involves adjusting the VNS settings. Reducing the stimulation intensity and duration can mitigate its impact on cardiac function while still providing seizure control. In this case, although adjustments were made, the cardiac pauses persisted, indicating that the patient's heart was highly sensitive to even lower levels of VNS.

Given the continued presence of significant pauses and the risk of prolonged asystole, the decision to implant a cardiac pacemaker was justified. Pacemaker implantation in pediatric patients requires careful consideration of the child's growth and long-term management. The pacemaker ensures continuous adequate heart rates and prevents potentially life-threatening pauses, thereby significantly improving the patient's quality of life and safety.

Implications for Future Practice

This case highlights several key points for clinical practice:

1. Vigilant Monitoring: Continuous ECG monitoring in patients with VNS is crucial, especially when new or unexplained symptoms arise.

2. Multidisciplinary Approach: Collaboration among specialists is essential for the comprehensive management of patients with complex conditions like epilepsy and cardiac arrhythmias.

3. Individualized Care: Each patient's response to VNS is unique, necessitating personalized adjustment of therapy and, when needed, the implementation of additional interventions like pacemaker therapy.

4. Awareness and Education: Educating caregivers about the potential cardiac side effects of VNS can help in early identification and intervention, preventing serious complications.

Conclusion

This case of an 11-year-old with epilepsy and VNS-induced AV block underscores the delicate balance between therapeutic benefits and side effects of VNS. It also illustrates the importance of integrated care approaches and the potential need for additional cardiac interventions in managing complex pediatric patients. The successful outcome following pacemaker implantation highlights the efficacy of this approach in ensuring patient safety and well-being.

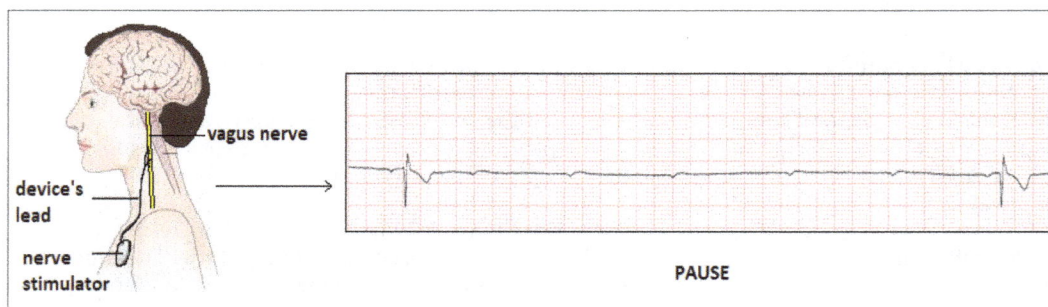

Figure 7.7 Schematic representation vagal nerve stimulation-induced pauses.

BIBLIOGRAPHY

1. Epilepsy Foundation. Vagus Nerve Stimulation (VNS) Therapy. Available at: Epilepsy Foundation https://www.epilepsy.com/treatment/devices/vagus-nerve-stimulation-therapy

2. Hamza M, Carron R, Dibué M, Moiraghi A, Barrit S, Filipescu C, Landré E, Gavaret M, Domenech P, Pallud J, Zanello M. Right-sided vagus nerve stimulation for drug-resistant epilepsy: A systematic review of the literature and perspectives. *Seizure.* 2024 April; 117: 298–304.

3. Cantarín-Extremera V, Ruíz-Falcó-Rojas ML, Tamaríz-Martel-Moreno A, García-Fernández M, Duat-Rodriguez A, Rivero-Martín B. Late-onset periodic bradycardia during vagus nerve stimulation in a pediatric patient. A new case and review of the literature. *Eur J Paediatr Neurol.* 2016 July; 20(4): 678–683.

4. Gandhi H, Ippoliti M, Iqbal F, Shah A. Bradyarrhythmia secondary to vagus nerve stimulator 7 years after placement. *BMJ Case Rep.* 2020 Jun. 30; 13(6):e235514. doi: 10.1136/bcr-2020-235514. PMID: 32606132; PMCID: PMC7328739.

5. Hotta H, Lazar J, Orman R, Koizumi K, Shiba K, Kamran H, Stewart M. Vagus nerve stimulation-induced bradyarrhythmias in rats. *Auton Neurosci.* 2009 Dec. 3; 151(2): 98–105. doi: 10.1016/j.autneu.2009.07.008. Epub 2009 Aug 3. PMID: 19651541.

6. Amark P, Stödberg T, Wallstedt L. Late onset bradyarrhythmia during vagus nerve stimulation. *Epilepsia.* 2007 May; 48(5):1023–1024. doi: 10.1111/j.1528-1167.2007.01023.x. Epub 2007 Mar 22. PMID: 17381444.

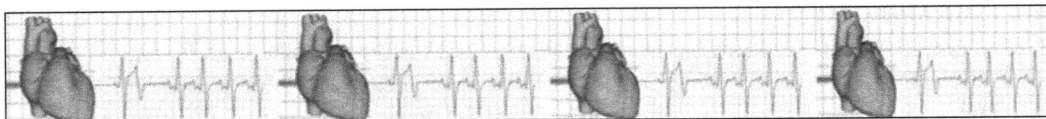

Case 8 Complete AV Block in a 12-Year-Old Girl

Cecilia Lazea, Alexandra Popa, and Gabriela Kelemen

CLINICAL CASE

A 12-year-old girl with no history of heart disease was referred to the Emergency Department by her family doctor after suffering from dyspnea following an argument with a friend. She did not display syncope, lightheadedness, or vertigo. The physical examination showed no signs of heart failure. The heart rate was 50 bpm and the blood pressure 110/70 mm Hg. The electrocardiogram (ECG) revealed complete atrioventricular (AV) block. A transthoracic echocardiography was conducted which showed normal results. Testing for autoimmune disease was negative, and diagnoses of both systemic lupus erythematosus and Sjoegren's syndrome were excluded. No reversible cause of AV block was found. The patient had a very good tolerance to exercise. A Holter ECG is presented below.

Ritm cardiac		
Total bătăi	62 520	(0% paced)
HR max / min	**98 / 36 bpm**	
Media HR	**Ø 50 bpm**	
HR Max / Min Sinus	98 / 36 bpm	
Media HR (Treaz/Adormit)	53 / 46 bpm	
Index circadian	1,15	
Tahicardie / Bradicardie	- % / 72 %	

Pauze		
RR Max	**1 738 ms**	
Pauze (>2000ms)	**0**	

Fibrilaţie atrială / Flutter atrial		
Total AF	-	
AF HR Max	0 bpm	
Cel mai lung AF	-	

Bradicardie		
Cea mai mică	Ø 42 bpm	00:52:38
Cea mai mare	Ø 43 bpm	01:01:24

ST		
St ridicare max	0,53 mV	aVR
ST depresurizare max	-0,40 mV	V5

Ectopie ventriculară		
V Total	0	(< 1%)
V / Ora Max	0	pe oră
Episoade Tahicardie V		-
Cea mai rapidă Tahicardie V		-
V Cea mai lungă secvenţă		-
Triplete / Execută		0 Σ 0 bătăi
Cuplete		0 Σ 0 bătăi
Bigeminism		0 Σ 0 bătăi
Trigeminism		0 Σ 0 bătăi

Ectopie supraventriculară		
S Tot	0	(< 1%)
Episoade Tahicardie SV		-
Cea mai rapidă Tahicardie SV		-
S Cea mai lungă secvenţă		-
Triplete / Execută		0 Σ 0 bătăi
Cuplete		0 Σ 0 bătăi

Figure 8.1 This chart presents a summary of the events observed on the Holter ECG. The total number of beats for the recording period is low: 62520/24 hours. The minimum rate was 36 bpm, while the maximum was 98 bpm. The mean heart rate is low at 53 bpm while awake, although it exceeds the 50 bpm threshold indicated in the cardiac pacing guidelines. No PACs or PVCs were documented.

DOI: 10.1201/9781003545040-8

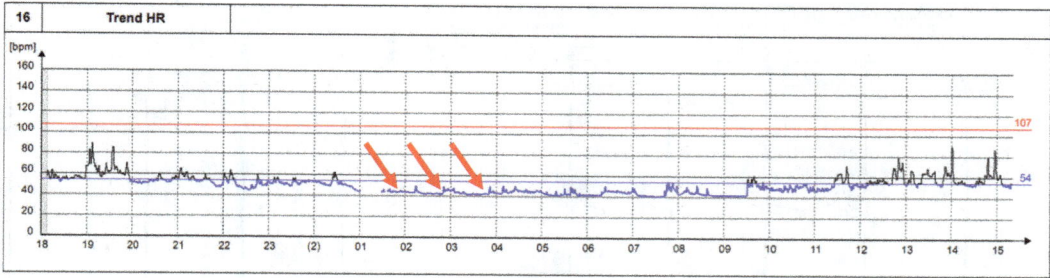

Figure 8.2 The HR trend shows low rates during sleep, close to a mean of 40 bpm. Bradycardia is indicated by a blue line at 54 bpm, while tachycardia is indicated by a red line at 107 bpm. Rates below 54 bpm are marked by a blue curve.

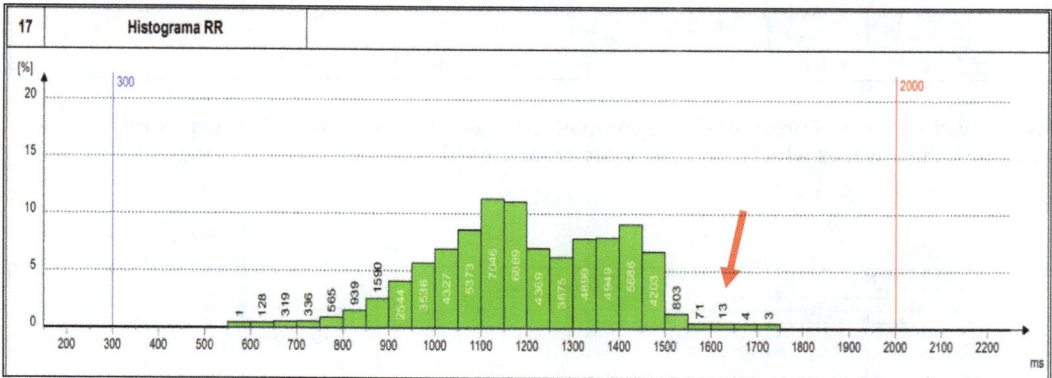

Figure 8.3 The RR histogram shows intervals marked with green line between 300 and 2000 ms. The longest intervals have 1500–1700 ms.

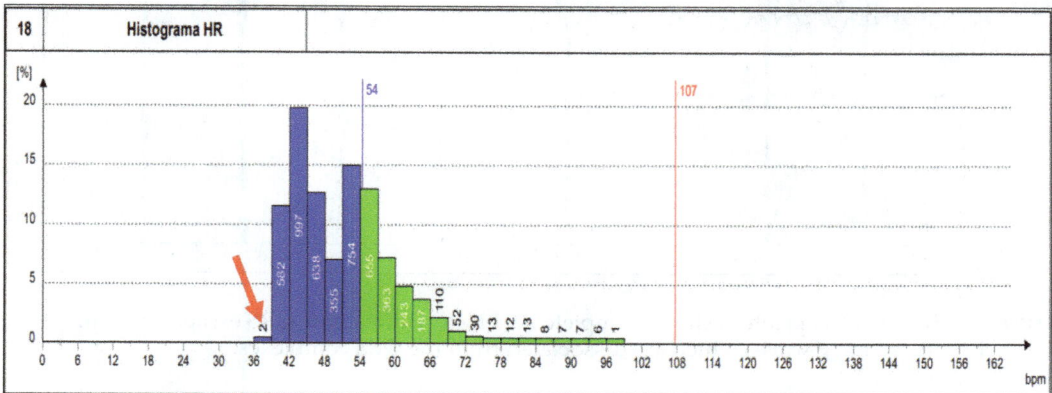

Figure 8.4 The HR histogram shows rates between 54 and 107 bpm marked with green bars and rates below 54 bpm marked with blue bars. The lowest rates were 36 bpm.

57

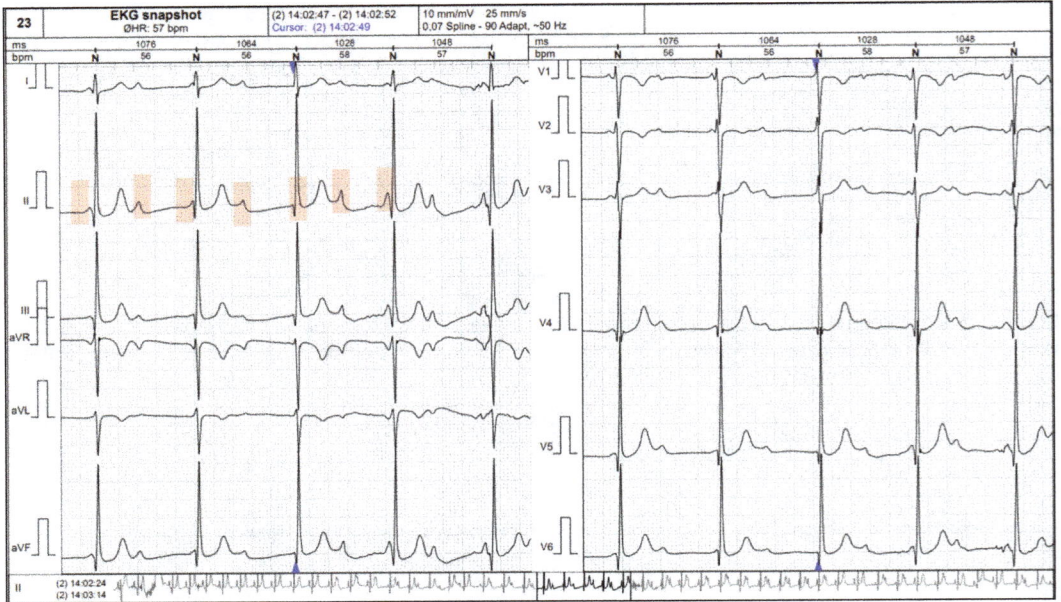

Figure 8.5 The ECG printout shows complete AV block with narrow QRS escape rhythm. Red bars mark the P waves which are dissociated from the QRS complexes.

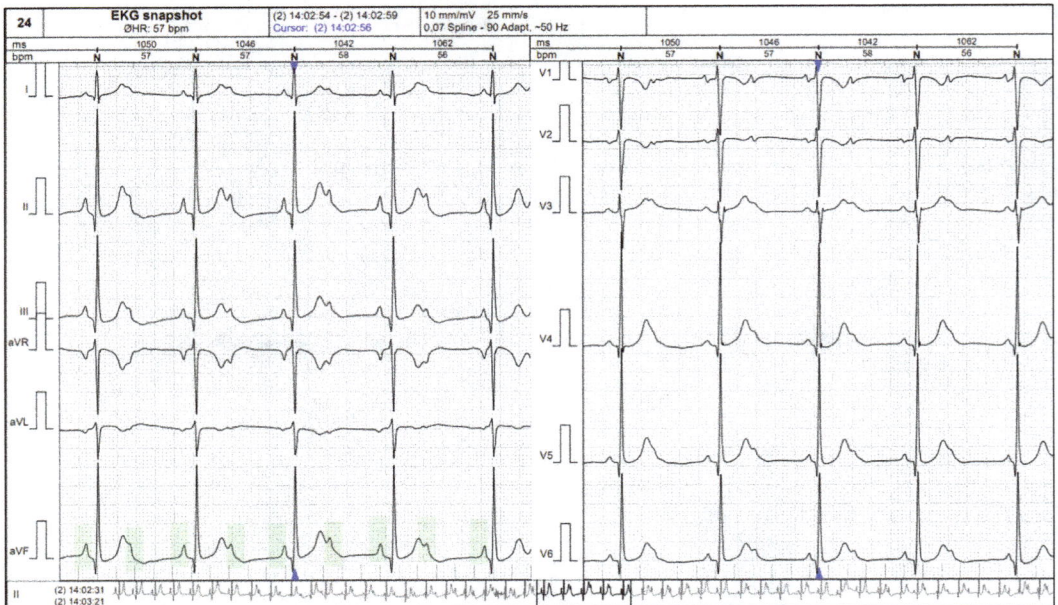

Figure 8.6 The ECG printout shows complete AV block with narrow QRS escape rhythm. Green bars mark the P waves which are dissociated from the QRS complexes.

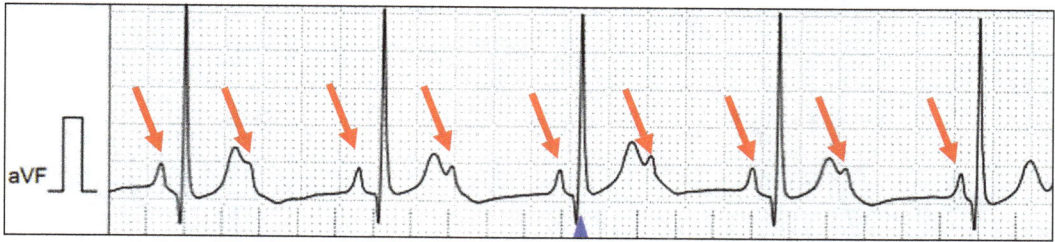

Figure 8.7 The ECG printout of lead avF shows complete AV block with narrow QRS escape rhythm. Red arrows mark the P waves which are dissociated from the QRS complexes.

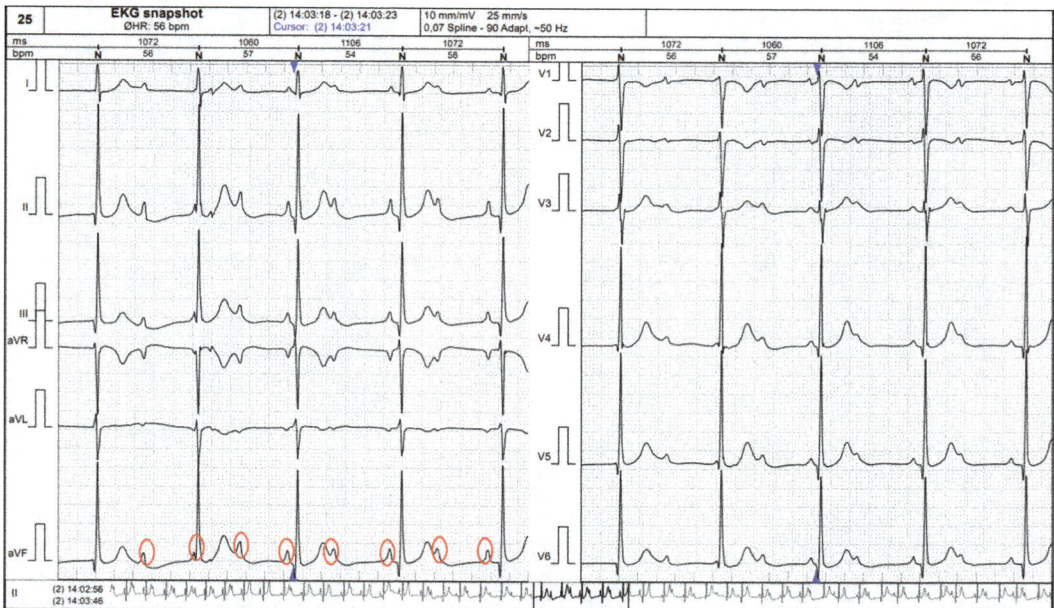

Figure 8.8 The ECG printout shows complete AV block with narrow QRS escape rhythm. Red circles mark the P waves which are dissociated from the QRS complexes.

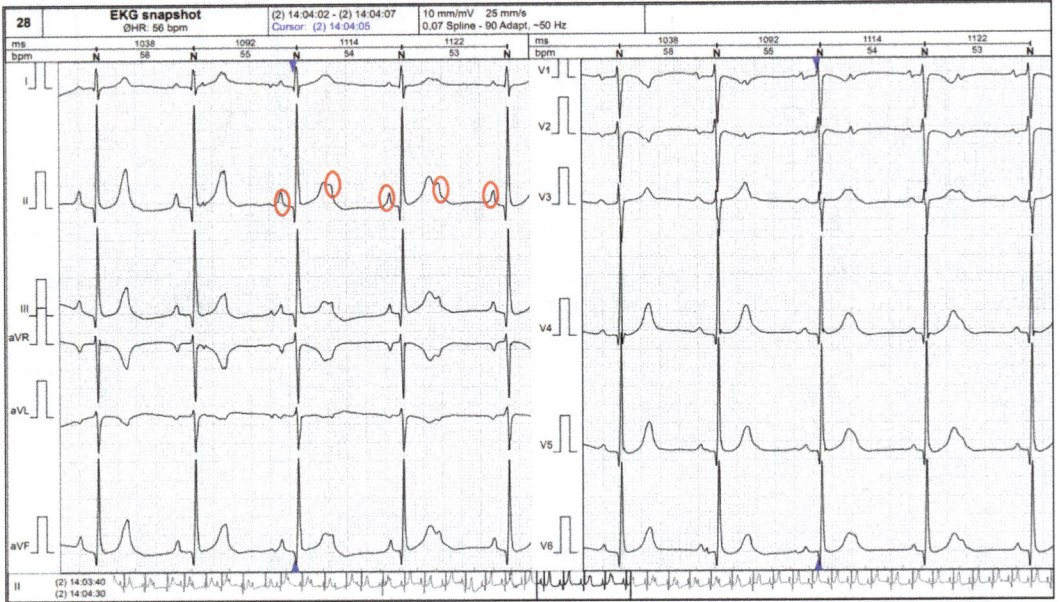

Figure 8.9 The ECG printout shows complete AV block mimicking 1:1 conduction from atria to ventricles. However, red circles mark the P waves which are dissociated from the QRS complexes.

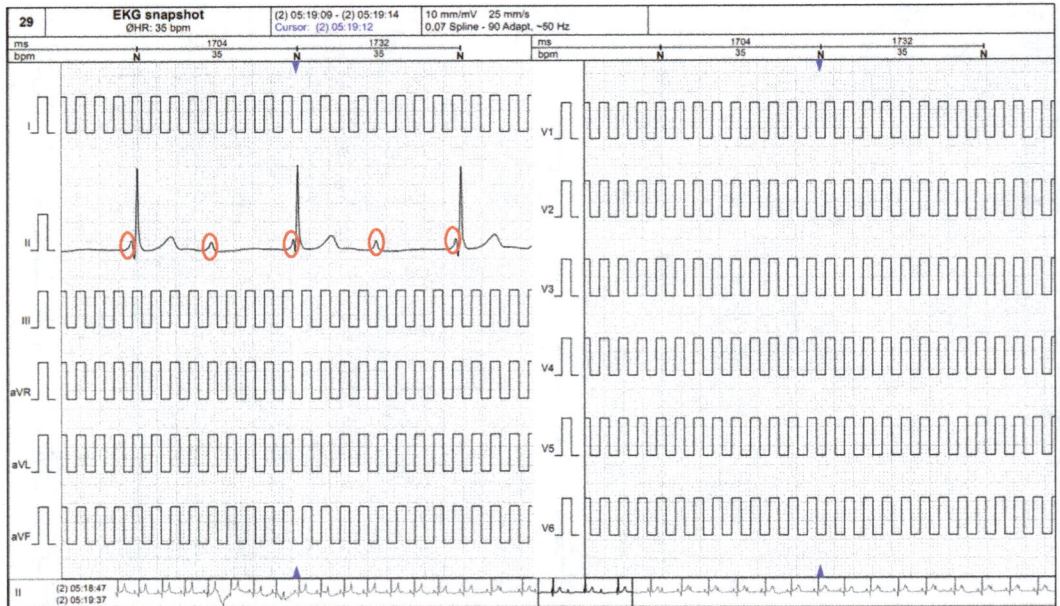

Figure 8.10 The ECG printout shows complete AV block with red circles marking the P waves which are dissociated from the QRS complexes. Only lead I has good quality electrical signal, the other leads having electrical artifacts.

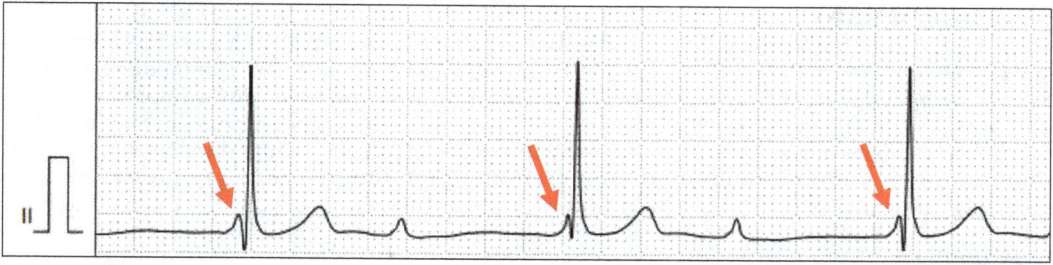

Figure 8.11 The ECG printout shows complete AV block mimicking ventricular preexcitation. Nonetheless, the wave shown by a red arrow is not a delta wave but rather a P wave, preceding the QRS complex.

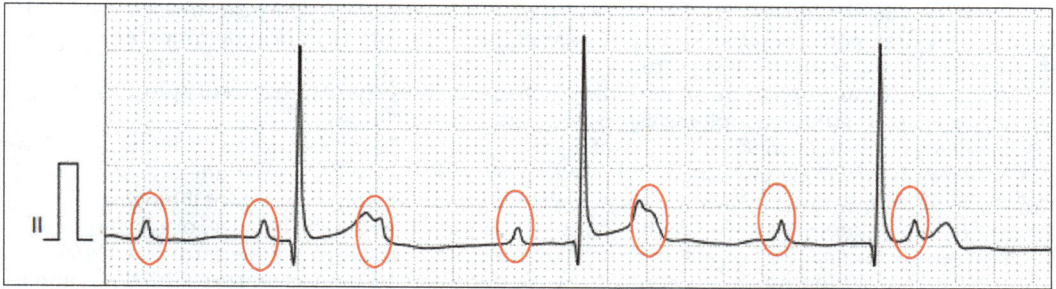

Figure 8.12 The ECG printout shows complete AV block with P waves dissociated from the QRS complexes.

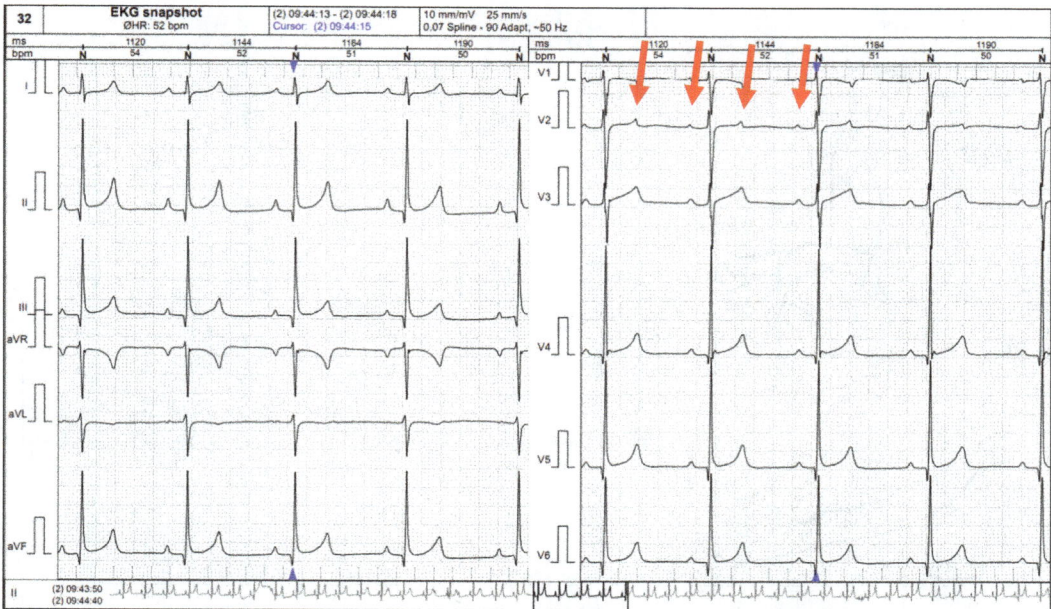

Figure 8.13 The ECG printout shows complete AV block mimicking 1:1 conduction from atria to ventricles. However, the sharp T wave, which is not present on other Holter traces, actually hides a blocked P wave within it.

HOLTER SUMMARY

The total number of beats for a 12-year-old pediatric patient is low: 62520/24 hours. The minimum rate was 36 bpm, while the maximum was 98 bpm. The mean heart rate was 53 bpm during the day and 46 bpm during the night hours. No premature atrial contractions (PACs) or premature ventricular contractions(PVCs) were documented. No ventricular escape rhythm or complex PVCs were seen. The patient was asymptomatic, exhibiting normal left ventricular dimensions, a normal ejection fraction, and no mitral regurgitation, therefore eliminating the need for a permanent pacemaker implantation.

DISCUSSION

Complete heart block, or third-degree atrioventricular block, is a bradyarrhythmia characterized by the absence of transmission of electrical impulses from the atria to the ventricles resulting from anatomical or functional anomalies of the cardiac conduction system. The abnormality os localized at the atrioventricular junction or below it. Complete AV block can appear in a structurally normal heart or may coexist with a congenital heart disease. It may be transient or permanent. Congenital heart block is defined as an AV block diagnosed in utero, at birth, or within the first month of life. The diagnosis of pediatric AV block is made when complete heart block is detected between the first month and the eighteenth year of life. The primary indication for pacemaker implantation is the presence of symptoms.

Patients may be asymptomatic or have diminished exercise capacity, recurrent episodes of syndrope, or heart failure symptoms associated with low heart rates.

Complete AV block in children can result from various etiologies, including viral (mononucleosis) or bacterial infections associated with myocarditis, infiltrative diseases of the myocardium, metabolic disorders, myotonic dystrophies, severe forms of hypothyroidism, pathological neurocardiogenic processes affecting the sympathetic-parasympathetic balance, or congenital coronary artery anomalies. It is also observed in acute rheumatic fever, Lyme carditis, Chagas disease, sarcoidosis and Kawasaki disease. The AV node may be injured by myocardial inflammation and infiltration during a viral infection, but the most frequent cause of permanent acquired atrioventricular block in children is direct trauma of the AV node during surgical intervention for congenital heart disease. The second most prevalent etiology is congenital heart disease

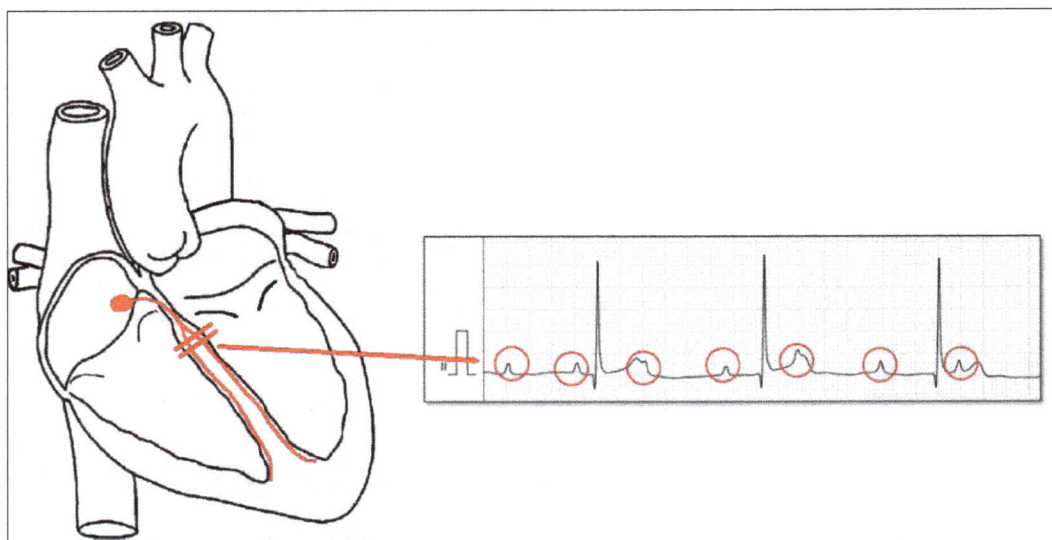

Figure 8.14 Complete AV block refers to a blockage in the conduction of electrical impulses from the atria to the ventricles. It may be situated above or below His. The resultant pattern shows several P waves dissociated from the QRS complexes.

associated with atrial or ventricular septal defect and complete AV block: transposition of great vessels, double-outlet right ventricle, heterotaxy syndrome and atrio-ventricular canal defects.

In third-degree AV block, the atria and ventricles depolarize independently, resulting in a ventricular rate that is generally slower than the atrial rate. The surface electrocardiogram may display either narrow or wide QRS complexes, dependent upon the site of the block and the place of the escape rhythm. The QRS is narrow when the escape rhythm originates in the supra-His region, and it is large when the escape rhythm arises from the intra-His or infra-His region. Escape ventricular rhythm with narrow QRS complexes may exhibit greater stability than that with large QRS complexes which has lower rates with higher risk of asystole.

Michaëlsson et al. have shown that children with complete AV block, develop during the 4th or 5th decade of life progressive left ventricular dysfunction and mitral regurgitation if pacemaker implantation is delayed for several decades. Therefore one of the recommendations for pacemaker implantation in children is complete AV block associated with left ventricular dysfunction of LV dilatation or severe mitral regurgitation.

Recommendations for pacing in congenital complete AV block:

1. **If complete AV block is associated with symptoms.**

2. In case of a wide QRS escape rhythm, complex ventricular ectopy.

3. If AV block is associated with left ventricular dysfunction.

4. Mean ventricular rate < 50 bpm.

5. AV block associated with LV dilatation with significant mitral regurgitation or LV systolic dysfunction.

6. If pauses or severe bradycardia associates with ventricular tachycardia.

7. If second degree AV block advances to third degree AV block with excercise.

BIBLIOGRAPHY

1. Michaëlsson M, Engle MA. Congenital complete heart block; an international study of the natural history *Cardiovasc Clin*. 1972; 4:85–101.

2. Gonzalez Corcia MC, Remy LS, Marchandise S. Exercise performance in young patients with complete atrioventricular block: The relevance of synchronous atrioventricular pacing. *Cardiol Young*. 2016; 26:261066–261071.

3. Rossano J, Bloemers B, Sreeram N. Efficacy of implantable loop recorders in establishing symptom-rhythm correlation in young patients with syncope and palpitations. *Pediatrics*. 2003; 112:e228–e233.

4. Dionne A, Mah D, Son MF. Atrio-ventricular block in children with multisystem inflammatory syndrome. *Pediatrics*. 2020; 146, e2020009704.

5. Forrester JD, Mead P. Third-degree heart block associated with lyme carditis: review of published cases. *Clin Infect Dis*. 2014; 59:996–1000.

6. Shen WK, Sheldon RS, Benditt DG. ACC/AHA/HRS guidelines for the evaluation and management of patients with syncope. *Circulation*. 2017; 136:e60–e122.

7. Wahbi K, Meune C, Porcher R. Electrophysiological study with prophylactic pacing and survival in adults with myotonic dystrophy and conduction system disease. *JAMA*. 2012; 307:1292–1301.

8. Di Mambro C, Tamborrino PP, Silvetti MS. Progressive involvement of cardiac conduction system in paediatric patients with Kearns-Sayre syndrome: How to predict occurrence of complete heart block and sudden cardiac death? *Europace*. 2021; 6:948–957.

9. Jaeggi ET, Hornberger LK, Smallhorn JF Prenatal diagnosis of complete atrioventricular block associated with structural heart disease: Combined experience of two tertiary care centers and review of the literature. *Ultrasound Obstet Gynecol*. 2005; 26:16–21.

10. Gross GJ, Chiu CC, Hamilton RM. Natural history of postoperative heart block in congenital heart disease: Implications for pacing intervention. *Heart Rhythm*. 2006; 3:601–604.

11. Aziz PF, Serwer GA, Bradley DJ. Pattern of recovery for transient complete heart block after open heart surgery for congenital heart disease: Duration alone predicts risk of late complete heart block. *Pediatric Cardiol.* 2012; 34:999–1005.

12. Romer AJ, Tabbutt S, Etheridge SP. Atrioventricular block after congenital heart surgery: Analysis from the Pediatric Cardiac Critical Care Consortium. *J Thorac Cardiovasc Surg.* 2019; 157:1168–1177.

13. Yandrapalli S, Harikrishnan P, Ojo A. Exercise induced complete atrioventricular block: Utility of exercise stress test. *J Electrocardiol.* 2018; 51:153–155.

14. Udink ten Cate F, Breur JM, Cohen MI. Dilated cardiomyopathy in isolated congenital complete atrioventricular block: Early and long term risk in children. *J Am Coll Cardiol.* 2001; 37:1129–1134.

15. Dewey RC, Capeless MA, Levy AM. Use of ambulatory electrocardiographic monitoring to identify high-risk patients with congenital complete heart block. *N Engl J Med.* 1987; 316:835–839.

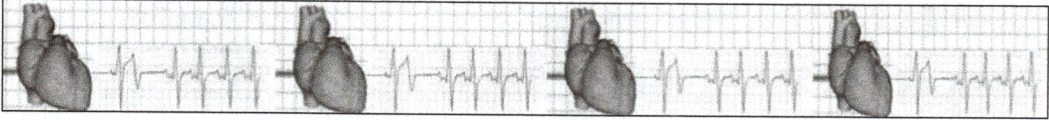

Case 9 Prolonged Sinus Pause in a Child with Breath-Holding Spells

Marta Rotella, Alessandra Grison, and Massimo Spanghero

CLINICAL CASE

A young boy manifested breath-holding spells at 1 year of age; after 10 months, the episodes become more frequent (up to twice a day). He had an otherwise silent clinical history, with normal psychomotor development. He underwent EEG, negative for epileptic seizures, and ECG Holter; the latter showed a prolonged sinus pause during loss of consciousness in the setting of one episode of breath-holding spell. The echocardiography and the baseline ECG were normal. There was no familiar history of sudden cardiac death or arrhythmia. He underwent a course of iron supplementation and with time the episodes became more and more sporadic. Given the spontaneous drop in frequency of the episodes and the natural history of breath-holding spells, the patient did not undergo pacemaker implantation or any other invasive treatment.

Sommario Statistiche

TUTTI I BATTITI	ECTOPICO VENTRICOLARE	SOPRAVENTRICOLARE ECTOPICO
Totali QRS:138602	Battiti Ventricolari:0	Prematurità:25%
Numero Battiti:137474	Singoli:0	Battiti Sopraventricolari:2
Battiti Sconosciuti:984	Coppie:0	Battiti Aberranti:0
Battiti BBB:0	Run:0	Singoli:2
Battiti di fusione:0	Run più veloce:0 alle 08:41:51	Coppie:0
Battiti Sopraventricolari:2	Run più lento:0 alle 11:36:05	Run:0
	Run più lungo:0 alle 08:42:15	Run più veloce:--- alle ---
Durata originale: 22 h 31 min	Battiti R su T:0	Run più lento:--- alle ---
Durata Registrazione:22 h 31 min	Battiti Interpolati:0	Run più lungo:--- alle ---
Durata Analisi:22 h 10 min	Battiti Isolati:0	SVR/1000:0
Durata Artefatti:0:17:58	VE/1000:0	Media SV/h:0
EPISODI FC	Media V/h:0	
Min/Max FC:Tutti i battiti		RITMO SOPRAVENTRICOLARE
Pause Escluse:No	RITMO VENTRICOLARE	Tachicardia Sopraventricolare:0
Min FC:53 BPM alle 11:35:59	Tachicardia Ventricolare:0	Freq. Sopravent.:> 100 BPM Battiti:> 3
FC Max:255 BPM alle 11:35:25	Freq. Vent.:> 100 BPM Battiti:> 3	Episodi bigeminismo:0
FC Media:112 BPM	Episodi bigeminismo:0	Battiti Bigemini:0
Tachicardia:> 120 BPM	Battiti Bigemini:0	Durata Bigeminismo:0:00:00
Bradicardia:< 50 BPM	Durata Bigeminismo:0:00:03	Episodi Trigemini:0
Durata Tac/Bra:> 0:03:00	Episodi Trigemini:0	Battiti Trigemini:0
Tachicardia più lunga:1:55:40, 145Media BPM alle08:14:46	Battiti Trigemini:0	Durata Trigemini:0:00:00
Tachicardia più veloce:0:12:03, 151Media BPM alle17:17:42	Durata Trigemini:0:00:00	
Bradicardia più lunga:---, ---Media BPM alle---		Percentuale FA:---
Bradicardia più lenta:---, ---Media BPM alle---		Frequenza Max FA:---

Figure 9.1 The Holter summary reveals a minimum heart rate recorded of 53 bpm, with no PVCs, and PACs < 1%. No episodes of supraventricular or ventricular tachycardia.

DOI: 10.1201/9781003545040-9

PAUSE: (Tutti i battiti)	STIMOLATI	ALTRI EPISODI RITMICI
Pause >2000ms: 3	Battiti PM Atriali (%): 0 (0%)	Definito da Utente 1 : — (—%)
RR più lungo:12,7 s alle 17:29:20	Battiti Vent. Condotti (%):0 (0%)	Definito da Utente 2 : — (—%)
	Battiti Doppi PM (%):0 (0%)	Definito da Utente 3 : — (—%)

Variabilità RR (Normale)	ANALISI QT (Formula QTc:Bazett; QTc RR:RRc)
pNN50:13%	Min. QT:216 ms alle 18:11:33
RMSSD:68 ms	Max QT:362 ms alle 04:01:30
SDANN:128 ms	QT Medio:298 ms
Indice SDANN:54 ms	Min. QTc:304 ms alle 19:40:28
SDANN:118 ms	Max QTc:555 ms alle 19:46:18
Indice Triangolare:28 ms	QTc Medio:401 ms

Figure 9.2   The same page reveals three pauses lasting more than 2 seconds, the longest being 12.7 seconds.

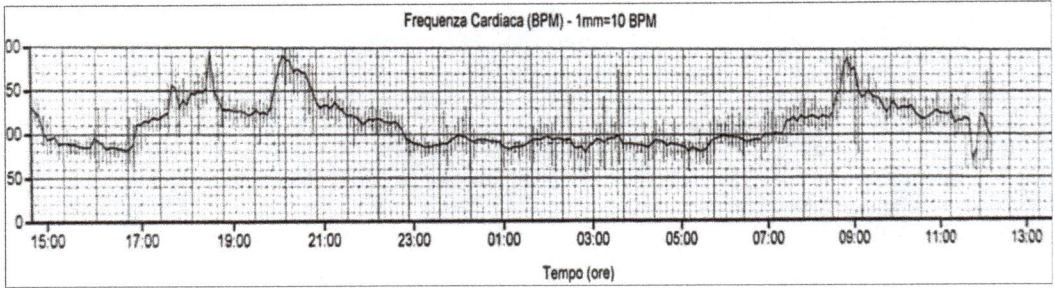

Figure 9.3   The heart rate chart shows a mean heart rate around 110 bpm, with normal variation for a 2-year-old boy.

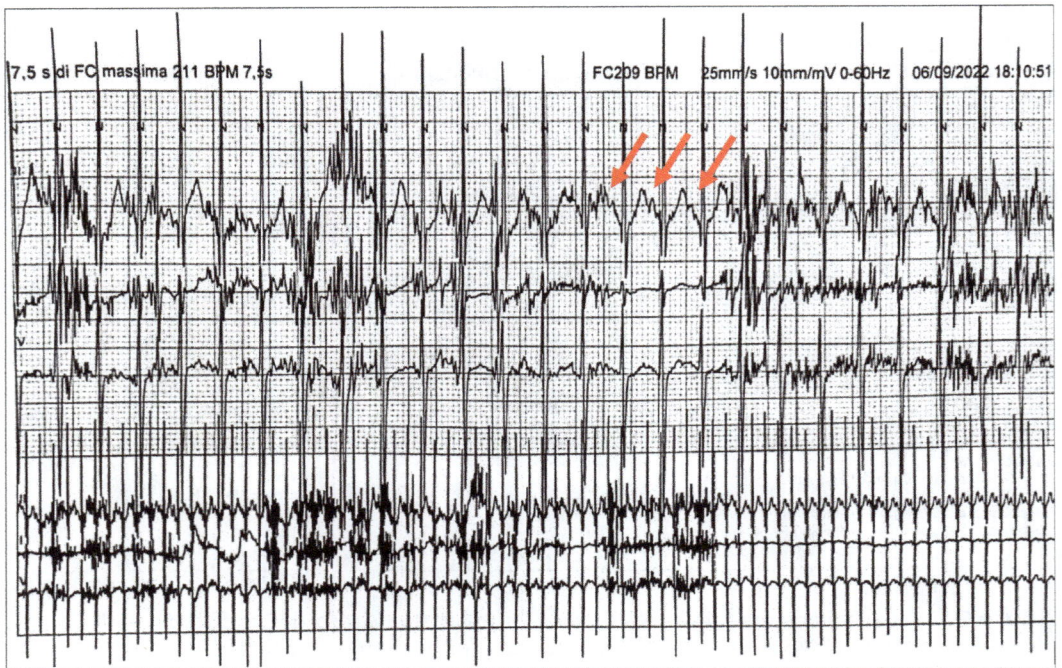

Figure 9.4   The image depicts the highest heart rate recorded (211 bpm). The strip is full of artifacts; however, the P illustrated by the arrows confirms it is sinusal tachycardia; in addition, the symptoms diary tells us that the young boy was crying.

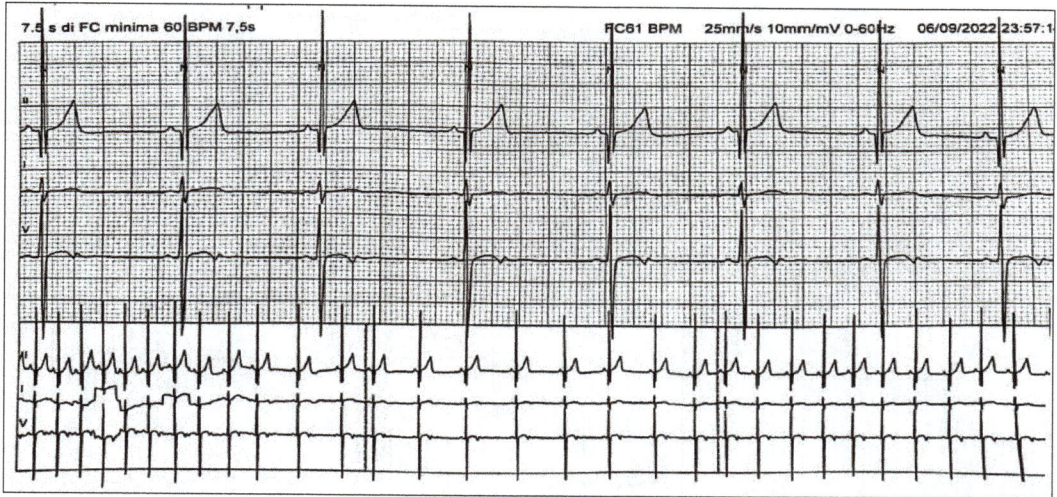

Figure 9.5 Minimum heart rate (around 60 bpm) during sleep: the trace shows a P wave preceding every QRS; there are no signs of atrioventricular block (PR interval duration of 100 ms which is normal for age, no PR interval prolongation or missing QRS). From the positive axis it can be assumed that it is a sinusal P (even though only three derivations are recorded).

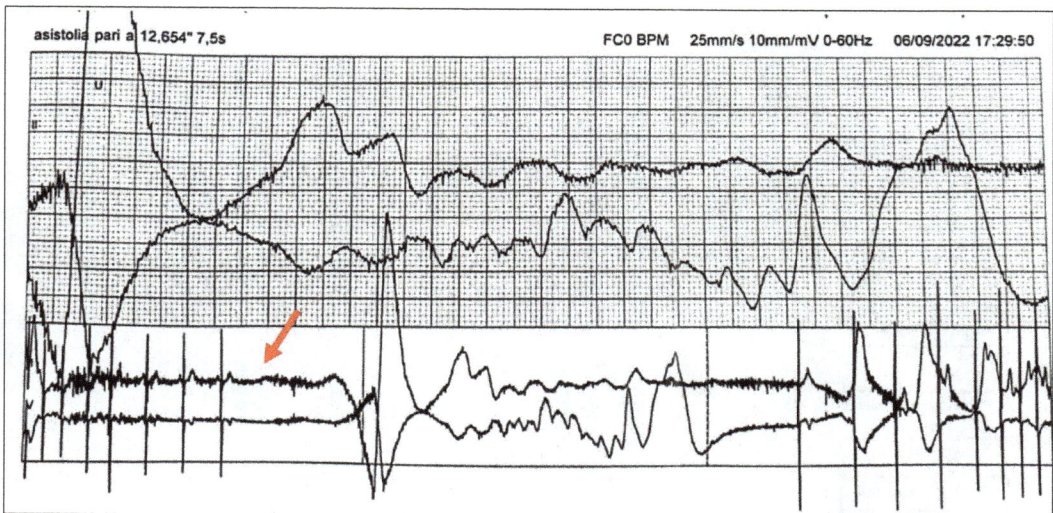

Figure 9.6 Long asystolic pause (12.7 seconds) registered during syncope in the setting of an episode of cyanotic spell. The child had a minor trauma and started crying aloud, holding his breath to the point that he lost consciousness. The artifact shown in the tracing is due to the resuscitation attempts held by the parents. The episode had a spontaneous resolution (a proper cardiopulmonary resuscitation was not performed as the parents were not trained at that moment). The arrow shows no blocked P wave, suggesting it's a sinusal pause.

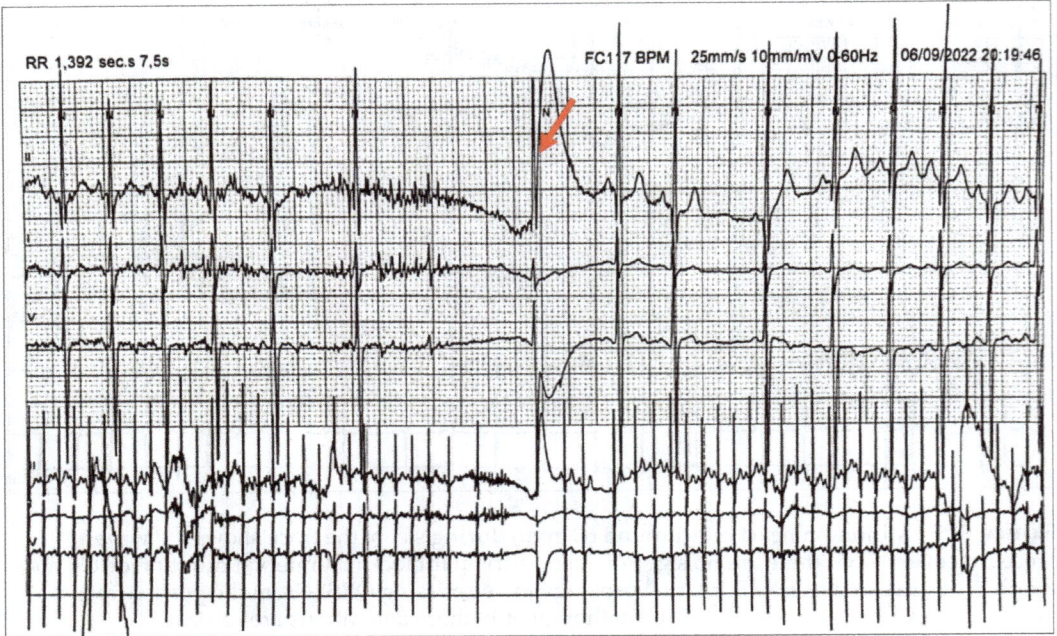

Figure 9.7 A shorter sinusal pause (1.4 seconds) during another episode of a breath-holding spell, without loss of consciousness documented. Arrow shows a junctional beat interrupting the asystole.

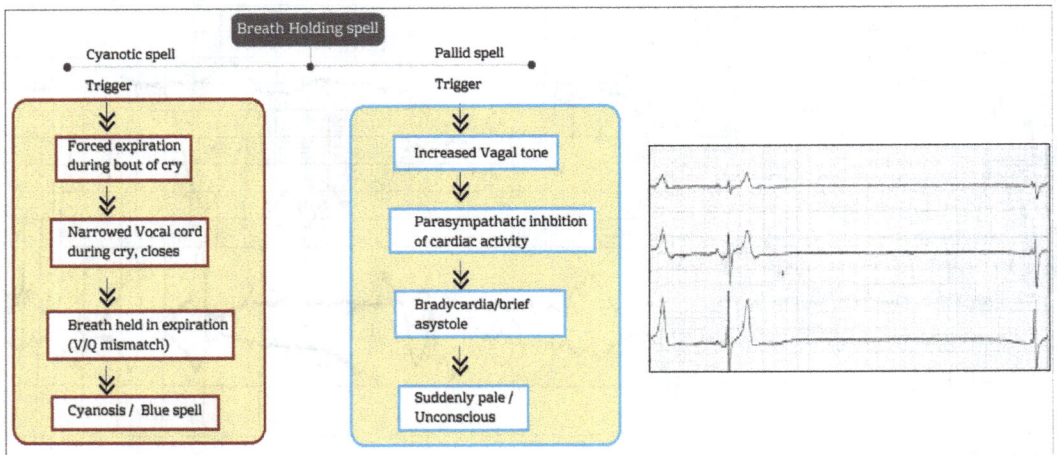

Figure 9.8 Schematic depiction of the pathogenesis in breath-holding spells.

HOLTER SUMMARY

The maximum heart rate reached was 211 beats per minute, and the minimum heart rate was 53 beats per minute during sleep; the average heart rate was 112 beats per minute. The recording shows a normal sinus rhythm with a prolonged asystolic pause of 12 seconds, recorded during loss of consciousness. Only two PACs were registered, with no PVC or other types of arrhythmias.

DISCUSSION

This case represents an example of sinus node dysfunction. The ECG trace shows a prolonged sinusal pause, with complete absence of electrical activity after a sinus beat, and it is interrupted by the recovery of normal sinus rhythm. It must be differentiated from AV blocks: in second-degree AV block Mobitz type I there is a progressive lengthening of the PR interval followed by one non conducted P, whereas Mobitz type II is characterized by intermittent sudden failure of AV conduction. Complete AV block is due to the absence of conduction from the atria to the ventricles. In the atrioventricular node dysfunction generally the sinus node keeps working and the ECG is characterized by P waves at a normal rate for age, with a different relationship with the QRS depending on the type of block.

Sinus node dysfunction is rare in the pediatric population and is generally either seen after surgical repair of cardiac defects or associated with structural heart disease. Altered sinus node function might be a secondary phenomenon in children, as in breath-holding spells.

This phenomenon, also called reflex asystolic syncope or reflex anoxic seizures, is a form of neurocardiogenic syncope that generally affects preschool children, typically before the age of two years.

According to the change in skin color during the event, breath-holding spells have been traditionally divided into two different types: cyanotic and pallid. These two clinical forms were originally thought to be due to different physiopathological sequences, both of which lead to cerebral hypoxia and subsequent loss of consciousness: in cyanotic breath-holding spells, initial violent crying causes hypocapnia, leading to hypoventilatory cerebral and systemic hypoxemia (cyanosis); by contrast, a marked bradycardia due to pain or distress-induced excessive vagal discharge has been considered responsible for pallid breath-holding spells. This distinction should be less rigid, however; the two sequences might overlap in mixed breath-holding spells. The syncope is generally brief and with spontaneous resolution and iron-deficiency anemia is thought to be part of the pathogenetic mechanisms.

Breath-holding spells have a good prognosis, even if they can be perceived as frightening for parents, and tend to resolve spontaneously by school age.

Anyway, in a small percentage of cases breath-holding spells are complicated by the occurrence of post-anoxic convulsions or trauma due to loss of muscle tone.

In the vast majority of cases pacemaker implantation is not required; in those patients where recurrent syncopal events may significantly alter the quality of life and in whom conservative treatments fails, pacemaker therapy may be useful. In these patients a clear relationship between symptoms and bradycardia should be established before pacemaker implantation, highlighting the importance of Holter monitoring and the comparison between the ECG trace and the symptoms diary. Given the spontaneous resolution and the benign behavior of breath-holding spells, pacing outcomes should be balanced against the complications of pacemaker implantation and chronic pacing.

BIBLIOGRAPHY

1. Silvetti MS, Colonna D, Gabbarini F, Porcedda G, Rimini A, D'Onofrio A, Leoni L. New guidelines of pediatric cardiac implantable electronic devices: What is changing in clinical practice? *J Cardiovasc Dev Dis.* 2024; 11:99.

2. Shah MJ, Silka MJ, Silva JNA, Balaji S, Beach CM, Benjamin MN, Berul CI, Cannon B, Cecchin F, Cohen MI, et al. 2021 PACES expert consensus statement on the indications and management of cardiovascular implantable electronic devices in pediatric patients. *Heart Rhythm.* 2021; 18:1888–1924.

3. Sartori S, Nosadini M, Leoni L. Pacemaker in complicated and refractory breath-holding spells: When to think about it? *Brain Dev.* 2014; 37(1):2–12.

4. Colina KF, Abelson HT. Resolution of breath-holding spells with treatment of concomitant anemia. *J Pediatr.* 1995; 126:395–397.

5. Daoud AS, Batieha A, Al-Sheyyab M, Abuekteish F, Hijazi S. Effectiveness of iron therapy on breath-holding spells. *J Pediatr.* 1997; 130:547–550.

6. Mocan H, Yildiran A, Orhan F, Erduran E. Breath holding spells in 91 children and response to treatment with iron. *Arch Dis Child.* 1999; 81:261–262.

7. Yilmaz O, Ciftel M, Ozturk K, Kilic O, Kahveci H, Laloğlu F, Ceylan O. Assessment of heart rate variability in breath holding children by 24 hour Holter monitoring. *Cardiol Young.* 2015 Feb.; 25(2):317–323. doi: 10.1017/S1047951113002333. Epub 2013 Dec 19. PMID: 24351939.

8. DiMario FJ Jr. Breath-holding spells in childhood. *Am J Dis Child.* 1992 Jan.; 146(1):125–131. doi: 10.1001/archpedi.1992.02160130127035. PMID: 1736640.

9. DiMario FJ Jr, Bauer L, Volpe J, Baxter D. Respiratory sinus arrhythmia in children with severe cyanotic breath-holding spells. *J Child Neurol.* 1997 Jun.; 12(4):260–262. doi: 10.1177/088307389701200408. PMID: 9203068.

10. Leung AKC, Leung AAM, Wong AHC, Hon KL. Breath-Holding Spells in Pediatrics: A Narrative Review of the Current Evidence. *Curr Pediatr Rev.* 2019; 15(1):22–29. doi: 10.2174/157 3396314666181113094047. PMID: 30421679; PMCID: PMC6696822.

11. DiMario FJ Jr, Bauer L, Baxter D. Respiratory sinus arrhythmia in children with severe cyanotic and pallid breath-holding spells. *J Child Neurol.* 1998 Sep.;13(9):440–442. doi: 10.1177/088307389801300905. PMID: 9733290.

12. Al-Shahawy A, El Amrousy D, Abo Elezz A. Evaluation of Heart Rate Variability in Children With Breath-Holding Episodes. *Pediatr Neurol.* 2019 Apr.; 93:34–38. doi: 10.1016/j.pediatrneurol. 2018.10.016. Epub 2018 Nov 22. PMID: 30594526.

13. Villain E, Lucet V, Do Ngoc D, Bonnet D, Fraisse A, Kachaner J. Stimulation cardiaque dans les spasmes du sanglot de l'enfant [Cardiac pacing in children with breath-holding spells]. *Arch Mal Coeur Vaiss.* 2000 May; 93(5):547–552. French. PMID: 10858851.

14. Kelly AM, Porter CJ, McGoon MD, Espinosa RE, Osborn MJ, Hayes DL. Breath-holding spells associated with significant bradycardia: successful treatment with permanent pacemaker implantation. *Pediatrics.* 2001 Sep.; 108(3):698–702. doi: 10.1542/peds.108.3.698. PMID: 11533339.

15. Sartori S, Nosadini M, Leoni L, de Palma L, Toldo I, Milanesi O, Cerutti A, Suppiej A. Pacemaker in complicated and refractory breath-holding spells: when to think about it? *Brain Dev.* 2015 Jan.; 37(1):2–12. doi: 10.1016/j.braindev.2014.02.004. Epub 2014 Mar. 12. PMID: 24630493.

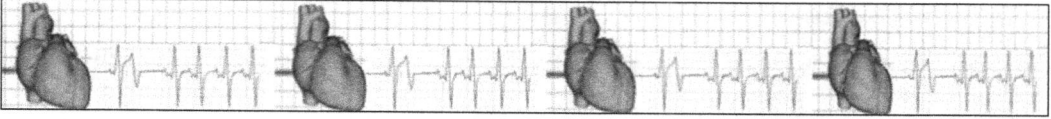

Case 10 A Newborn with Progressive Atrioventricular Block

Ayse Sulu

CLINICAL CASE

A newborn, who was being monitored in the neonatal intensive care unit due to a history of postnatal fetal mitral insufficiency, was found to have 2:1 block on the electrocardiogram taken due to intermittent bradycardia. Holter monitoring showed a maximum heart rate of 150 bpm, a minimum of 78 bpm, and an average of 98 bpm. A first-degree block and second-degree type 1 block, and occasionally a second-degree type 2:1 block were observed when the atrial rate increased. The patient, who had no complaints or hemodynamic deterioration during the eight-day observation and no block other than first-degree block on daily electrocardiography checks and monitoring, was put under outpatient follow-up. On the 28th day of follow-up, Holter monitoring showed first-degree and second-degree type 1 blocks, and rarely 2:1 block. The heart rate was a maximum of 124 bpm, a minimum of 76 bpm, and an average of 88 bpm. Complete AV block was observed in Holter monitoring performed at 3 months postnatally, with a maximum heart rate of 61 bpm, a minimum of 45 bpm, and an average of 52 bpm. The patient, who was asymptomatic and had no escape ventricular beats or pauses on Holter recording, was put under close observation. At 4 months, Holter monitoring showed an average heart rate of 45 bpm, and the patient underwent epicardial pacemaker implantation. During this period, the antibody levels measured in the mother were found to be high.

Graphs

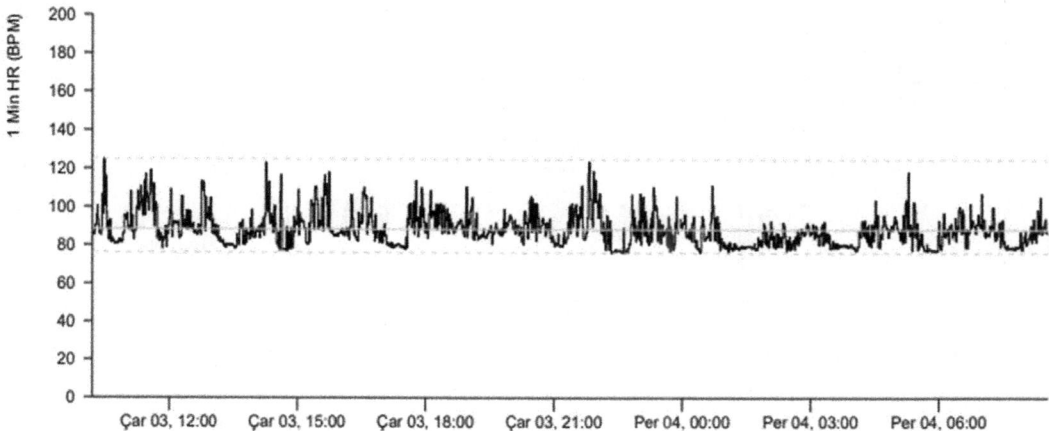

Figure 10.1   First postnatal day heart rate graph monitoring shows a mean rate of 98 bpm.

DOI: 10.1201/9781003545040-10

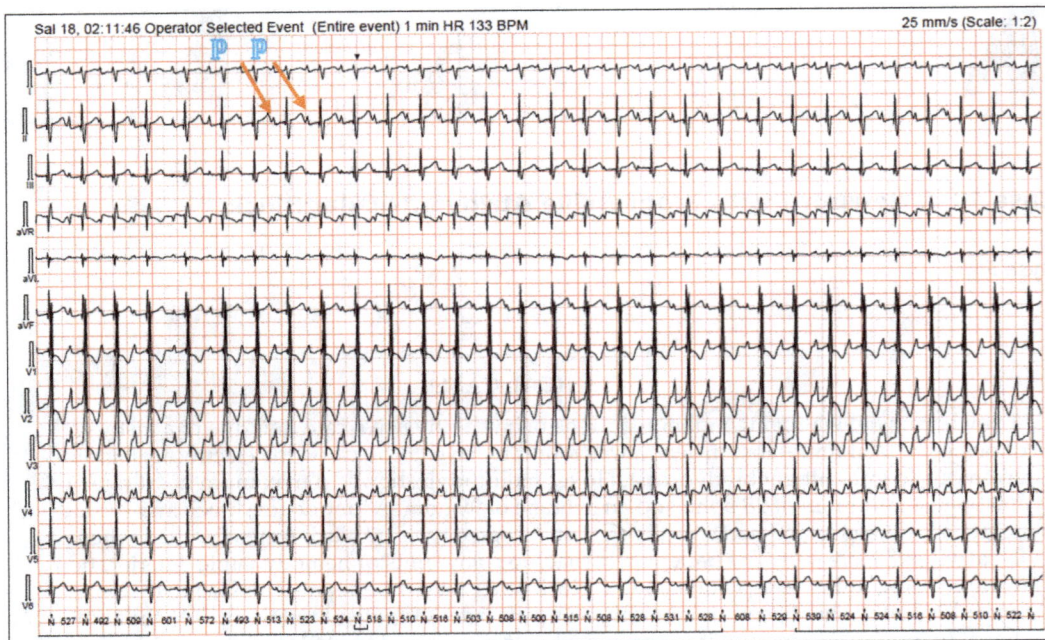

Figure 10.2 First-degree AV block, PR interval: 230 ms.

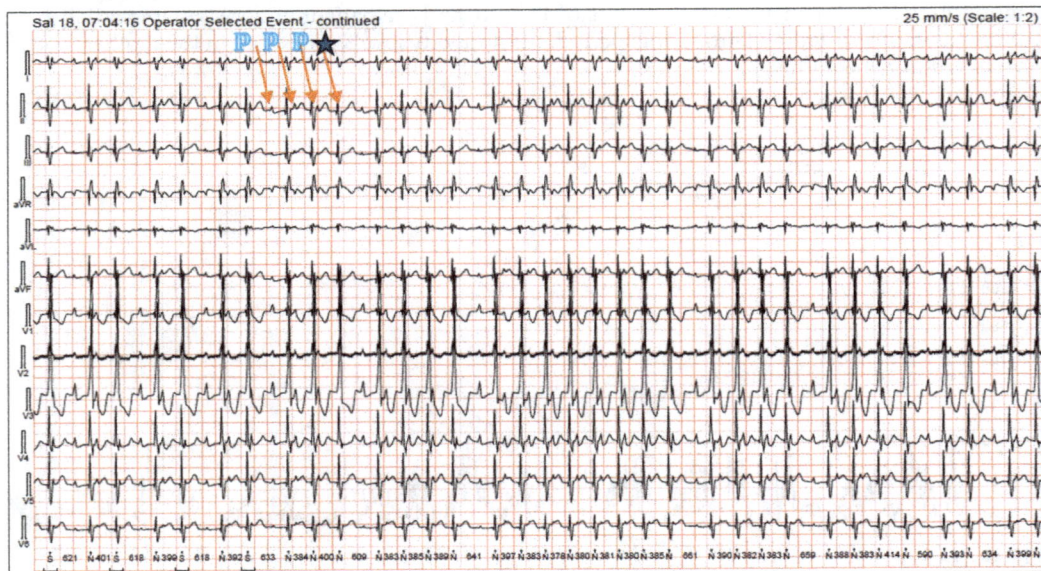

Figure 10.3 The PR interval progressively lengthens until a P wave is not conducted.

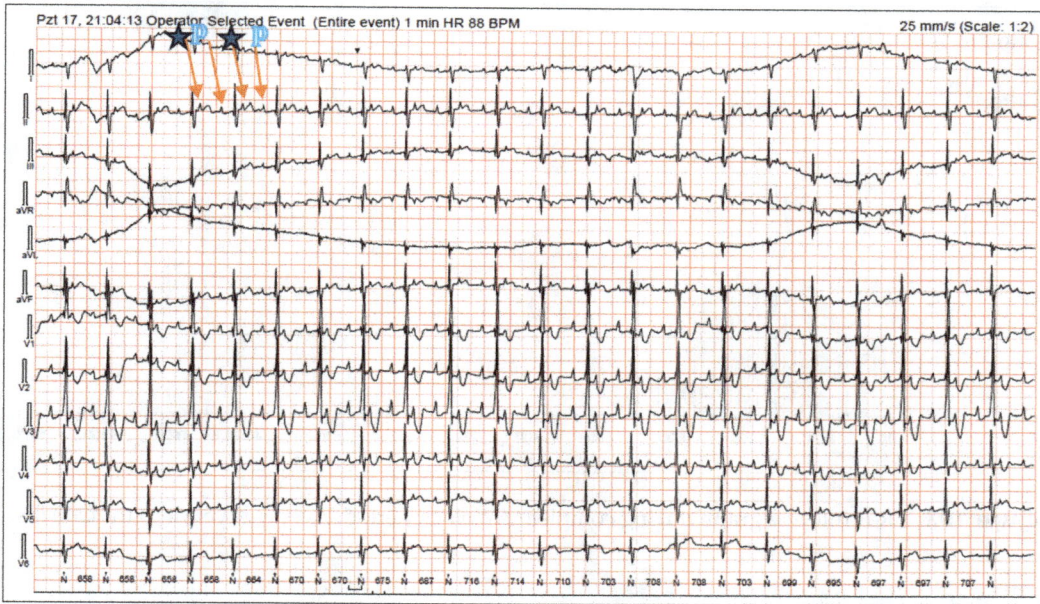

Figure 10.4 Second-degree Type 2 AV block (2:1 AV block). Every other P wave is not conducted (marked with a star).

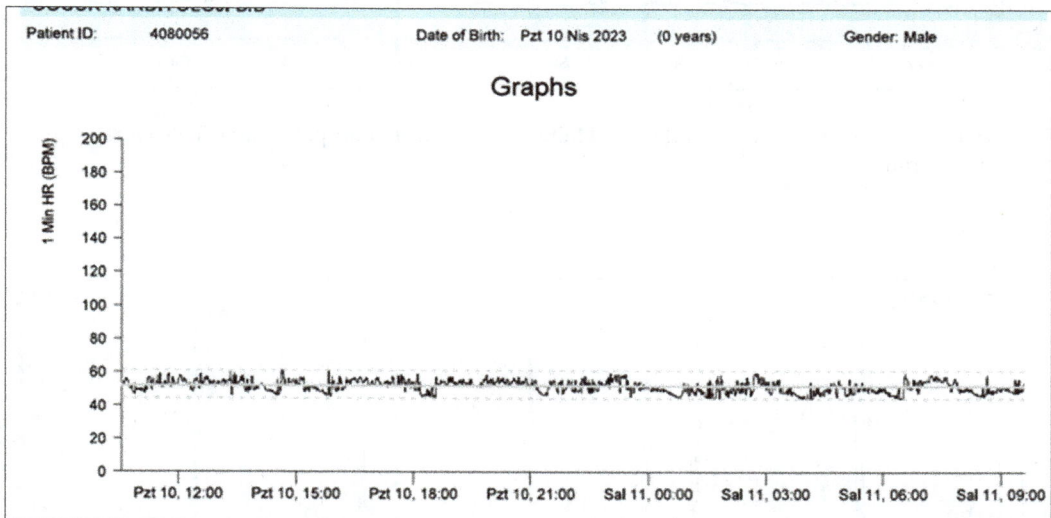

Figure 10.5 Heart rate graph during complete AV block period. Average heart rate: 52 bpm.

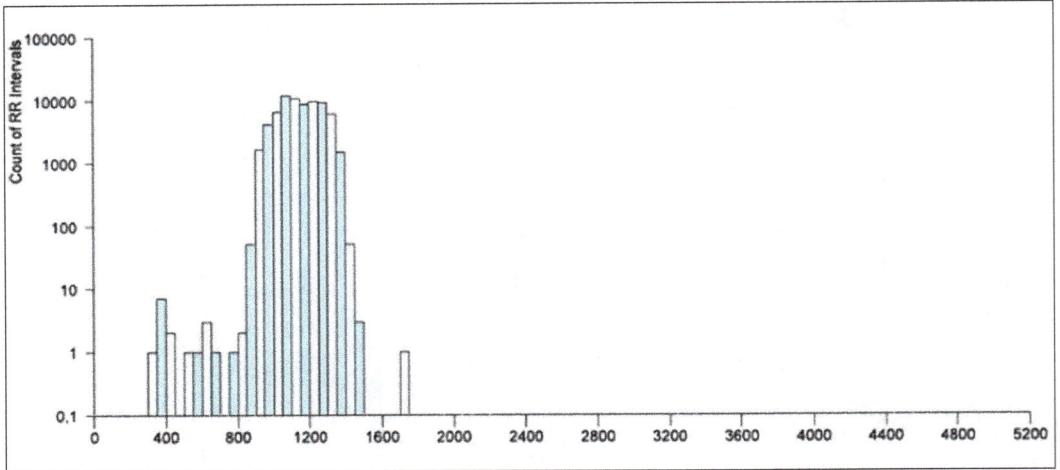

Figure 10.6 R-R interval graph during complete AV block period. Average cycle length: 1200 ms.

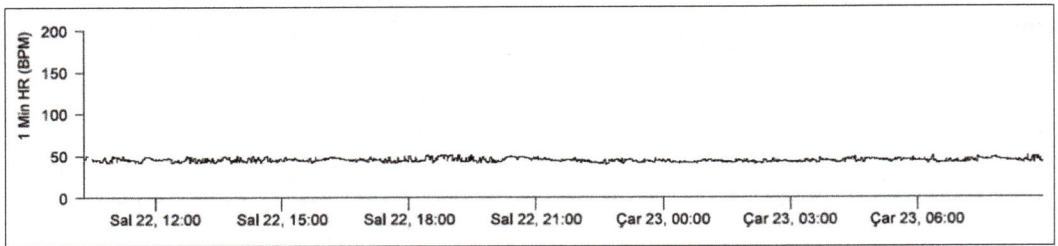

Figure 10.7 Heart rate graph on the last Holter before pacemaker placement. The average heart rate was 45 bpm.

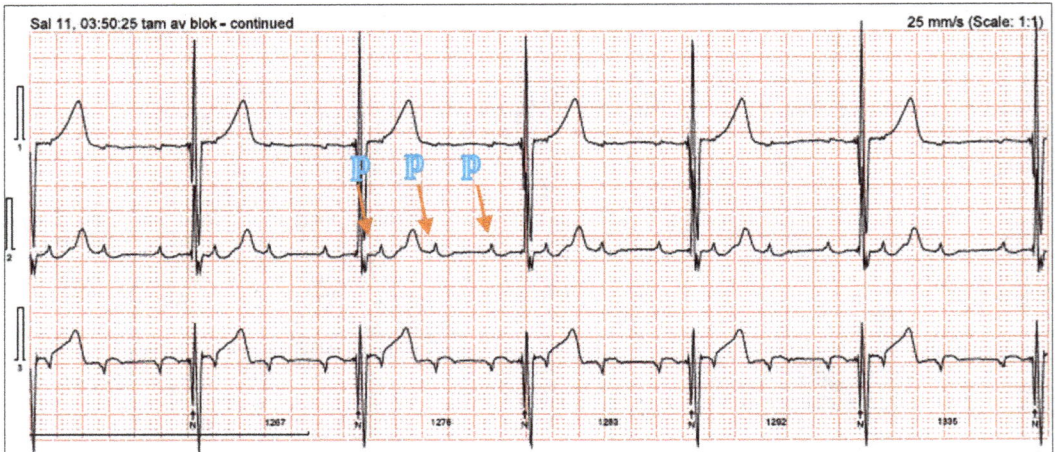

Figure 10.8 Holter monitoring during complete AV block. The P and QRS waves are regular within themselves.

TABLE 10.1 Criteria for the Diagnosis of Atrioventricular Block Types

First-degree AV block		1- PR prolongation. 2- P–QRS relationship remains 1:1.
Second-degree AV block	Type 1(Wenckebach)	1- Progressive prolongation of the PR interval 2- The first PR interval is the shortest. 3- The most significant prolongation is between the first and second PR intervals. 4- Progressive shortening of the RR interval. 5- The interval between the last conducted P wave and the first conducted P wave after the pause is 2x the PP interval. 6- Exercise, increased sympathetic tone, and atropine reduce or correct the degree of block, while carotid sinus massage increases the block.
	Type 2	1- Every other P wave is not conducted, without prolongation of the PR interval. 2- The QRS can be widened.
Complete AV block		1- Complete AV dissociation is present. 2- Often there is a nodal escape rhythm. 3- PP and RR intervals are equal, but there is no AV relationship.

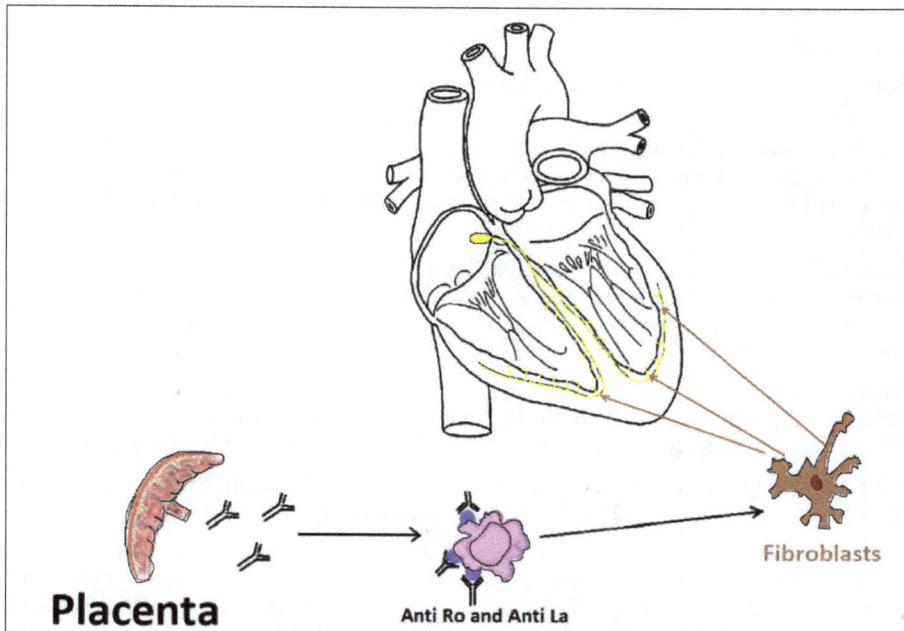

Figure 10.9 Schematic depiction of the effects of maternal antibodies on the conduction system, which produce fibrosis and degeneration.

HOLTER SUMMARY

The patient underwent regular Holter monitoring until reaching 4 months of age. Grade 1 AV block and relatively low average heart rates were initially observed. Subsequent monitoring revealed a deterioration of the conduction disorder, progressing to a grade 2 block and ultimately a grade 3 one, with average rates over 24 hours that were too low, requiring permanent cardiostimulation.

DISCUSSION

Congenital AV block is a rare disease often associated with maternal antibodies. Its prevalence varies between 1/15,000 and 1/22,000. In addition to AV block, neonatal lupus can be associated with endocardial fibroelastosis, heart failure, myocarditis, and dilated cardiomyopathy. Maternal anti-Ro/SSA and/or anti-La/SSB antibodies, which pass through the placenta into the fetal circulation, trigger an inflammatory response in the fetus, leading to fibrosis in the conduction system and causing AV block. It is known that mortality is higher in patients who develop dilated cardiomyopathy. Progressive AV block is often observed in the prenatal period, but cases of progression in the postnatal period have also been reported. While there are recommendations for the use of fluorinated steroids and IVIG treatment for fetuses diagnosed prenatally, studies have shown mixed results regarding their impact on disease progression. Additionally, although there are case reports of IVIG treatment in postnatally diagnosed patients, our patient's mother's diagnosis was confirmed at a later stage, and no treatment was administered as the patient already had third-degree block at that time.

Complete AV block in children can also be associated with congenital heart diseases such as left atrial isomerism, as well as acquired diseases such as acute rheumatic fever, myocarditis, and Lyme disease. Rarely, progressive blocks due to myopathies and genetic disorders can also be observed. The most common cause of block in children is postoperative AV block. All patients in the risk group should be monitored intermittently, and the potential for block progression should be kept in mind.

BIBLIOGRAPHY

1. Song MK, Kim NY, Bae EJ, Kim GB, Kwak JG, Kim WH, et al. Long-term follow-up of epicardial pacing and left ventricular dysfunction in children with congenital heart block. *Ann Thorac Surg*. 2020; 109:1913–1921.

2. Freidman RA, Fenrich AL, Kertesz NJ. Congenital complete atrioventricular block. *Pace*. 2001; 24:1681–1688.

3. Villain E, Coastedoat-Chalumeau N, Marijon E, Boudjemline Y, Piette JC, Bonnet D. Presentation and prognosis of complete atrioventricular block in childhood, according to maternal antibody status. *J Am Coll Cardiol*. 2006 October 17; 48(8):1682–1687. doi: 10.1016/j.jacc.2006.07.034

4. Ruffatti A, Cerutti A, Tonello M, Favaro M, Del Ross T, Calligaro A, Grava C, Zen M, Hoxha A, Di Salvo G. Short and long-term outcomes of children with autoimmune congenital heart block treated with a combined maternal–neonatal therapy. A comparison study. *J Perinatol*. 2022 September; 42(9):1161–1168. doi: 10.1038/s41372-022-01431-4

5. Di Mauro A, Caroli Casavola V, Favia Guarnieri G, Calderoni G, Cicinelli E, Laforgia N. Antenatal and postnatal combined therapy for autoantibody-related congenital atrioventricular block. *BMC Pregnancy Childbirth*. 2013 November 29; 13:220. doi: 10.1186/1471-2393-13-220

6. Mond HG, Vohra J. The electrocardiographic footprints of Wenckebach block. *Heart Lung Circ*. 2017 December; 26(12):1252–1266. doi: 10.1016/j.hlc.2017.06.718

7. Baruteau AE, Pass RH, Thambo JB, Behaghel A, Le Pennec S, Perdreau E, Combes N, Liberman L, McLeod CJ. Congenital and childhood atrioventricular blocks: pathophysiology and contemporary management. *Eur J Pediatr*. 2016 Sep; 175(9):1235–1248. doi: 10.1007/s00431-016-2748-0. Epub 2016 Jun 28. PMID: 27351174; PMCID: PMC5005411.

8. Swaminathan S, Parthiban A. Progressive fetal atrioventricular block in heterotaxy syndrome. *Cardiol Young*. 2007 Aug.; 17(4):432–434. doi: 10.1017/S1047951107000868. Epub 2007 Jun 18. PMID: 17572927.

9. Jaeggi ET, Silverman ED, Laskin C, Kingdom J, Golding F, Weber R. Prolongation of the atrioventricular conduction in fetuses exposed to maternal anti-Ro/SSA and anti-La/SSB antibodies did not predict progressive heart block. A prospective observational study on the effects of maternal antibodies on 165 fetuses. *J Am Coll Cardiol*. 2011 Mar. 29; 57(13):1487–1492. doi: 10.1016/j.jacc.2010.12.014. PMID: 21435519.

10. Friedman D, Duncanson LJ, Glickstein J, Buyon J. A review of congenital heart block. *Images Paediatr Cardiol*. 2003 Jul.; 5(3):36–48. PMID: 22368629; PMCID: PMC3232542.

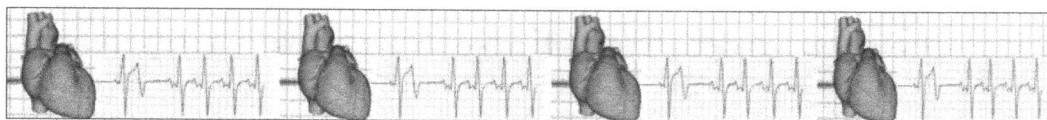

Case 11 Complete AV Block with Dizziness

Cismaru Gabriel, Radu Rosu, Gabriel Gusetu, Ioan Alexandru Minciuna, and Dana Pop

CLINICAL CASE

A 15-year-old female patient came to the Cardiology Department complaining of dizziness. She was diagnosed with first-degree AV block by a pediatrician and then referred to the pediatric cardiologist. Three weeks prior to her presentation, she experienced dizziness during a sports tournament, which recurred several days later. An ECG revealed second-degree AV block with Wenckebach phenomena; hence, a Holter ECG was requested. Following 24 hours of Holter monitoring, she was referred to our arrhythmology department and underwent implantation of a dual-chamber pacemaker.

Concluzie

Ritm cardiac		
Total bătăi	56 513	(0% paced)
HR max / min	**93 / 28 bpm**	
Media HR	**Ø 42 bpm**	
HR Max / Min Sinus	93 / 28 bpm	
Media HR (Treaz/Adormit)	45 / 37 bpm	
Index circadian	1,22	
Tahicardie / Bradicardie	- % / 92 %	

Pauze		
RR Max	**3 392 ms**	
Pauze (>2000ms)	**157**	

Fibrilaţie atrială / Flutter atrial		
Total AF	-	
AF HR Max	0 bpm	
Cel mai lung AF	-	

Bradicardie		
Cea mai mică	Ø 34 bpm	00:43:32
Cea mai mare	Ø 35 bpm	02:37:44

ST		
St ridicare max	1,95 mV	V2
ST depresurizare max	-3,52 mV	V2

Ectopie ventriculară		
V Total	11	(< 1%)
V / Ora Max	8	pe oră
Episoade Tahicardie V	-	
Cea mai rapidă Tahicardie V	-	
V Cea mai lungă secvenţă	-	
Triplete / Execută	0	Σ 0 bătăi
Cuplete	0	Σ 0 bătăi
Bigeminism	1	Σ 8 bătăi
Trigeminism	0	Σ 0 bătăi

Ectopie supraventriculară		
S Tot	0	(< 1%)
Episoade Tahicardie SV	-	
Cea mai rapidă Tahicardie SV	-	
S Cea mai lungă secvenţă	-	
Triplete / Execută	0	Σ 0 bătăi
Cuplete	0	Σ 0 bătăi

Figure 11.1 The summary page shows low rhythm during the monitoring period (lowest 28 bpm and highest 93 bpm), although the girl practiced physical activity during monitoring, and the longest pause was 3.39 seconds. A low percentage of PVCs (< 1%) was detected.

DOI: 10.1201/9781003545040-11

2	Bradicardii					Primele 5 episoade cu media HR > 54 bpm
Începe de la	Ritm	HR Media	HR Min		HR Max	Durata
(2) 04:59:30	Bradicardie	34	30		51	00:43:32
(2) 00:11:54	Bradicardie	34	28		57	01:10:50
(2) 03:49:28	Bradicardie	34	31		53	01:09:40
(2) 01:49:42	Bradicardie	34	28		53	01:46:14
(2) 05:43:04	Bradicardie	35	28		55	02:37:44
3	Tahicardii					Primele 5 episoade cu media HR > 107 bpm
Începe de la	Ritm	HR Media	HR Min		HR Max	Durata
4	Secventa V					secvența cea mai lungă 5
Începe de la	Ritm	HR Media	HR Min		HR Max	Durata
5	Secventa S					Primele 5 cele mai lungi secvențe
Începe de la	Ritm	HR Media	HR Min		HR Max	Durata
6	Episoadele V Tach					Toate episoadele cu media HR > 107 bpm
Începe de la	Ritm	HR Media	HR Min		HR Max	Durata

Figure 11.2 The table shows the lowest rate detected during monitoring: 28 bpm at 1:49 during the night, and at 5:43 in the morning.

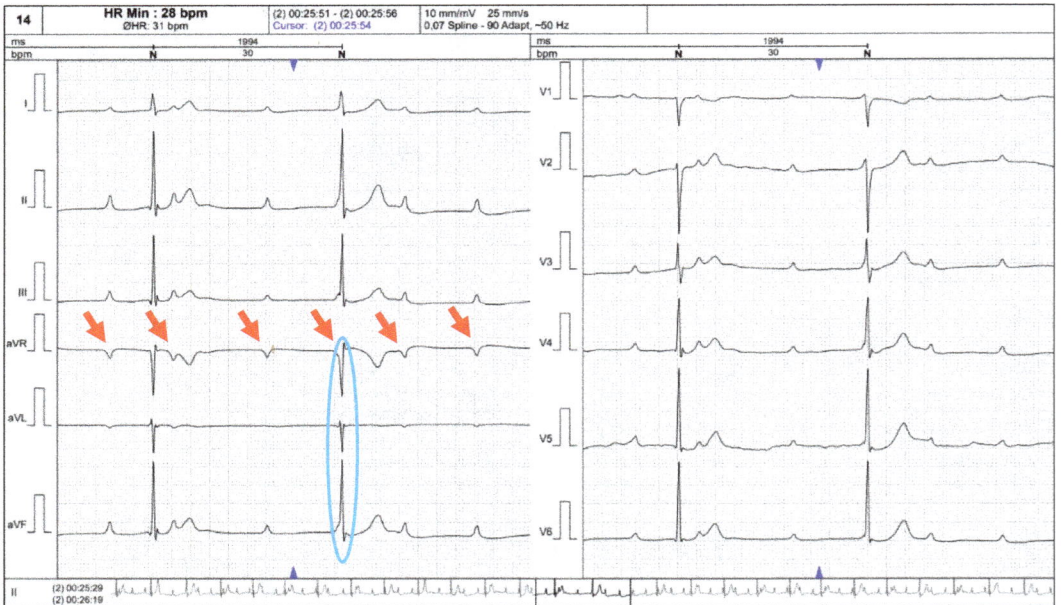

Figure 11.3 The image shows a complete AV block. There is no relationship between P waves and the narrow QRS complex.

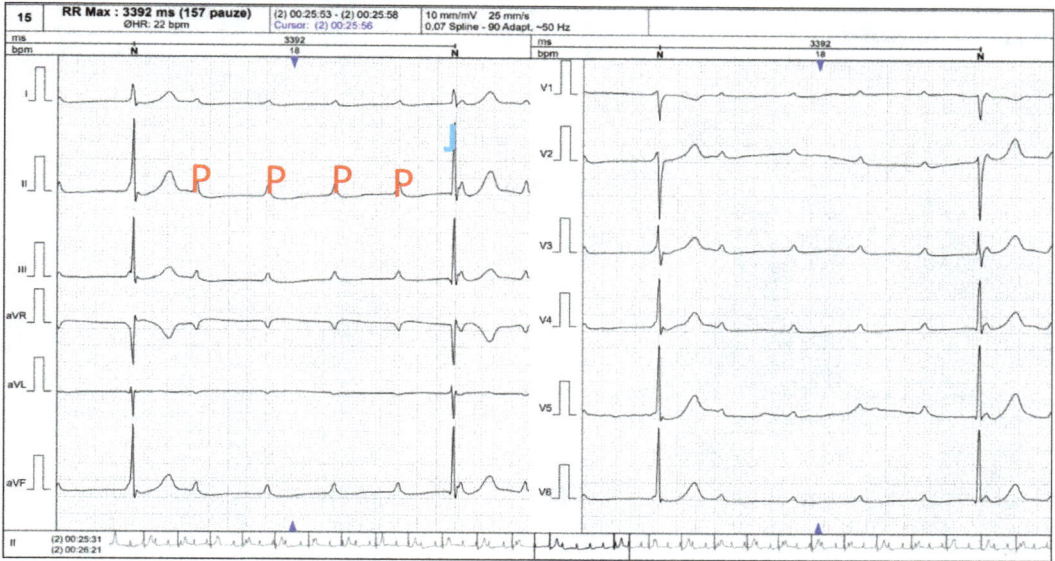

Figure 11.4 High-degree AV block. Multiple block P waves are followed by one junctional escape beat.

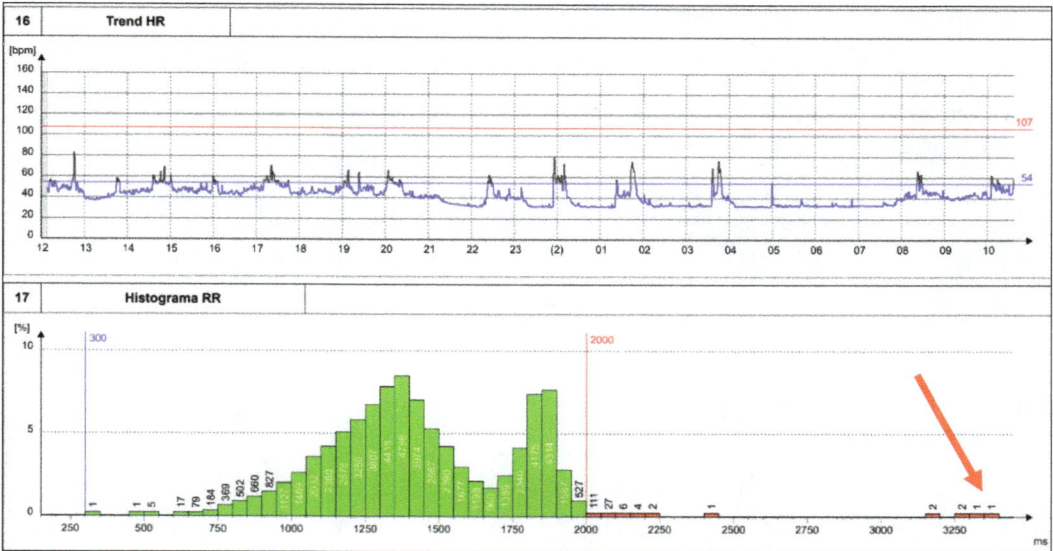

Figure 11.5 Heart rate trend and RR histogram. Heart rate trend shows chronotropic insufficiency with rates between 28 and 93 bpm during intense physical activity leading to dyspnea and dizziness. RR histogram shows long RR intervals (> 3.2 seconds) due to high-degree AV block (red arrow).

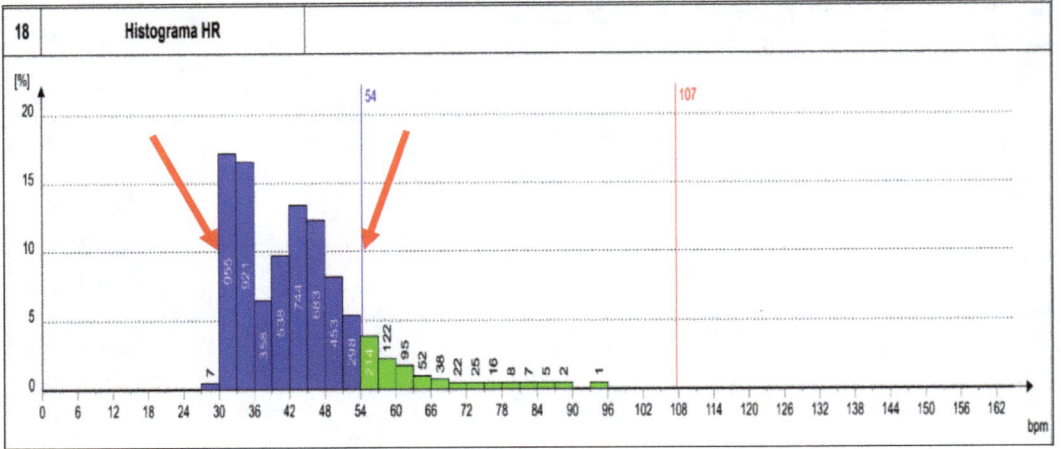

Figure 11.6 Heart rate histogram shows rates between 28 and 93 bpm, most of the rates being between 30 and 55 bpm (red arrow), which is too low for a 15-year-old girl.

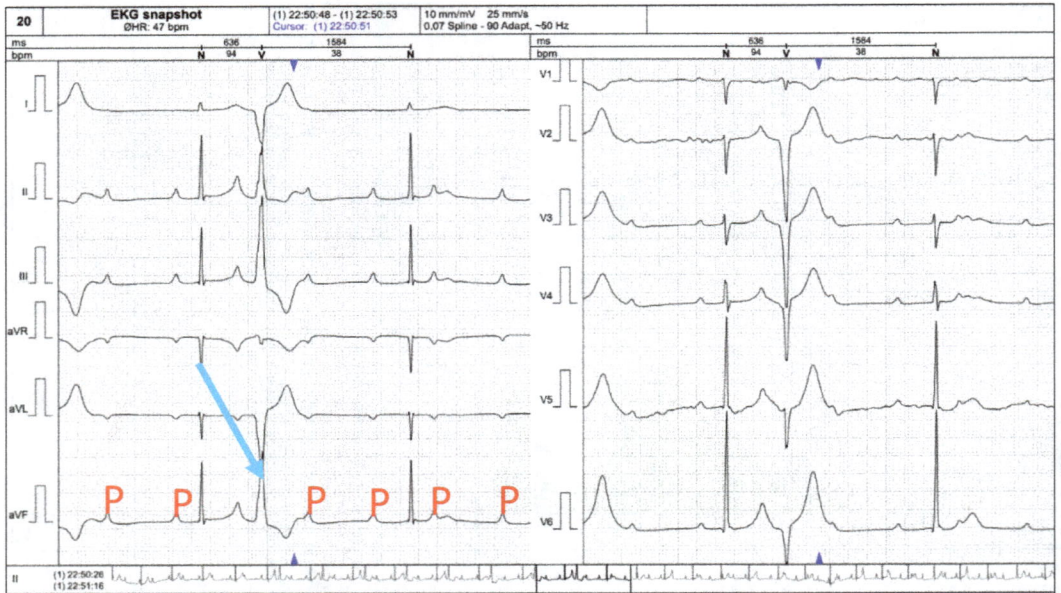

Figure 11.7 The image shows complete AV block (P waves are dissociated from QRS complexes – red arrows) with one premature ventricular contraction (blue arrow).

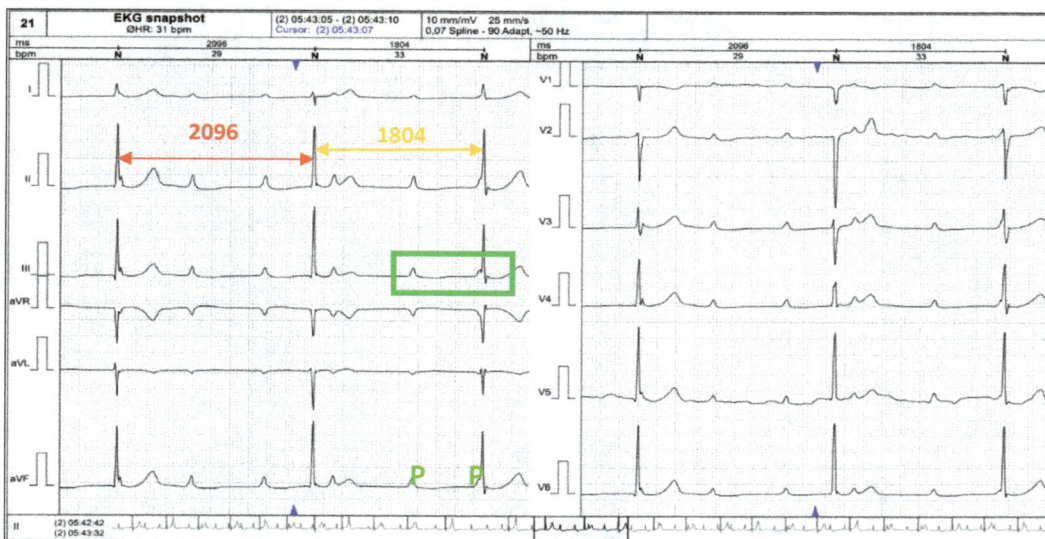

Figure 11.8 AV block grade 2 demonstrated by the different RR interval (2096 ms compared to 1804 ms). The long PR interval of 750 ms, depicted with a green square, indicates a P wave conducted from the atrium to the ventricles.

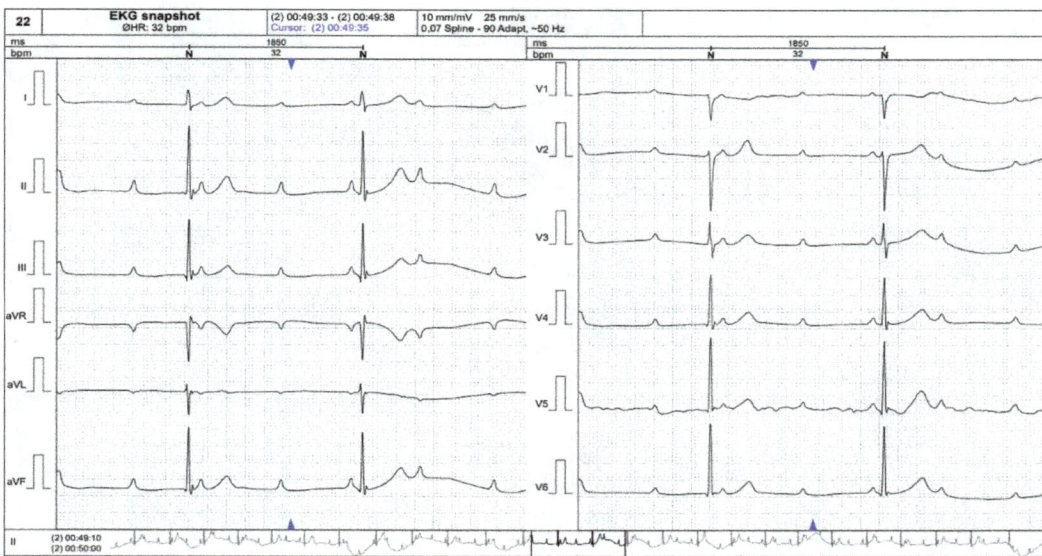

Figure 11.9 Complete AV block. There is no relationship between P waves and QRS complexes.

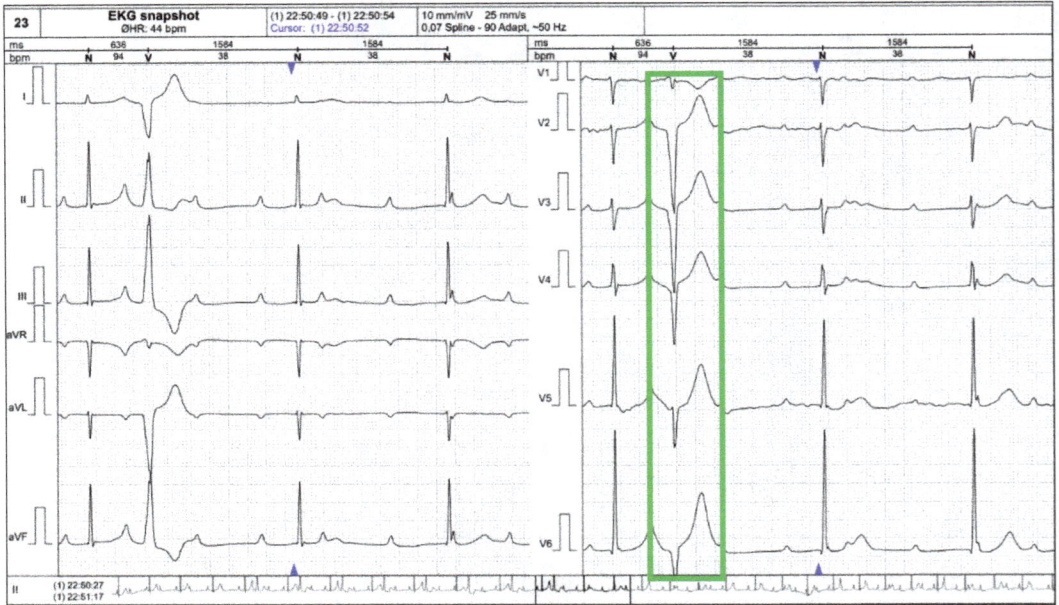

Figure 11.10 One PVC is observed on the trace; it exhibits identical morphology to the other PVCs observed in the other tracings.

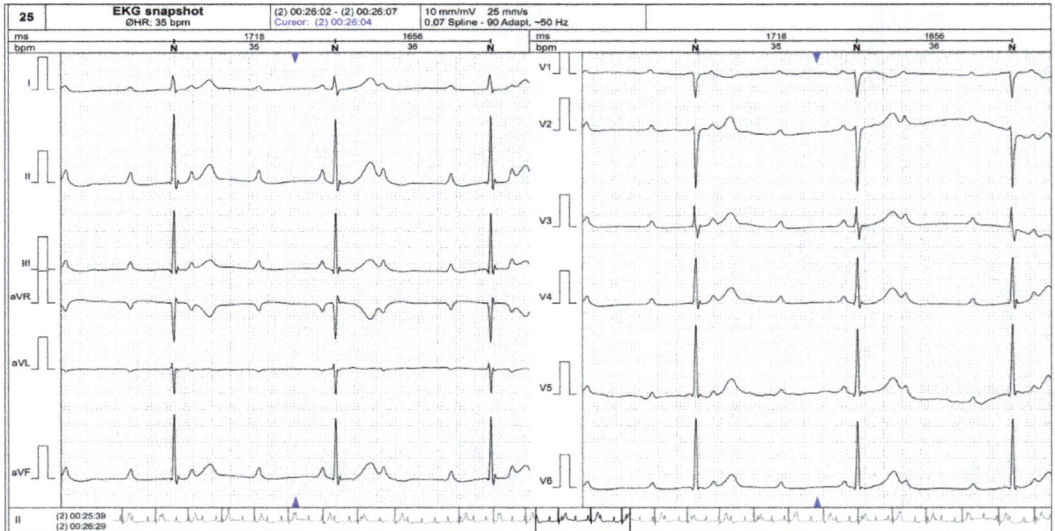

Figure 11.11 Complete AV block. There is no relationship between P waves and QRS complexes.

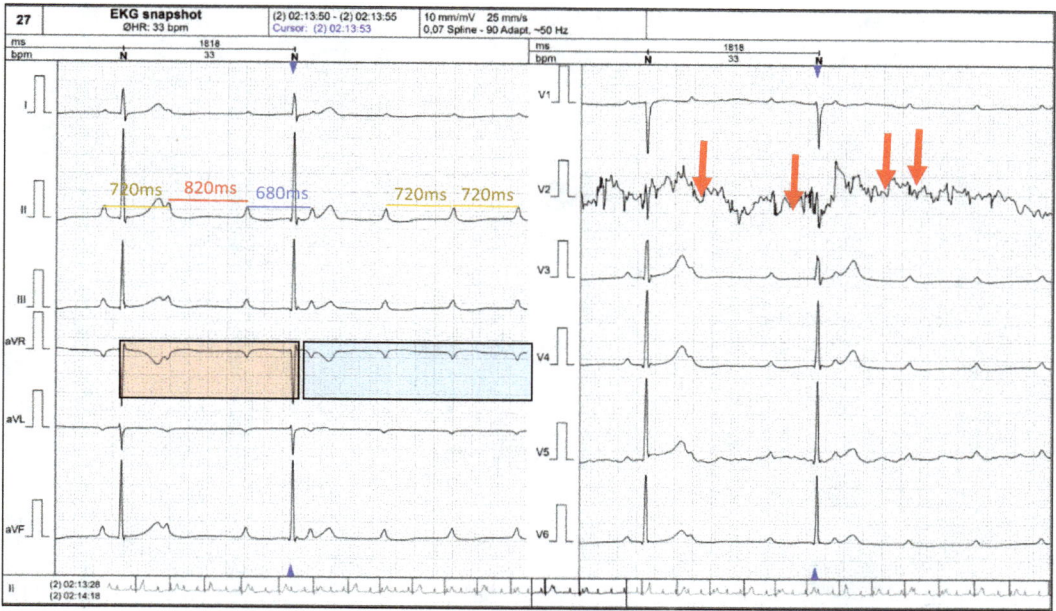

Figure 11.12 Second-degree AV block (red square) followed by high-degree AV block (blue square). The red arrows show electrical artifacts due to loose V2 electrode–skin connection.

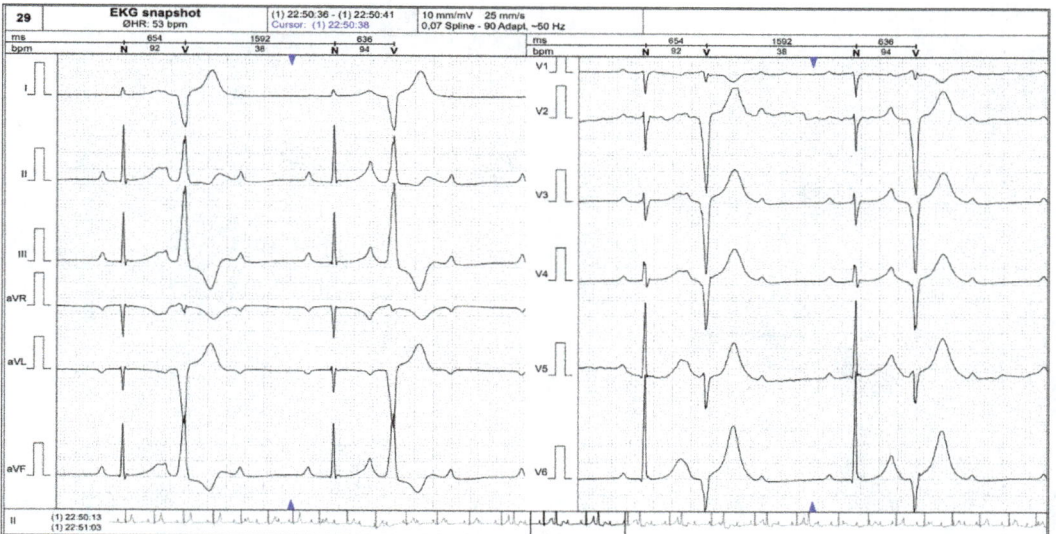

Figure 11.13 Complete AV block with 2 premature ventricular contractions.

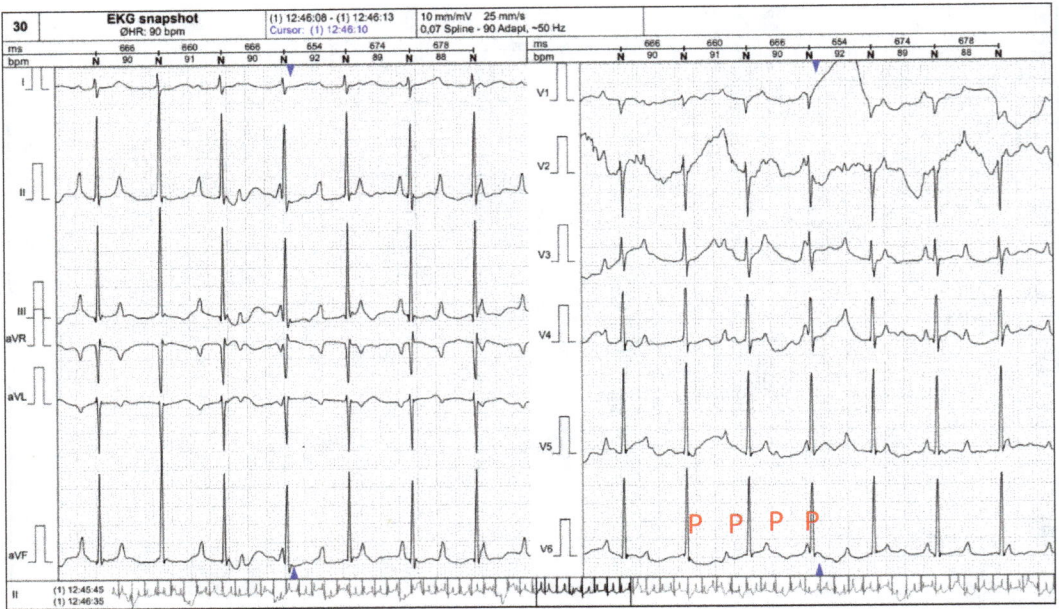

Figure 11.14 The highest rate during physical activity shows complete AV block with dissociation between P waves and QRS complexes. This is the highest rate detected during Holter monitoring.

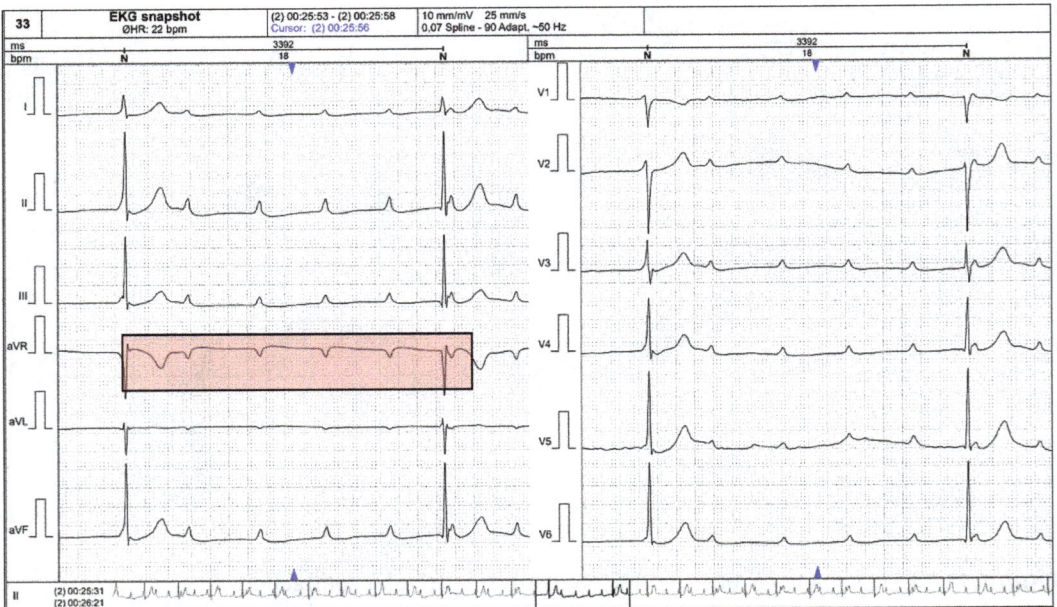

Figure 11.15 High-degree AV block. There are 5 P waves and only 1 corresponding QRS complex.

HOLTER SUMMARY

The monitoring revealed a complete AV block with a minimum rate of 28 bpm, a maximum rate of 93 bpm during physical activity and a pause of 3.4 seconds with multiple blocked P waves. As the patient was symptomatic with chronotropic insufficiency and complete AV block, a double chamber pacemaker was implanted.

DISCUSSION

Sinus node disease and atrioventricular block are uncommon disorders in newborns and children. It may manifest in a completely structurally normal heart or in conjunction with concurrent congenital heart disease. AV block is categorized as congenital if identified in utero, at birth, or within the initial month of life, whereas childhood AV block is diagnosed between the first month and the 18th year of life.

Congenital AV block may be passively acquired through an autoimmune mechanism affecting the developing heart, resulting from the transplacental transfer of maternal anti-Ro/SSA and/or anti-La/SSB autoantibodies. Upon entering the fetal circulation, they can directly bind to L-type calcium channels of fetal cardiomyocytes, resulting in apoptosis and cell death. Maternal autoantibodies are identifiable in more than 95% of fetuses or infants exhibiting atrioventricular (AV) block, primarily congenital AV block. Conversely, maternal autoantibodies are absent in infants diagnosed with AV block beyond the neonatal period, representing a separate and unique clinical entity. Nonetheless, certain isolated AV blocks identified beyond the neonatal period may also be immune-mediated, characterized by the delayed identification of maternal anti-Ro/SSA autoantibodies, indicating a late progressive congenital variant of immunological AV block.

Inherited progressive cardiac conduction disease is identified in young individuals who have unexplained progressive conduction abnormalities while having an otherwise structurally normal heart. Inherited conduction disorders in structurally normal hearts manifest as a main electrical disorder and has been associated with genetic polymorphisms in the ion channel genes SCN5A, SCN1B, SCN10A, TRPM4, and KCNK17, as well as in genes encoding cardiac connexin proteins.

The primary cause of permanent acquired complete AV block in infants is surgical intervention for congenital heart disease. The second most prevalent cause is congenital heart disease associated with complete atrioventricular block. Other causes of acquired AV block tend to be reversible and include digitalis intoxications, viral myocarditis, acute rheumatic fever, Lyme disease, and mononucleosis. In this case, AV blocks may be reversible.

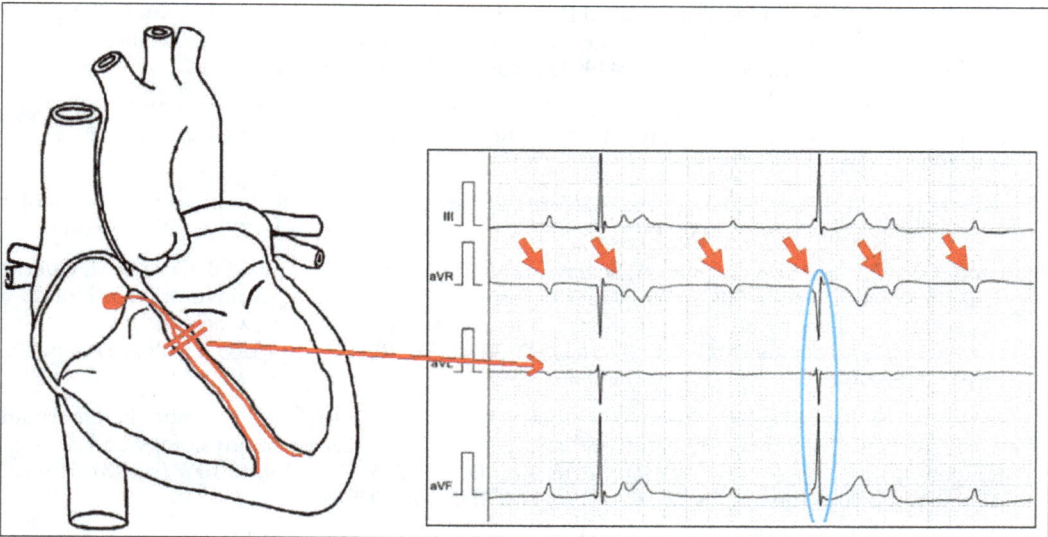

Figure 11.16 Complete AV block: P waves are dissociated from the QRS complexes.

If left untreated, congenital AV block lead to fetal and neonatal mortality rates of 14% to 34%. Fetal hydrops and ventricular escape rates below 55 bpm have been recognized as risk factors for mortality. The use of dexamethasone may substantially reduce fetal mortality; however, its administration is controversial due to potential impairment of fetal neurological development. Following the infant's delivery, intravenous administration of isoproterenol, atropine, epinephrine, norepinephrine, dobutamine and dopamine can be used. However, all symptomatic, irreversible AV node disorders necessitate the insertion of a permanent pacemaker. Pacing should also be evaluated in asymptomatic high-degree AV blockages with risk factors.

Our patient received a double chamber pacemaker with one lead placed inside the right atrium and the other on the septal aspect of the right ventricle.

BIBLIOGRAPHY

1. Brucato A, Jonzon A, Friedman D, Allan LD, Vignati G, Gasparini M, Stein JI, Montella S, Michaelsson M, Buyon J. Proposal for a new definition of congenital complete atrioventricular block. *Lupus*. 2003; 12:427–435. doi: 10.1191/0961203303lu408oa

2. Cuneo BF, Lee M, Roberson D, Niksch A, Ovadia M, Parilla BV, Benson DW. A management strategy for fetal immune-mediated atrioventricular block. *J Matern Fetal Neonatal Med*. 2010; 23:1400–1405. doi: 10.3109/14767051003728237

3. Gazes PC, Culler RM, Taber E, Kelly TE. Congenital familial cardiac conduction defects. *Circulation*. 1965;32:32–34. doi: 10.1161/01.CIR.32.1.32

4. Gheissari A, Hordof AJ, Spotnitz HM. Transvenous pacemakers in children: Relation of lead length to anticipated growth. *Ann Thorac Surg*. 1991; 52:118–121. doi: 10.1016/0003-4975(91)91431-T

5. Jaeggi ET, Hamilton RM, Silverman ED, Zamora SA, Hornberger LK. Outcome of children with fetal, neonatal or childhood diagnosis of isolated congenital atrio-ventricular block. *J Am Coll Cardiol*. 2002; 39:130–137. doi: 10.1016/S0735-1097(01)01697-7

6. Jaeggi ET, Fouron JC, Silverman ED, Ryan G, Smallhorn J, Hornberger LK. Transplacental fetal treatment improves the outcome of prenatally diagnosed complete atrioventricular block without structural heart disease. *Circulation*. 2004; 110:1542–1548. doi: 10.1161/01.CIR.0000142046.58632.3A

7. Janousek J, Kubus P. What's new in cardiac pacing in children? *Curr Opin Cardiol*. 2014; 29:76–82. doi: 10.1097/HCO.0000000000000025

8. Lazzerini PE, Capecchi PL, Laghi-Pasini F. Isolated atrioventricular block of unknown origin in adults and anti-Ro/SSA antibodies: Clinical evidence, putative mechanisms, and therapeutic implications. *Heart Rhythm*. 2015; 12:449–454. doi: 10.1016/j.hrthm.2014.10.031

9. Liberman L, Silver ES, Chai P, Anderson BR. Incidence and characteristics of heart block after heart surgery in pediatric patients: A multicenter study. *J Thorac Cardiovasc Surg*. 2016 doi: 10.1016/j.jtcvs.2016.03.081

10. Michaelsson M, Riesenfeld T, Jonzon A. Natural history of congenital complete atrioventricular block. *Pacing Clin Electrophysiol*. 1997; 20:2098–2101. doi: 10.1111/j.1540-8159.1997.tb03636.x

11. Cioffi GM, Gasperetti A, Tersalvi G, Schiavone M, Compagnucci P, Sozzi FB, Casella M, Guerra F, Dello Russo A, Forleo GB. Etiology and device therapy in complete atrioventricular block in pediatric and young adult population: Contemporary review and new perspectives. *J Cardiovasc Electrophysiol*. 2021 Nov.;32(11):3082–3094. doi: 10.1111/jce.15255. Epub 2021 Sep. 30. PMID: 34570400.

12. Baruteau AE, Pass RH, Thambo JB, Behaghel A, Le Pennec S, Perdreau E, Combes N, Liberman L, McLeod CJ. Congenital and childhood atrioventricular blocks: pathophysiology and contemporary management. *Eur J Pediatr*. 2016 Sep.; 175(9):1235–1248. doi: 10.1007/s00431-016-2748-0. Epub 2016 Jun. 28. PMID: 27351174; PMCID: PMC5005411.

13. Clowse MEB, Eudy AM, Kiernan E, et al. The prevention, screening and treatment of congenital heart block from neonatal lupus: a survey of provider practices. *Rheumatology*. 2018; 57:V9–V17.

14. Bordachar P, Zachary W, Ploux S, Labrousse L, Haissaguerre M, Thambo JB. Pathophysiology, clinical course, and management of congenital complete atrioventricular block. *Heart Rhythm.* 2013; 10(5):760–766.

15. Saleh F, Greene EA, Mathison D. Evaluation and management of atrioventricular block in children. *Curr Opin Pediatr.* 2014 Jun.; 26(3):279–285. doi: 10.1097/MOP.0000000000000100. PMID: 24759228.

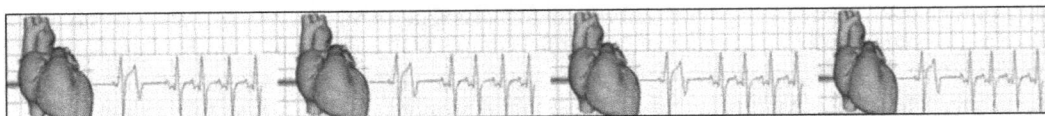

Case 12 Low Atrial Rhythm in a 12-Year-Old Girl

Cecilia Lazea and Gabriela Kelemen

CLINICAL CASE

A 12-year-old girl had thoracic pain and echocardiography revealed an interatrial septal aneurysm with a non-significant left to right shunt. Her ECG was normal, and her Holter ECG during the episodes of thoracic pain was also normal. However, during monitoring, an atrial rhythm with negative P waves was detected with a rate of 90–100 bpm.

Concluzie

Ritm cardiac		
Total bătăi	107 912	(0% paced)
HR max / min	**182 / 57 bpm**	
Media HR	**Ø 90 bpm**	
HR Max / Min Sinus	182 / 57 bpm	
Media HR (Treaz/Adormit)	98 / 81 bpm	
Index circadian	1,21	
Tahicardie / Bradicardie	22 % / - %	

Pauze	
RR Max	**1 350 ms**
Pauze (>2000ms)	0

Fibrilaţie atrială / Flutter atrial	
Total AF	-
AF HR Max	0 bpm
Cel mai lung AF	-

Bradicardie	
Cea mai mică	-
Cea mai mare	-

ST		
St ridicare max	0,17 mV	aVL
ST depresurizare max	-0,33 mV	III

Ectopie ventriculară		
V Total	0	(< 1%)
V / Ora Max	0	pe oră
Episoade Tahicardie V	-	
Cea mai rapidă Tahicardie V	-	
V Cea mai lungă secvenţă	-	
Triplete / Execută	0 Σ 0 bătăi	
Cuplete	0 Σ 0 bătăi	
Bigeminism	0 Σ 0 bătăi	
Trigeminism	0 Σ 0 bătăi	

Ectopie supraventriculară		
S Tot	0	(< 1%)
Episoade Tahicardie SV	-	
Cea mai rapidă Tahicardie SV	-	
S Cea mai lungă secvenţă	-	
Triplete / Execută	0 Σ 0 bătăi	
Cuplete	0 Σ 0 bătăi	

Figure 12.1   The summary page shows a maximum heart rate of 182 bpm and a minimum rate of 57 bpm. There was no PVC and no PAC. The maximum pause detected was 1.35 seconds.

DOI: 10.1201/9781003545040-12

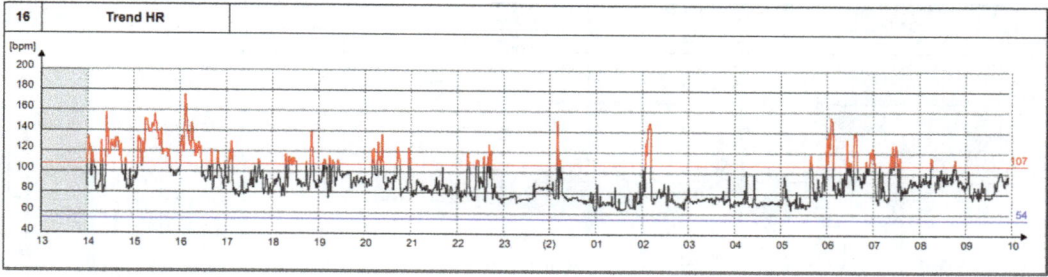

Figure 12.2   The heart rate histogram shows the mean rate over 24 hours of monitoring.

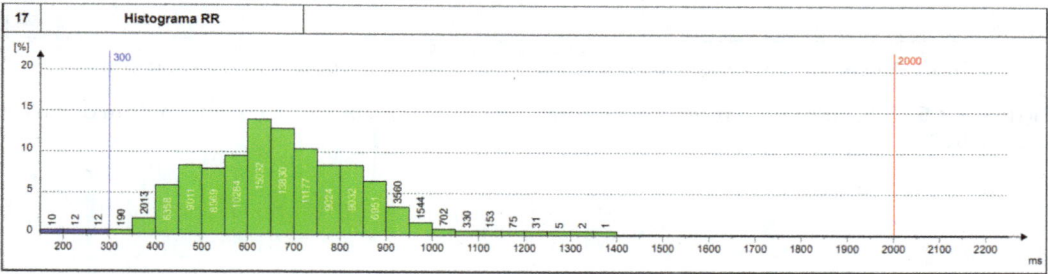

Figure 12.3   The RR histogram shows cycle length between 200 and 1350 ms. Minimal RR cycle lengths of 200 ms should be differentiated from artifacts.

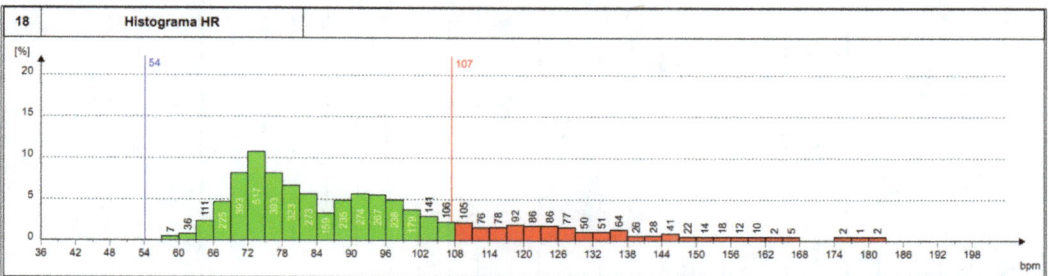

Figure 12.4   The HR histogram shows heart rates during 24 hours period of monitoring. The rate ranges from 57 to 182 bpm.

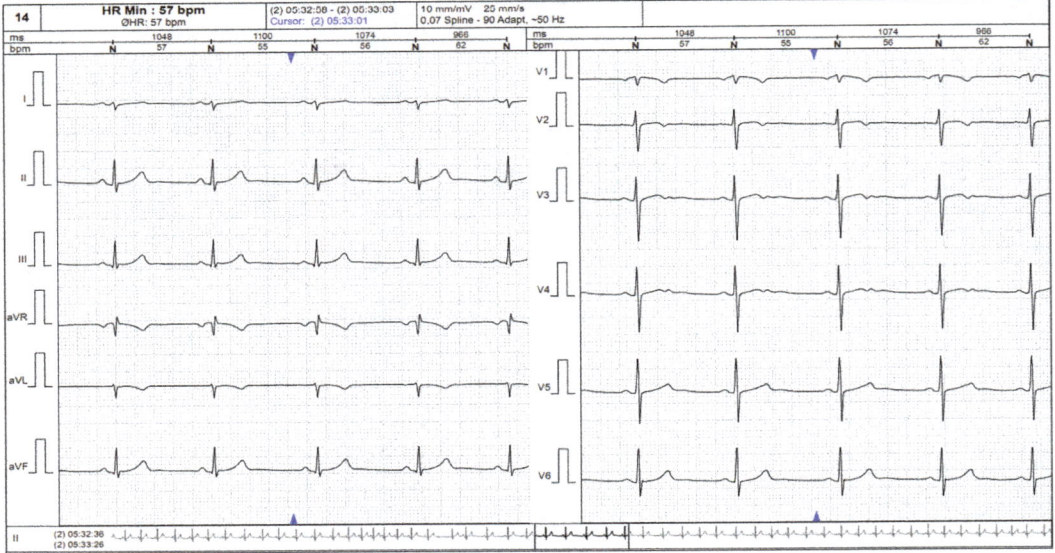

Figure 12.5   The minimum recorded heart rate was 57 bpm, with normal sinus rhythm during sleep at 5:32.

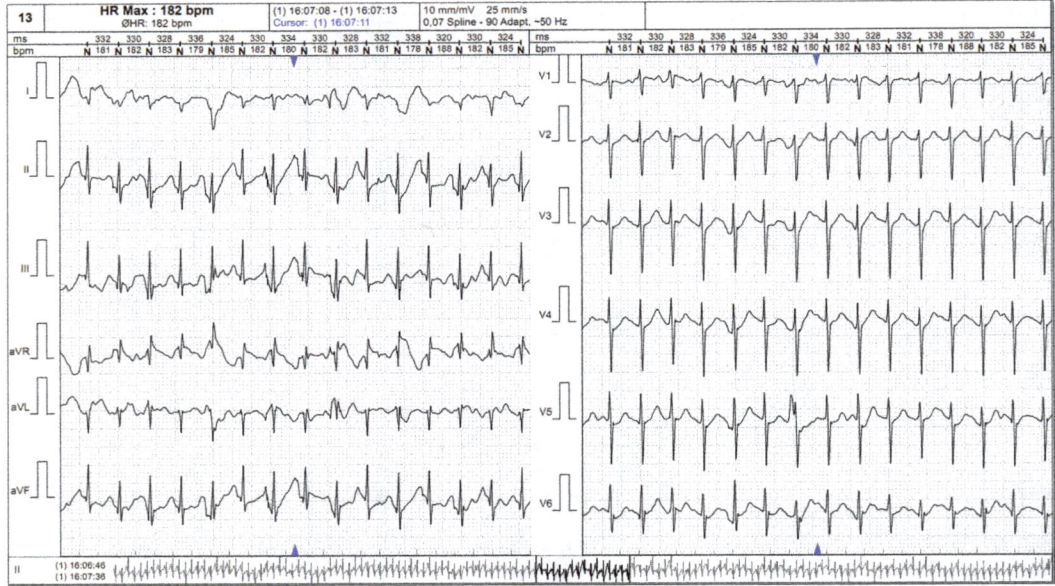

Figure 12.6   The maximum recorded heart rate was 182 bpm, due to sinus tachycardia.

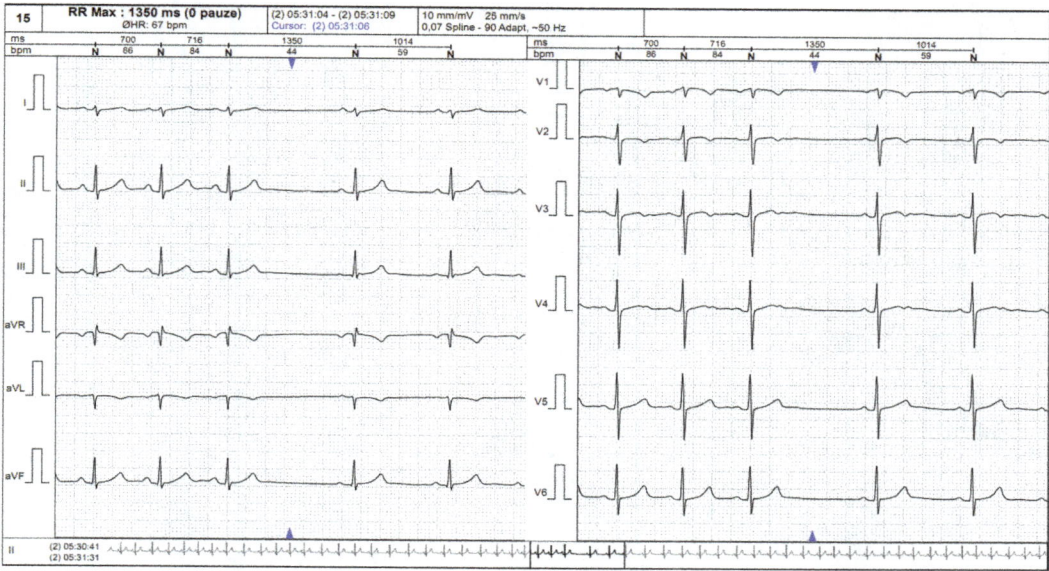

Figure 12.7   The tracing shows the maximum pause of 1.35 seconds, which is a physiological sinus pause.

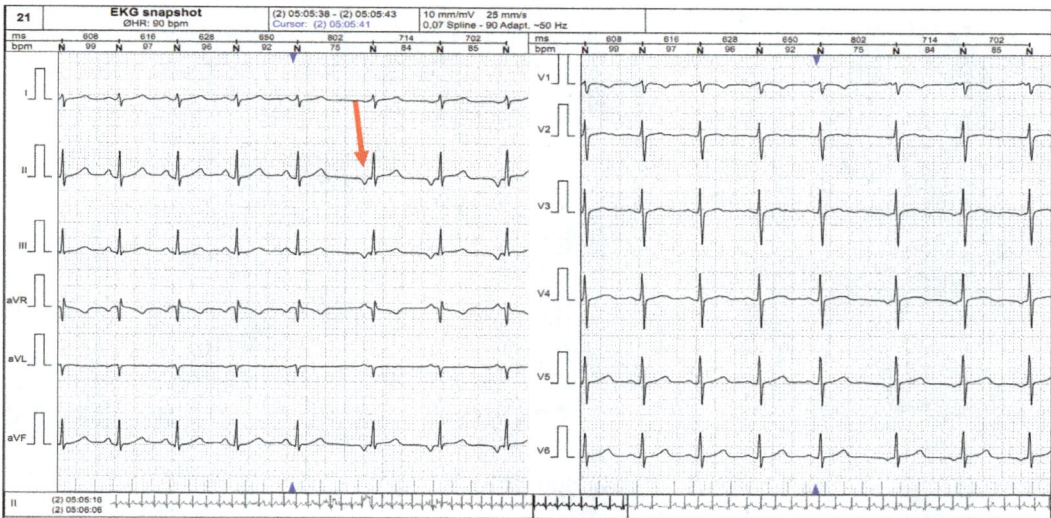

Figure 12.8   The tracing shows normal sinus rhythm (5 beats) alternating with low atrial rhythm (3 beats).

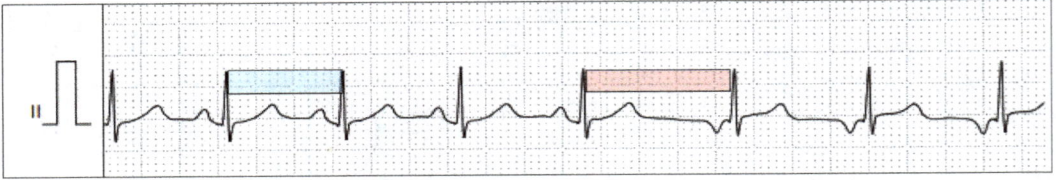

Figure 12.9 Lead II is magnified showing 5 sinus beats and 3 low atrial rhythm beats. The RR cycle length is longer during low atrial rhythm.

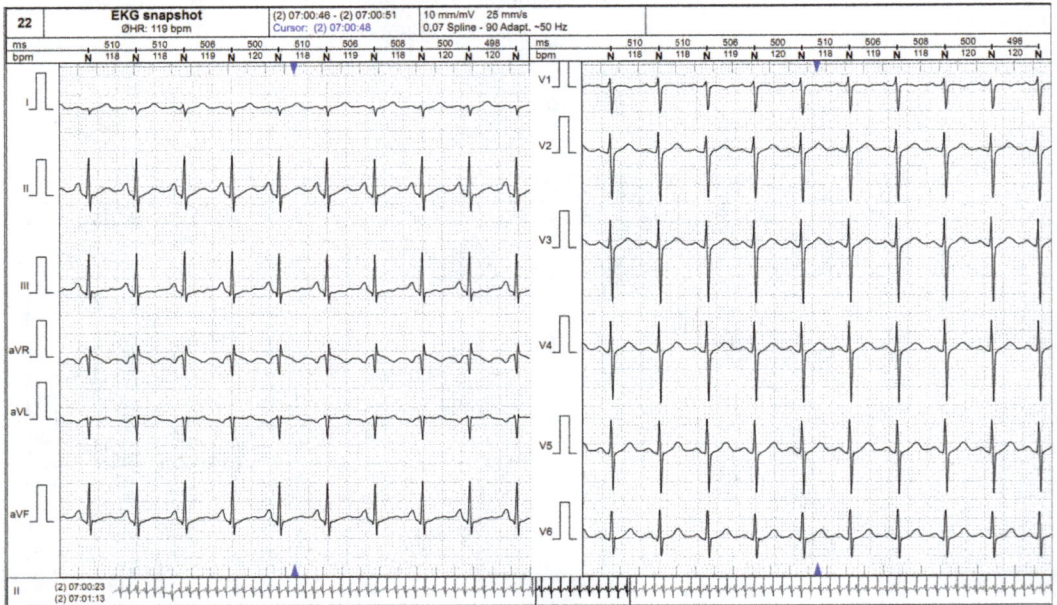

Figure 12.10 The tracing shows sinus rhythm with a rate of 119 bpm.

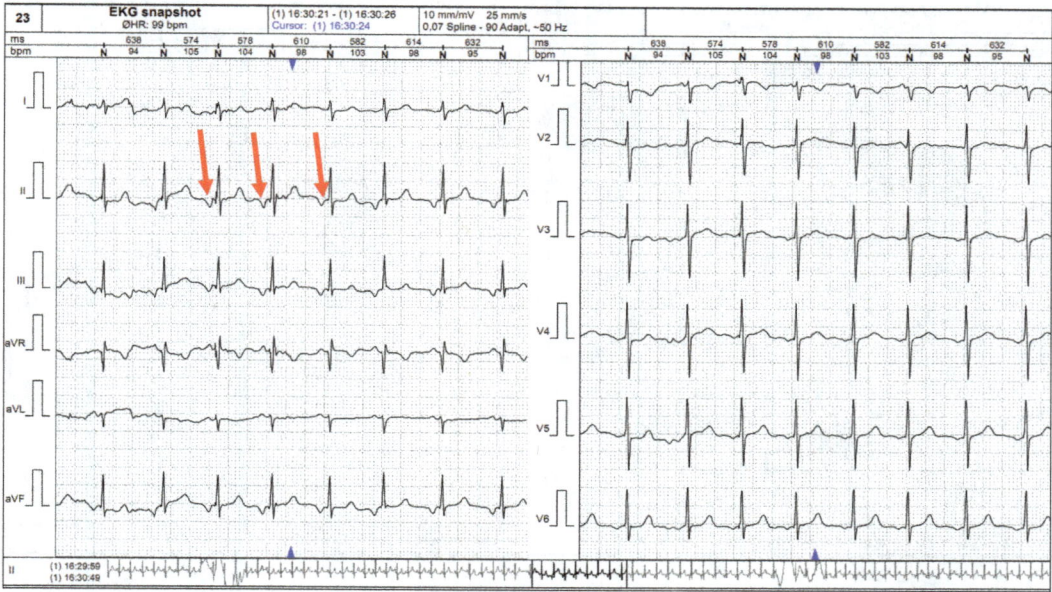

Figure 12.11   The tracing shows low atrial rhythm with a rate of 99 bpm.

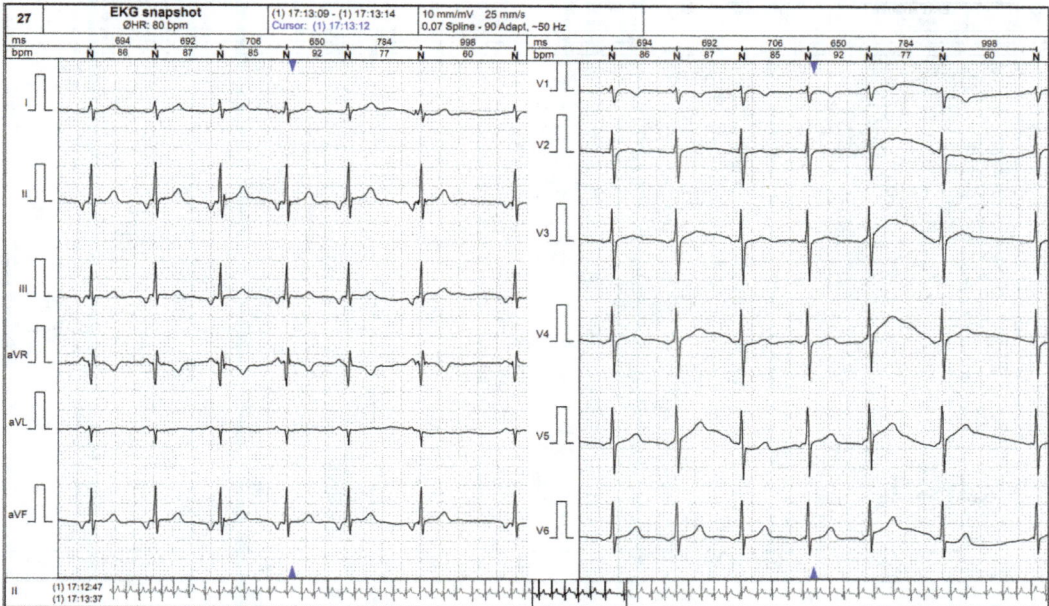

Figure 12.12   The tracing shows low atrial rhythm with a rate of 80 bpm with respiratory arrhythmia.

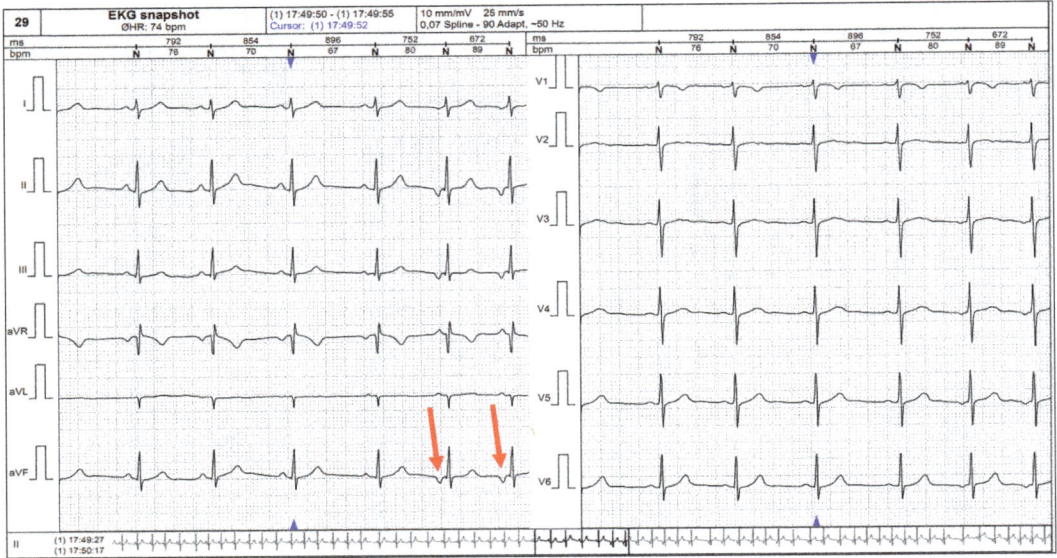

Figure 12.13 The tracing shows sinus rhythm alternating with low atrial rhythm with a rate faster than the sinus one.

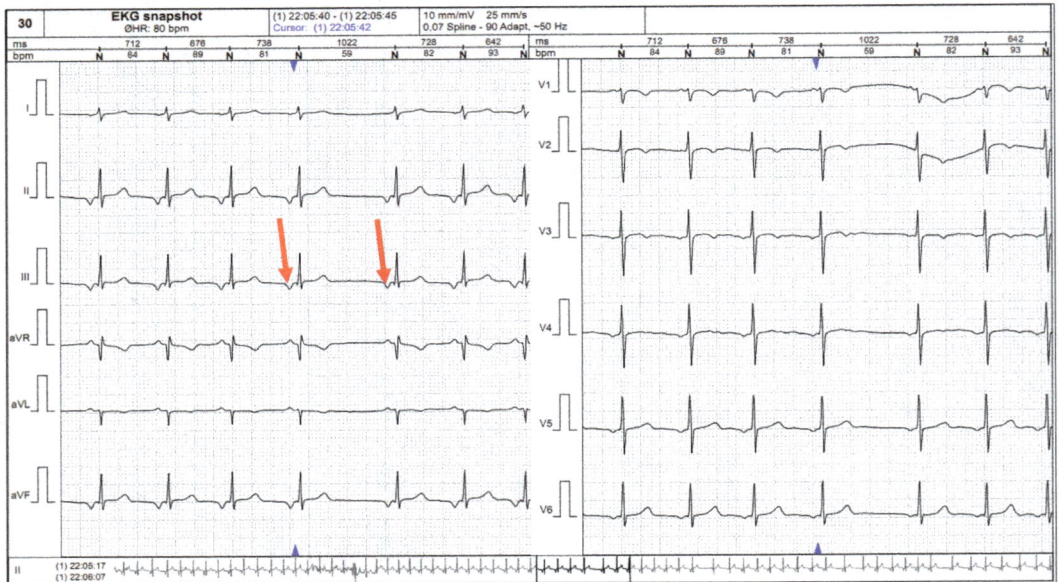

Figure 12.14 The tracing shows low atrial rhythm with a rate of 80 bpm with respiratory arrhythmia.

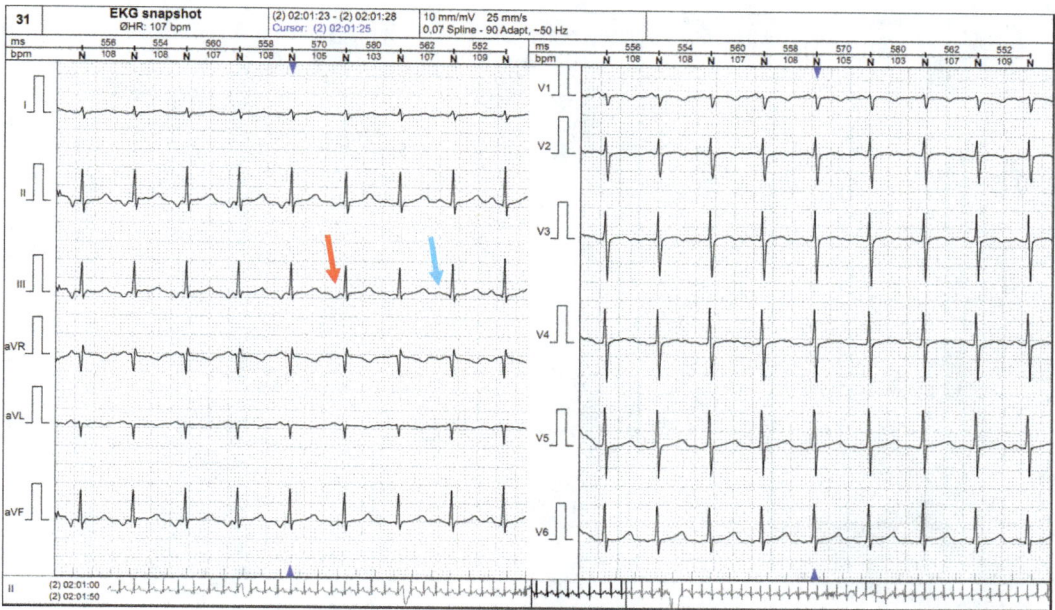

Figure 12.15 The tracing shows low atrial rhythm (red arrow) alternating with sinus rhythm (blue arrow) with similar rates.

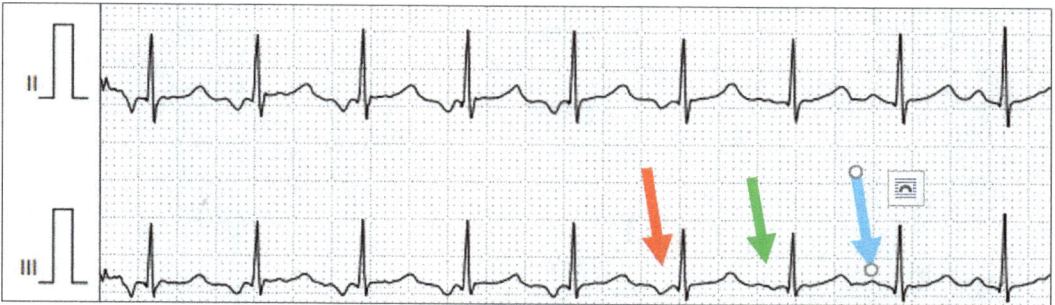

Figure 12.16 A magnified image on leads II and III shows an intermediate P wave morphology (green arrow) during the transition from low atrial rhythm to normal sinus rhythm.

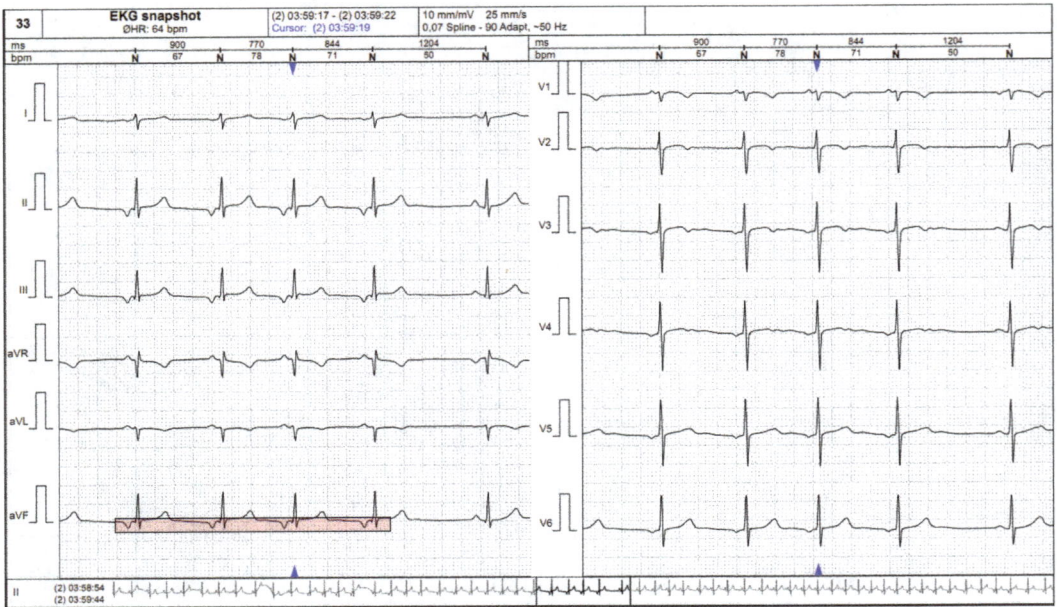

Figure 12.17 The tracing shows low atrial rhythm followed by a normal sinus beat.

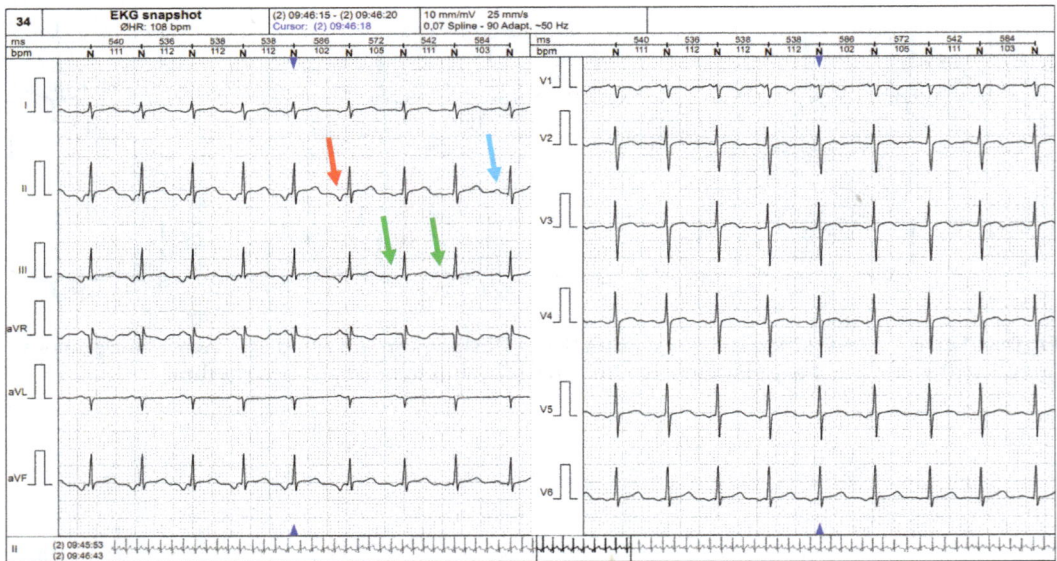

Figure 12.18 The tracing shows low atrial rhythm (red arrow) alternating with sinus rhythm (blue arrow) with similar rates. The green arrows mark 2 transition beats with a P wave morphology between sinus and low atrial.

HOLTER SUMMARY

The Holter monitoring shows normal sinus rhythm alternating with low atrial rhythm. No premature atrial or ventricular contractions were seen. Low atrial rhythm manifested at a rate inferior to that of the sinus rhythm, although it also exhibited a more rapid rate than sinus rhythm. Moreover, low atrial rhythm is influenced by the sympathetic/parasympathetic balance and the respiratory cycle (inspiration/expiration). The transition from low atrial rhythm to sinus rhythm is accomplished by a P wave morphology that is intermediate between sinus and low atrial morphology.

DISCUSSION

The low atrial rhythm is an ectopic rhythm observed in pediatric patients and athletes. It is considered physiological, a variation of normality. It is asymptomatic; however, accurate diagnosis is essential to distinguish it from potentially abnormal rhythms.

In low atrial rhythm, the sinus node is activated from the inferior region of the atrium instead of beginning activation from the above. The focus below the sinus node takes control by enhancing its own automaticity, or the sinus node gives up control by diminishing its own automaticity. Conduction from the atrial abnormal focus to the AV node is antegrade, while conduction to the sinus node is retrograde. Retrograde conduction to the sinus node results in inverted P waves in the inferior frontal leads, II, III, and AVF; and the QRS complex remains narrow, attributable to

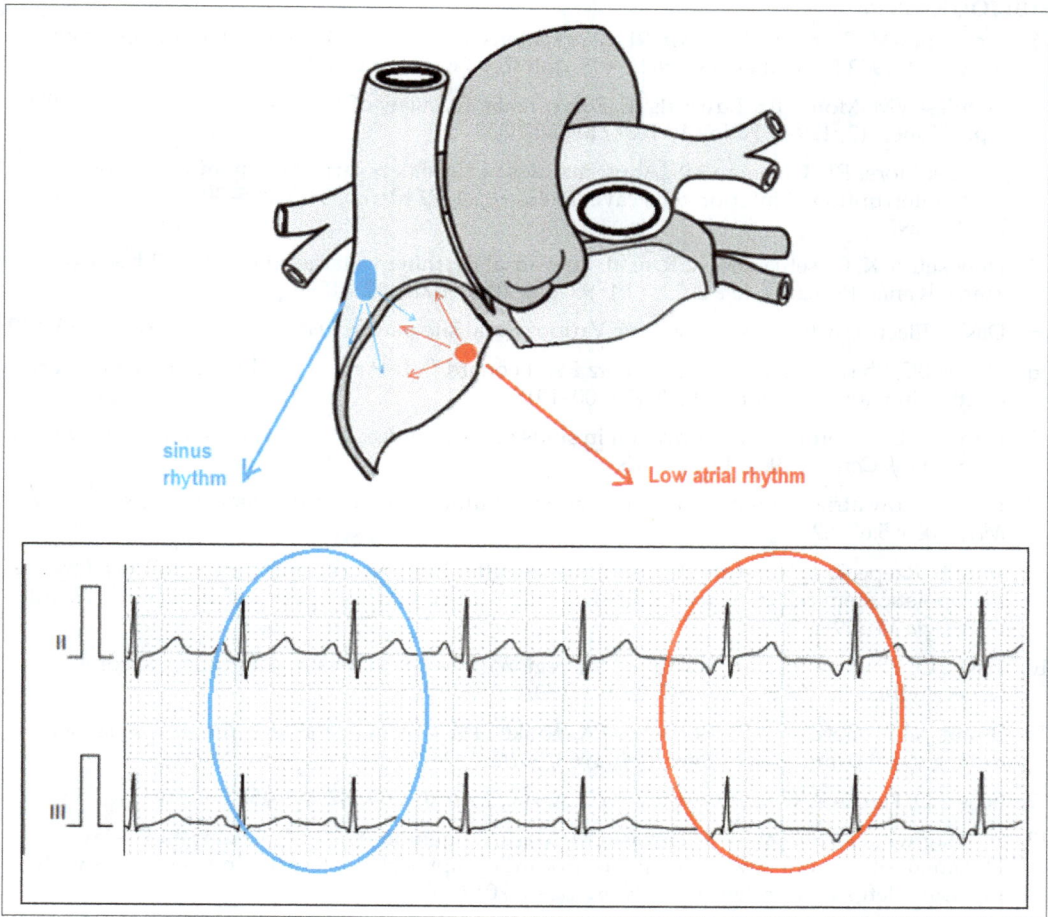

Figure 12.19 In sinus rhythm, the activation of the right atrium occurs in a superior-to-inferior direction (from the top to the bottom), resulting in a positive P wave in leads II, III, and aVF. During low atrial rhythm, atrial activation occurs in an inferior-to-superior direction, resulting in a negative P wave in leads II, III, and aVF.

normal activation via the AV node. A negative P wave in leads I and V6 indicates an origin within the left atrium. This arrhythmia manifests when the sinus node exhibits a deceleration, as observed in vagal circumstances.

The coronary sinus rhythm is a type of low atrial rhythm that develops at the ostium of the coronary sinus due to heightened automaticity.

Increased vagal tone during sleep in children produces a physiological junctional rhythm, which is normal and may present as negative P waves that can precede, follow, or be hidden within the QRS complex. Low atrial rhythm may associate with type sinus venosus atrial septal defect as the posterior part of the right atrium with the sinus node may be affected; in this condition alternate focus from the inferior right atrium gives the dominant rhythm. Pathological low atrial rhythm may occur during digitalis intoxication, or after cardiac surgery.

Meerakker et al. described a large family with an autosomal disorder associating low atrial rhythm with left atrial isomerism, two morphological left atria and left atrial appendages. This abnormality is characterized by hypoplasia, absence or ectopic localization of the sinus node. An anomaly of the 9q chromosome was documented in all family members.

Freedom et al. found a low atrial rhythm in 9 of 12 patients with polysplenia syndrome. The authors propose that polysplenia and low atrial rhythm are correlated with inferior vena cava malformations in the renal or hepatic regions, indicating that cardiac catheterization in these children should be conducted via the superior vena cava.

BIBLIOGRAPHY

1. Freedom RM, Schaffer MS, Rowe RD. Anomalous low insertion of right superior vena cava. *Br Heart J.* 1982 December; 48(6):601–603. doi: 10.1136/hrt.48.6.601

2. Peoples WM, Moller JH, Edwards JE. Polysplenia: A review of 146 cases. *Pediatr Cardiol.* 1983 April–June; 4(2):129–137. doi: 10.1007/BF02076338

3. Van der Horst RL, Gotsman MS. Abnormalities of atrial depolarization in infradiaphragmatic interruption of inferior vena cava. *Br Heart J.* 1972 March; 34(3):295–300. doi: 10.1136/hrt.34.3.295

4. Henckell A-K, Gusetu G, Rosu R, et al. Low atrial rhythm in a large cohort of children from Transylvania, Romania. *Life* 2022; 12:1895. doi: 10.3390/life12111895

5. Das A. Electrocardiographic features: Various atrial site pacing. *Indian Heart J.* 2017; 69:675–680.

6. Harris BC, Shaver JA, Gray S III, Kroetz FW, Leonard JJ. Left atrial rhythm. Experimental production in man. *Circulation.* 1968; 37:1000–1015.

7. Hancock EW. Coronary sinus rhythm in sinus venosus defect and persistent left superior vena cava. *Am. J. Cardiol.* 1964; 14:608–615.

8. Basis, F. Low atrial rhythm as a complication of buthotus judaicus envenomation. *Isr. J. Emerg. Med.* 2005; 5:60–62.

9. Mlot B, Rzepecki P. Heart rhythm disturbances after high-dose chemotherapy followed by haematopoietic stem cell transplantation in a patient with refractory germ cell cancer. *Wspolczesna Onkologia* 14:389–392.

10. Eliska O, Eliskova M. Morphology of the region of the coronary sinus in respect to coronary sinus rhythm. *Int. J. Cardiol.* 1990; 29:141–153.

11. Bouman LN, Gerlings ED, Biersteker PA, Bonke FIM. Pacemaker shift in the sino-atrial node during vagal stimulation. *Pflüg. Arch.* 1968; 302:255–267.

12. Scherf D, Harris R. Coronary sinus rhythm. *Am. Heart J.* 1946; 32:443–456.

13. Ito-Hagiwara K, Iwasaki Y-K, Hayashi M, Maru Y, Fujimoto Y, Oka E, Takahashi K, Hayashi H, Yamamoto T, Yodogawa K, et al. Electrocardiographic characteristics in the patients with a persistent left superior vena cava. *Heart Vessel.* 2019; 34:650–657.

14. Sánchez-García M, Arias-López I, Tomoiu IG, Delgado-Casado JA. Alteraciones electrocardiográficas: Ritmo auricular bajo Semergen. *Soc. Esp. Med. Rural Gen.* 2016; 42:e92–e93.

15. Mirowski M. Left atrial rhythm: Diagnostic criteria and differentiation from nodal arrhythmias. *Am J Cardiol.* 1966; 17(2):203–210.

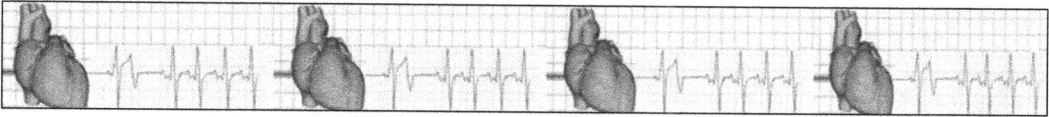

Case 13 Blocked P Waves and Focal Atrial Tachycardia

Cecilia Lazea, Gabriela Kelemen, Alexandra Cocoi, Alexandra Popa, and Crina Sufana

CLINICAL CASE

A 16-year-old girl experienced palpitations and dizziness that started 4 weeks before her presentation. No triggering event or infectious episode was identified. The ECG revealed premature atrial contractions. Echocardiography showed a minor left-to-right shunt in the interatrial septum, without hemodynamic significance. The Holter ECG is presented below. During monitoring she felt short episodes of 4–5 consecutive abnormal beats.

Concluzie

Ritm cardiac		
Total bătăi	109 755	(0% paced)
HR max / min	**151 / 42 bpm**	
Media HR	**Ø 74 bpm**	
HR Max / Min Sinus	151 / 42 bpm	
Media HR (Treaz/Adormit)	78 / 68 bpm	
Index circadian	1,15	
Tahicardie / Bradicardie	4 % / 10 %	

Pauze	
RR Max	**2 192 ms**
Pauze (>2000ms)	**5**

Fibrilaţie atrială / Flutter atrial	
Total AF	-
AF HR Max	0 bpm
Cel mai lung AF	-

Bradicardie		
Cea mai mică	Ø 48 bpm	14 sec
Cea mai mare	Ø 51 bpm	00:07:12

ST		
St ridicare max	1,36 mV	III
ST depresurizare max	-0,99 mV	aVL

Ectopie ventriculară		
V Total	0	(< 1%)
V / Ora Max	0	pe oră
Episoade Tahicardie V		-
Cea mai rapidă Tahicardie V		-
V Cea mai lungă secvenţă		-
Triplete / Execută		0 Σ 0 bătăi
Cuplete		0 Σ 0 bătăi
Bigeminism		0 Σ 0 bătăi
Trigeminism		0 Σ 0 bătăi

Ectopie supraventriculară		
S Tot	11314	(10%)
Episoade Tahicardie SV		8 Σ 00:01:56
Cea mai rapidă Tahicardie SV	Ø 128 bpm	9 sec
S Cea mai lungă secvenţă	Ø 80 bpm	00:01:08
Triplete / Execută	1353	Σ 6177 bătăi
Cuplete	971	Σ 1942 bătăi

Figure 13.1 The summary page shows a maximum heart rate of 151 bpm and a minimum rate of 42 bpm. The PAC burden is increased: 10% on 24 hours with an episode of atrial tachycardia of 9 seconds.

DOI: 10.1201/9781003545040-13

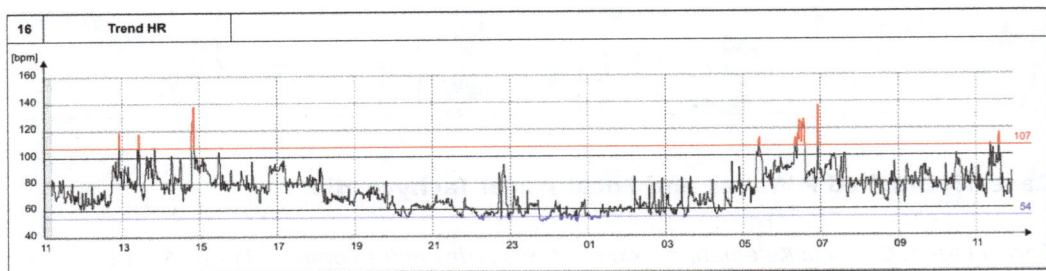

Figure 13.2 The heart rate trend shows the mean rate over 24 hours of monitoring with mean limits of 54 to 107.

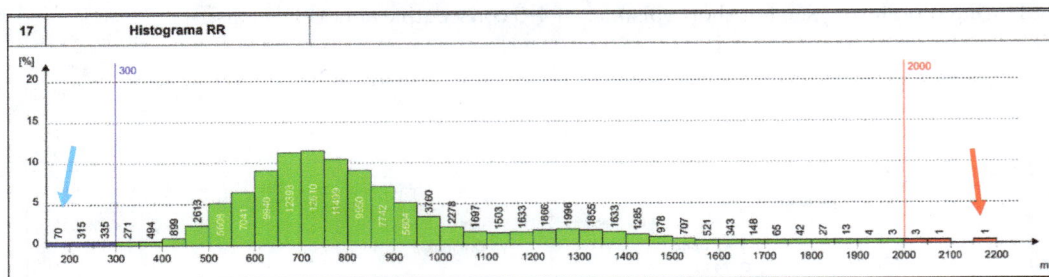

Figure 13.3 The RR histogram shows RR intervals up to 2200 ms which correspond to a postextrasystolic pause (red arrow) and short intervals of 70 ms (blue arrow) which are electrical artifacts as seen in Figure 13.10.

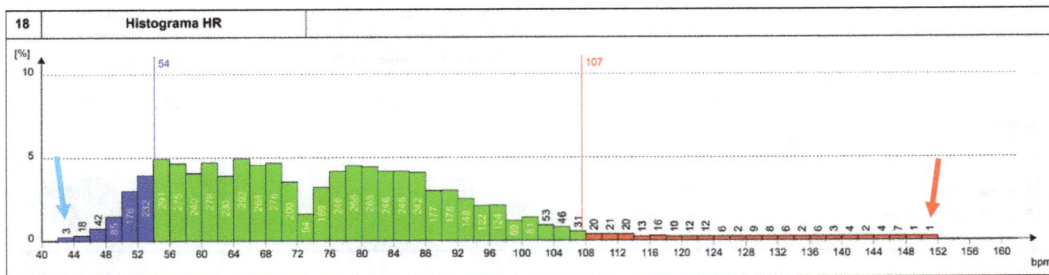

Figure 13.4 The HR histogram shows rates up to 151 bpm during tachycardia (red arrow) and slow rates of 40bpm seen at 3:35 during the night (blue arrow).

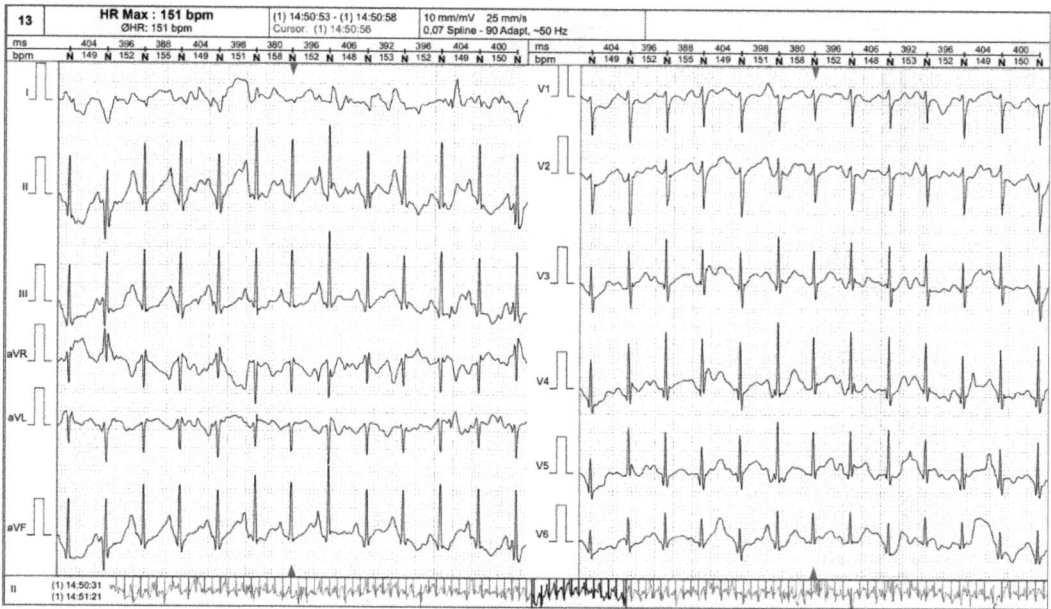

Figure 13.5 The image shows the fastest recorded rate, which is 151 bpm. Positive P waves in leads II, III and AVF as well as precordial leads confirm sinus tachycardia.

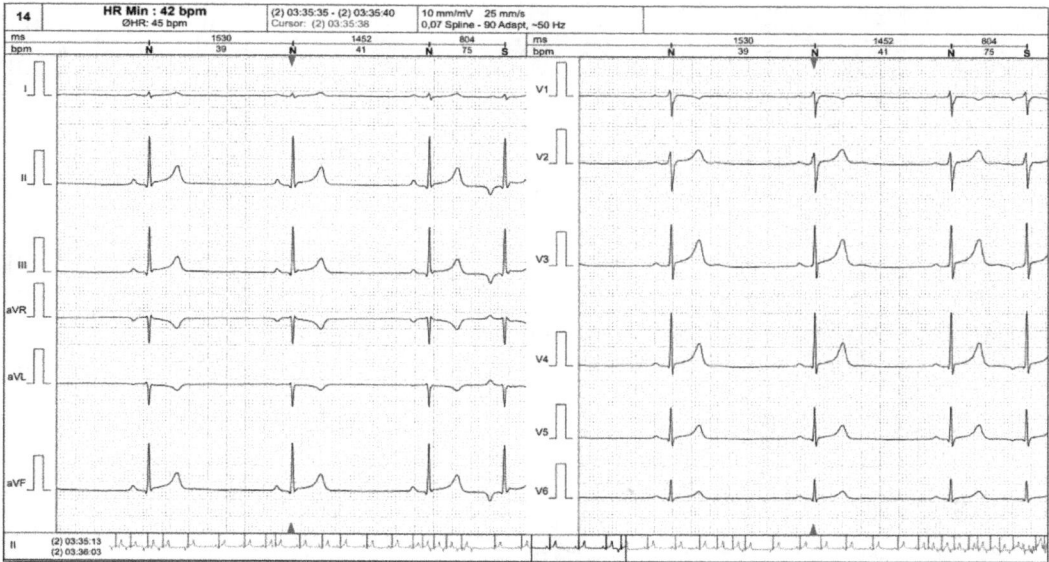

Figure 13.6 The image shows the lowest recorded rate, which is a sinus bradycardia occurring during night at 3:35.

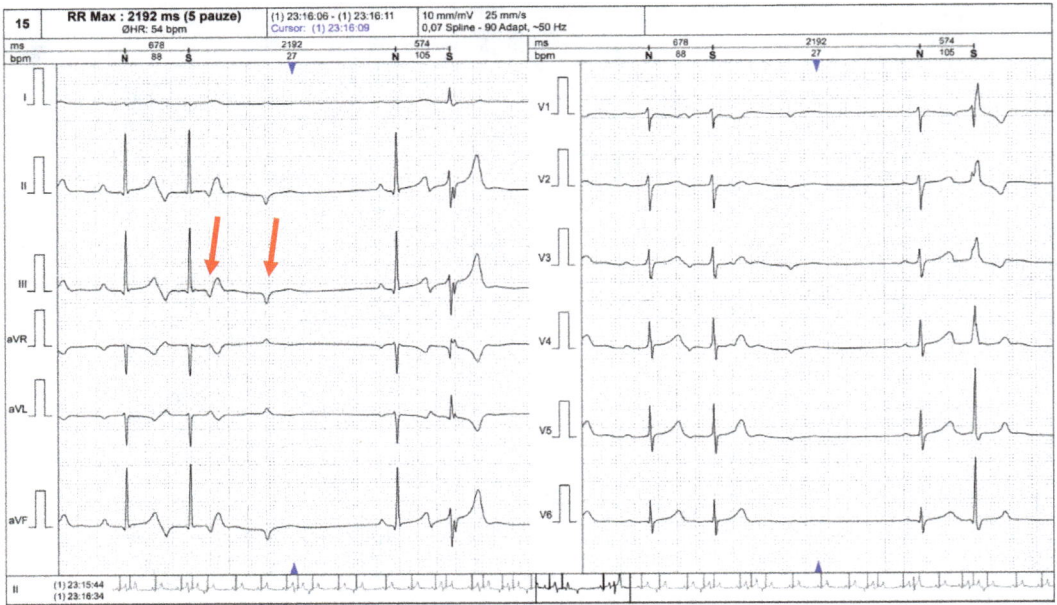

Figure 13.7 The tracing shows the longest pause of 2.19 seconds, which is a postextrasystolic pause. During this interval 2 blocked P waves are visible: the first P wave inside the T wave and the second wave after the T wave (red arrows).

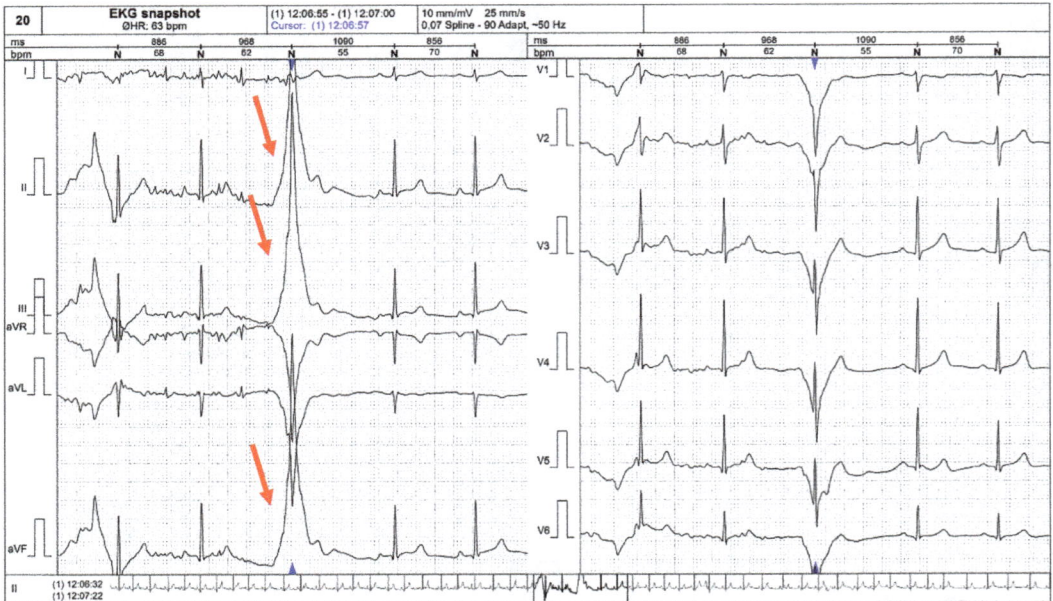

Figure 13.8 The tracing shows an electrical artifact which mimics a ventricular abnormal beat.

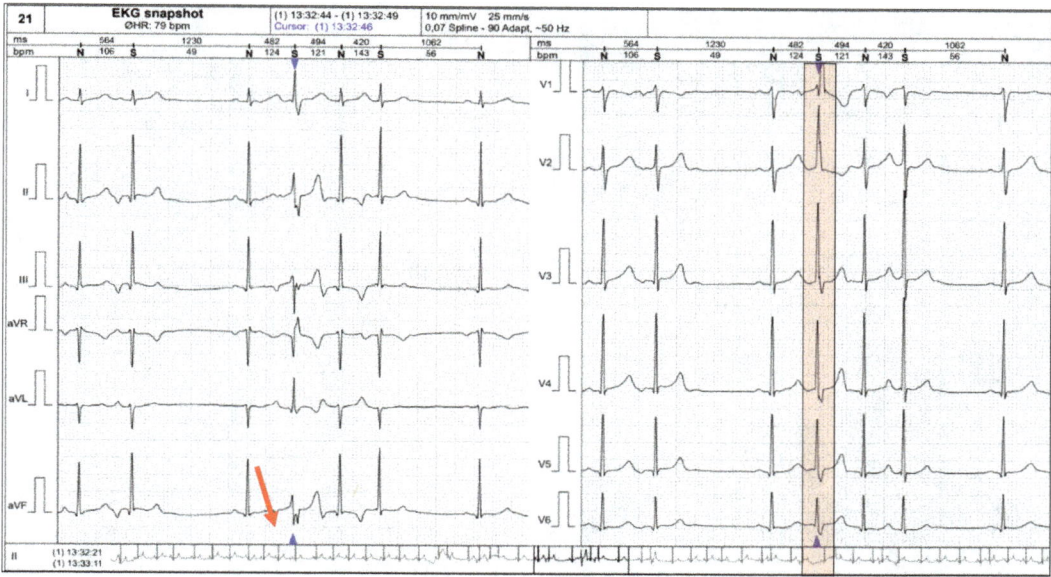

Figure 13.9 The tracing shows an atrial premature contraction with negative P wave in inferior leads (II, III and avF) (red arrow) with RBBB aberrancy (red square).

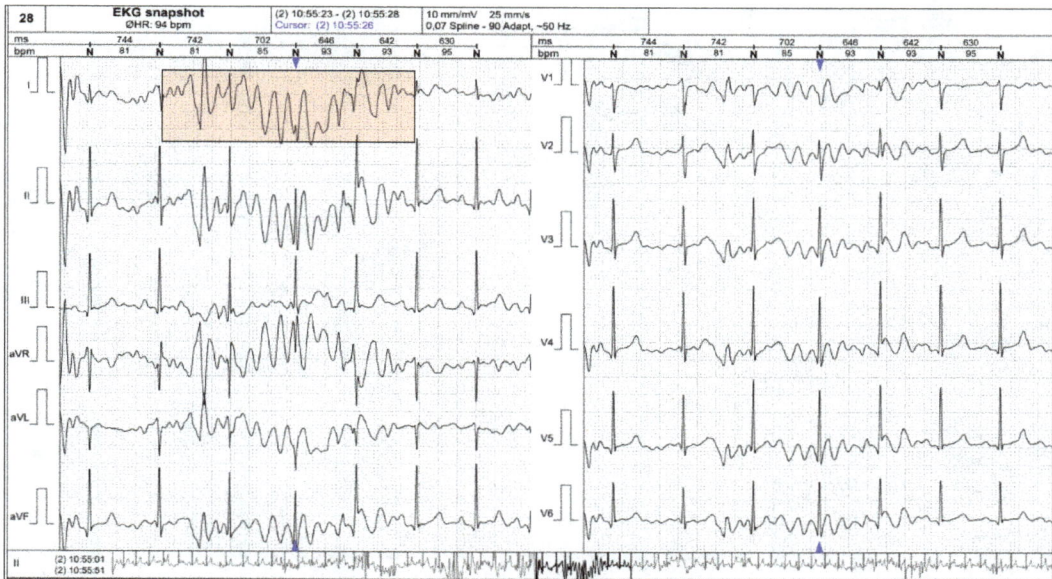

Figure 13.10 The tracing shows an electrical artifact mimicking a ventricular fast arrhythmia.

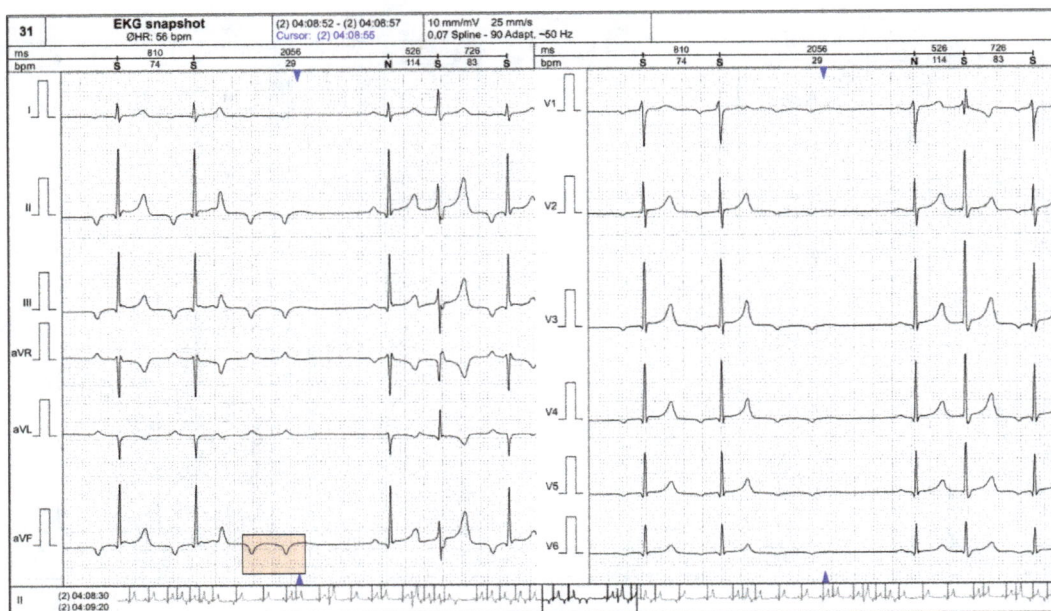

Figure 13.11 The tracing shows a pause of 2.05 seconds, with 2 blocked premature atrial contractions.

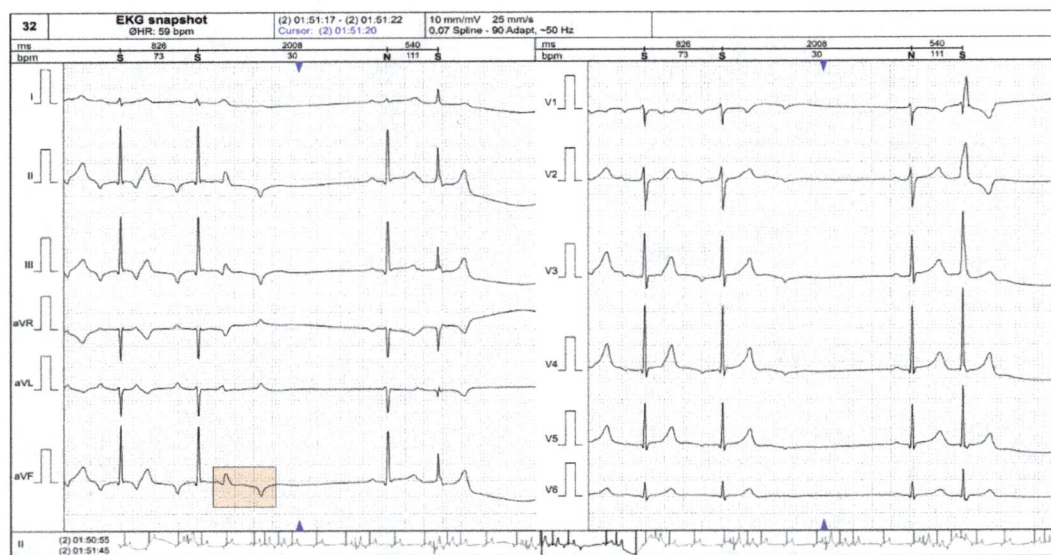

Figure 13.12 The tracing shows a pause of 2.0 seconds, with 2 blocked premature atrial contractions (one inside the T wave and the other after the T wave).

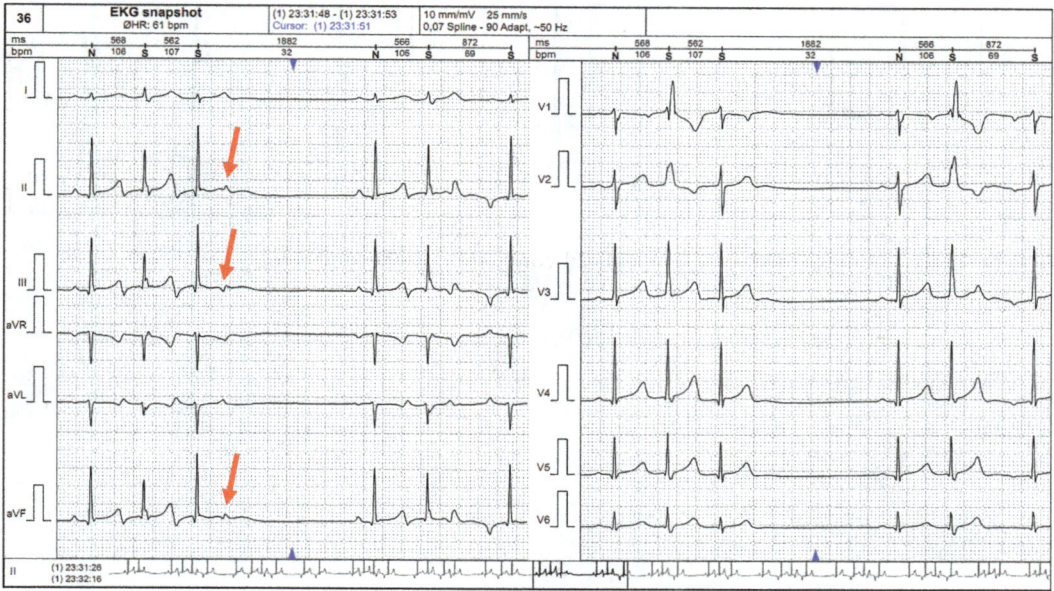

Figure 13.13 The tracing shows a pause of 1.88 seconds with a blocked premature atrial contraction.

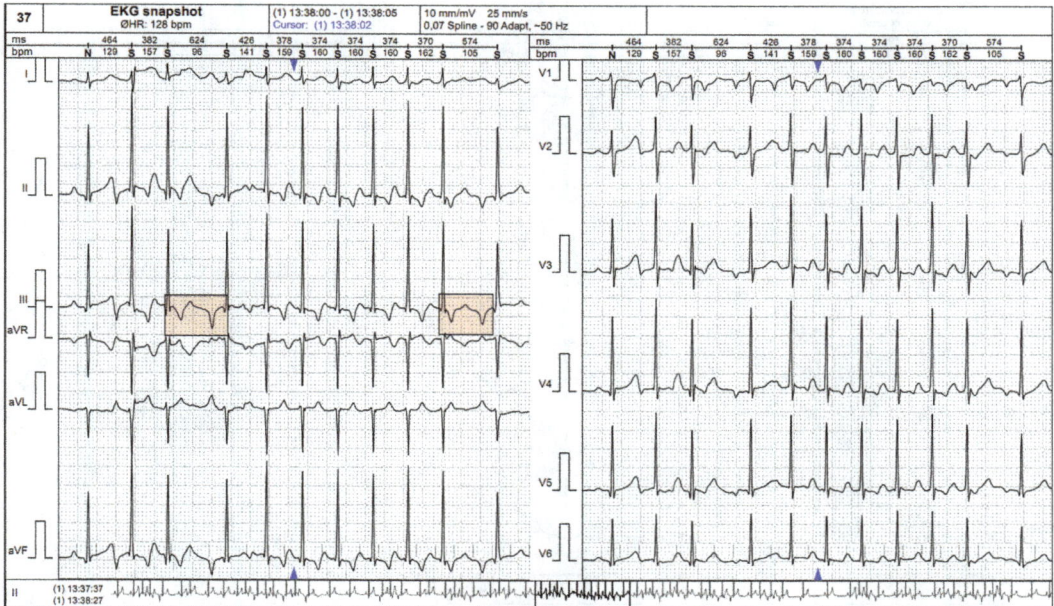

Figure 13.14 The tracing shows an episode of atrial tachycardia with 1:1 and 2:1 conduction to the ventricles. The red squares mark 2:1 conduction to the ventricles.

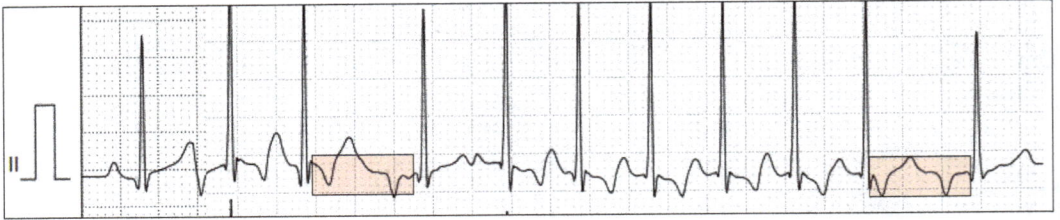

Figure 13.15   A magnified lead II reveals 2:1 conduction to the ventricles.

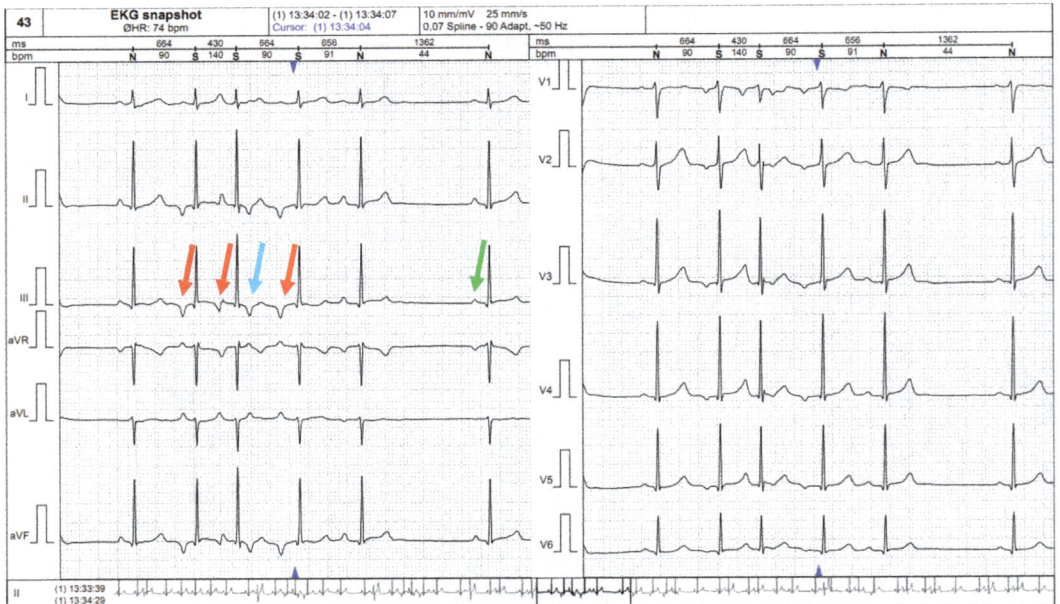

Figure 13.16   The tracing shows premature atrial contractions conducted to the ventricles (red arrow) or blocked in the AV node (blue arrow). The green arrow marks a normal sinus beat.

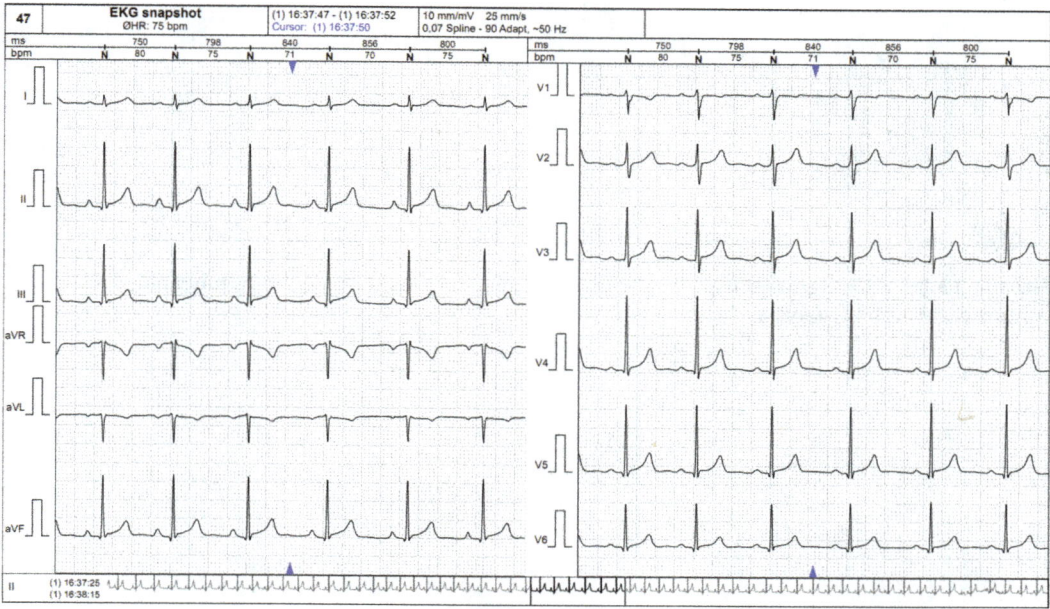

Figure 13.17 The image shows normal sinus rhythm with a rate of 75 bpm.

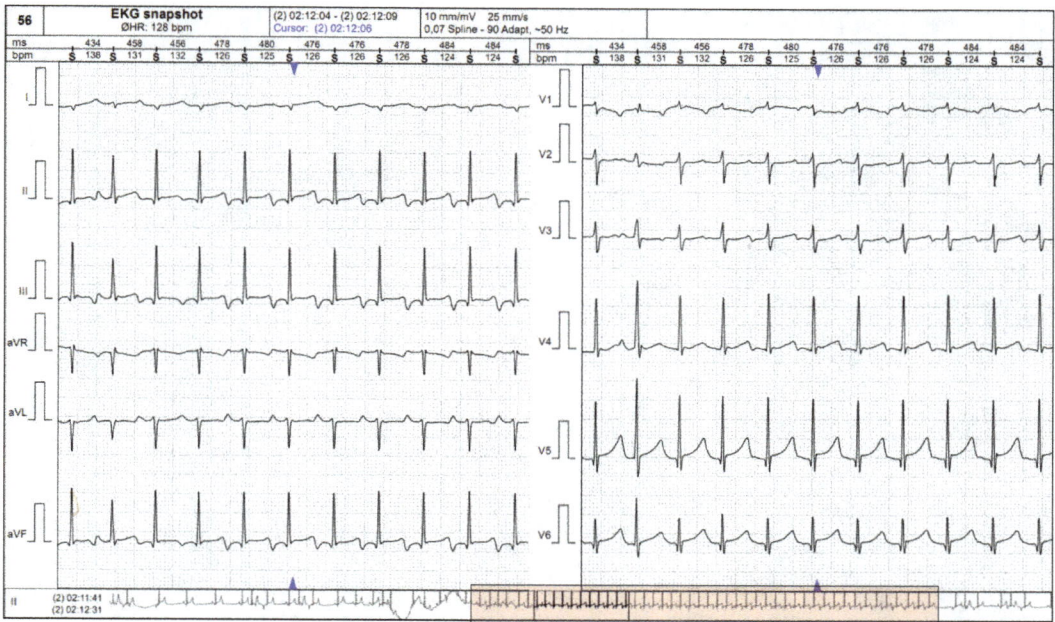

Figure 13.18 The image shows an episode of atrial tachycardia of 48 consecutive atrial beats (red square) with a rate of 128 bpm.

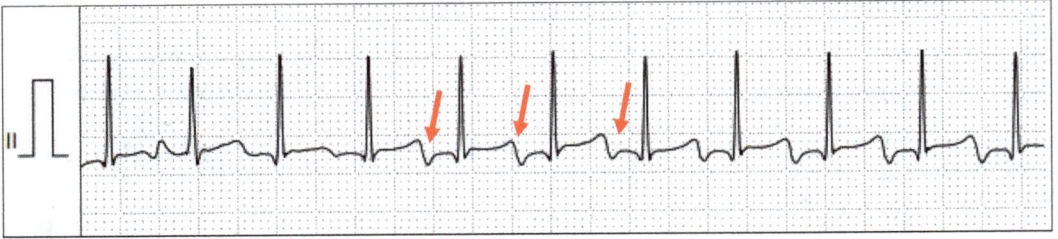

Figure 13.19 A magnified lead II reveals abnormal P waves with different morphology compared to sinus P waves.

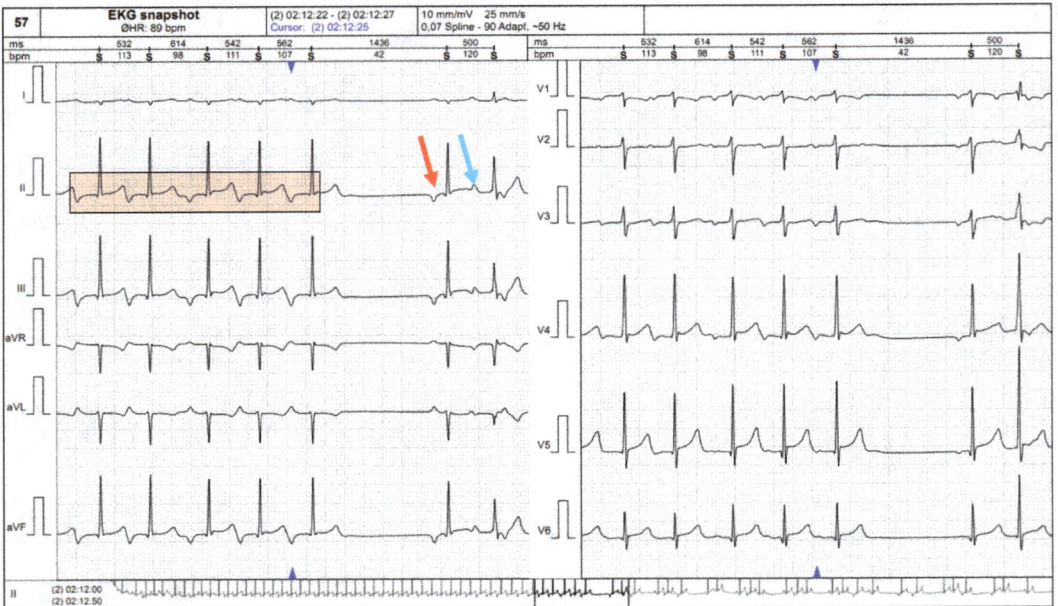

Figure 13.20 The episode of atrial tachycardia (red square) stops and is followed by an 2 atrial premature beats with different P wave morphology (red and blue arrows).

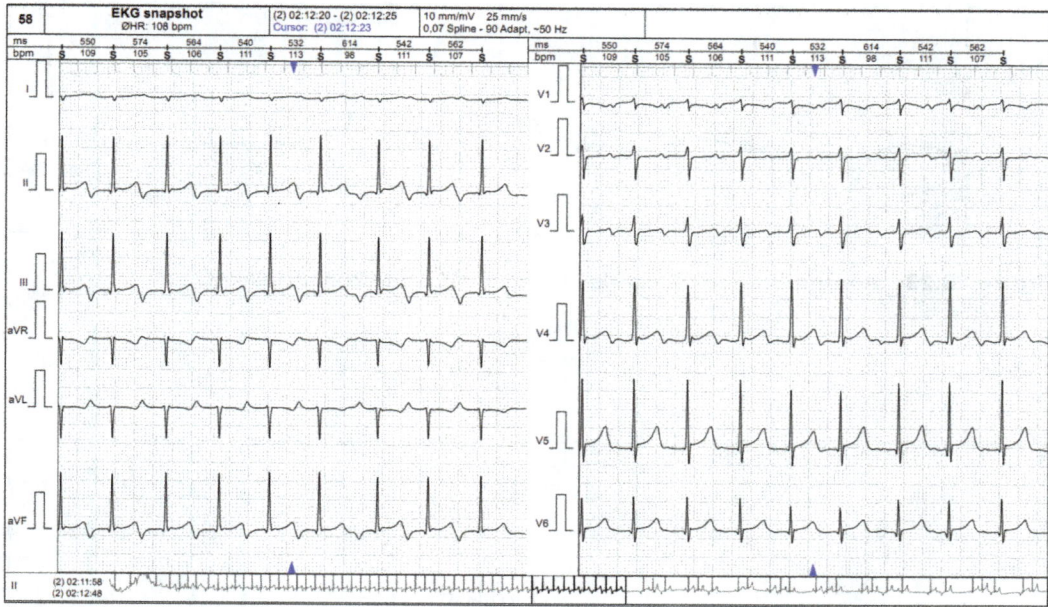

Figure 13.21   Episode of monomorphic atrial tachycardia.

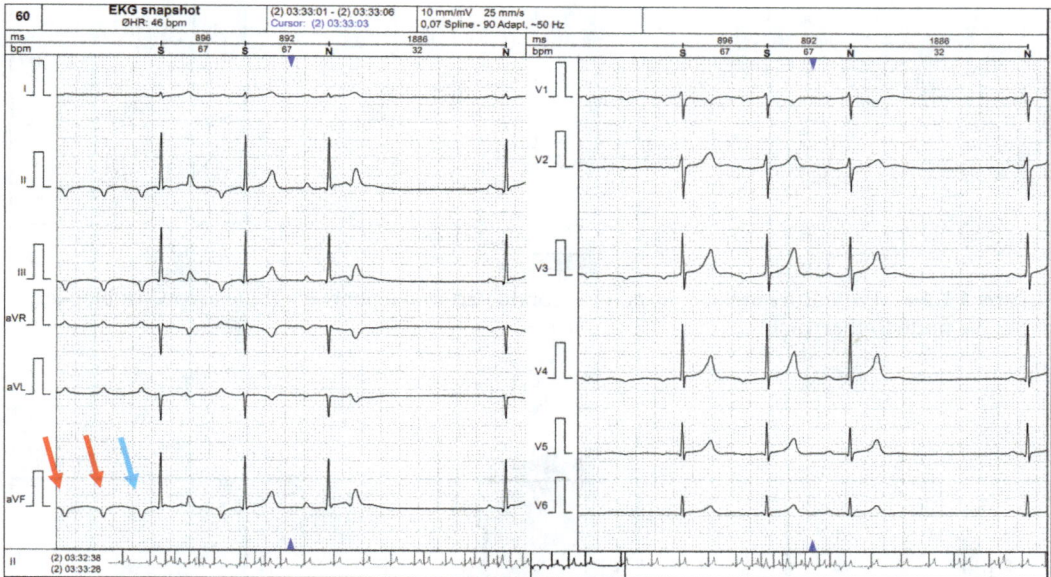

Figure 13.22   Premature atrial contractions conducted to the ventricle (blue arrow) or blocked in the AV node (red arrow).

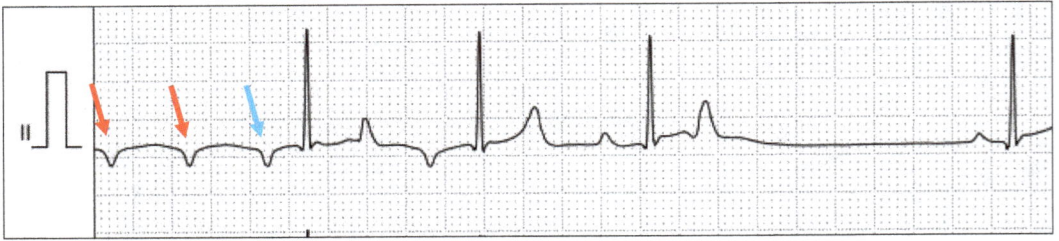

Figure 13.23 A magnified lead II reveals 2 blocked PAC and 1 conducted PAC.

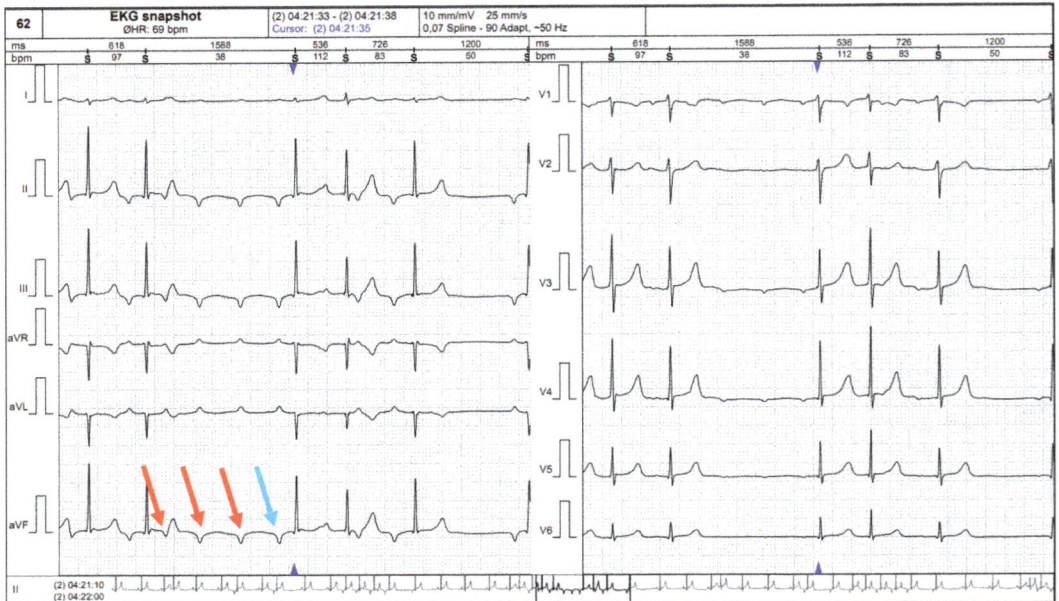

Figure 13.24 Premature atrial contractions conducted to the ventricle (blue arrow) or blocked in the AV node (red arrow).

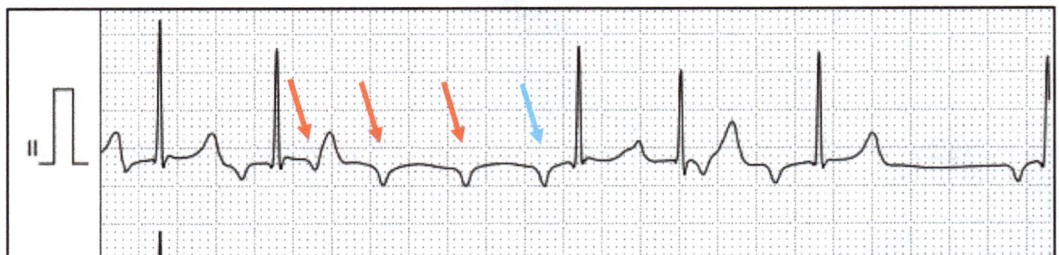

Figure 13.25 A magnified lead II reveals three blocked P waves with negative morphology (red arrow), followed by a conducted PAC (blue arrow).

HOLTER SUMMARY

During 24 hours of Holter monitoring 11.314 PACs were detected. Most of them were isolated, followed by a narrow QRS complex; some of them were conducted to the ventricles with an RBBB aberrancy. Blocked premature atrial contractions were also present. Short bursts of atrial tachycardia of 4 to 5 consecutive beats were felt by the patient. However, a longer episode of 48 consecutive beats occurred during the night at 2:12:04. The ventricular rate during atrial tachycardia was 125 to 150 bpm.

DISCUSSION

A premature atrial contraction emerges when a focus from the right or left atrium generates an action potential prior to the following spontaneous activation of the sinus node. There are 4 ECG characteristics of PACs:

1. They are premature, earlier than expected compared to the previous P–P interval.

2. They are ectopic with a different P wave morphology and PR interval.

3. They are followed by narrow QRS complexes. Since they activate the ventricles through the AV node, both LV and RV are depolarized at the same time. However, sometimes the right or left branch of the conduction system may be refractory which leads to RBBB or LBBB aberrancy.

4. They are followed by a pause after the PAC. It may be compensatory, noncompensatory or absent, in the function of the coupling interval between the PAC and the preceding beat.

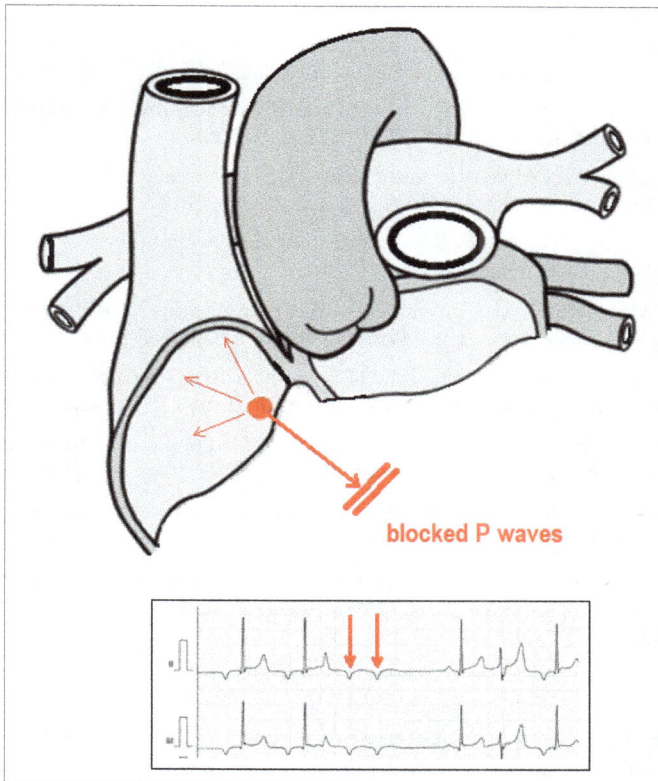

Figure 13.26   Atrial activation may block at the level of the AV node, preventing any further ventricular activation. This results in blocked P waves visible on the ECG. The negative morphology in inferior leads II, III, and avF suggests an inferior origin of atrial activation inside the atrium.

111

Premature atrial contractions are detected in 1–7% of fetuses between 36 to 41 weeks of gestation. They are not usually present between 30 to 35 weeks of gestation. The incidence of premature atrial contractions in neonates is similar to the incidence between 36 to 41 weeks, and usually disappears during the first year of life. Increased automaticity of the atrial focus may lead to focal atrial tachycardia. Current medical research indicates a very high rate of spontaneous resolution in children under 1 year of age, and a high rate in those aged 1 to 3 years.

Our patient experienced an episode of 48 consecutive atrial beats (focal atrial tachycardia) with identical morphology to the premature atrial beats. Treatment with 2 × 50 mg of Flecainide was ineffective in reducing PAC burden; therefore, it was increased to 2 × 100 mg daily. In the event of medication failure, targeted catheter ablation of the atrial focus will be recommended. The use of three-dimensional electroanatomic mapping systems improves the success rates of ablation in atrial tachycardia.

When atrial tachycardia is present in more than 50% of the recording time in Holter monitoring, this is termed incessant atrial tachycardia. It may lead to tachycardia-induced cardiomyopathy defined by an ejection fraction of less than 40% due to arrhythmia.

In the study of Kang et al. on 249 children with a median age of 7.2 years, the rate of spontaneous resolution was 89%; consequently, the authors advocate for medical therapy until the full resolution of the tachyarrhythmia, rather than catheter ablation.

Beta blockers and class Ic antiarrhythmic agents are primarily used for the management of focal atrial tachycardia, in contrast to other drugs such as Amiodarone, which demonstrates less efficacy.

Previous studies indicate reduced success rates and elevated complication rates linked to catheter ablation in young or small children; hence, numerous institutions do not routinely offer catheter ablation for children under three years of age or weighing less than 25 kg.

BIBLIOGRAPHY

1. Teuwen CP, Korevaar TIM, Coolen RL. Frequent atrial extrasystolic beats predict atrial fibrillation in patients with congenital heart defects. *Europace*. 2018; 20:25–32.

2. Conen D, Adam M, Roche F. Premature atrial contractions in the general population: Frequency and risk factors. *Circulation*. 2012; 126:2302–2308.

3. Lin CY, Lin YJ, Chen YY. Prognostic significance of premature atrial complexes burden in prediction of long-term outcome. *J Am Heart Assoc*. 2015; 4:e002192.

4. Southall DP, Richards J, Hardwick RA. Prospective study of fetal heart rate and rhythm patterns. *Arch Dis Child*. 1980; 55:506–511.

5. Nagashima M, Matsushima M, Ogawa A. Cardiac arrhythmias in healthy children revealed by 24-hour ambulatory ECG monitoring. *Pediatr Cardiol*. 1987; 8:103–108.

6. Southall DP, Johnston F, Shinebourne EA. 24-hour electrocardiographic study of heart rate and rhythm patterns in population of healthy children. *Br Heart J*. 1981; 45:281–291.

7. Scott O, Williams GJ, Fiddler GI. Results of 24 hour ambulatory monitoring of electrocardiogram in 131 healthy boys aged 10 to 13 years. *Br Heart J*. 1980; 44:304–308.

8. Southall DP, Richards J, Mitchell P. Study of cardiac rhythm in healthy newborn infants. *Br Heart J*. 1980; 43:14–20.

9. Gunda S, Akyeampong D, Gomez-Arroyo J. Consequences of chronic frequent premature atrial contractions: Association with cardiac arrhythmias and cardiac structural changes. *J Cardiovasc Electrophysiol*. 2019; 30:1952–1959.

10. Acharya T, Tringali S, Bhullar M. Frequent atrial premature complexes and their association with risk of atrial fibrillation. *Am J Cardiol*. 2015; 116:1852–1857.

11. Elliott AD, Linz D, Mishima R. Association between physical activity and risk of incident arrhythmias in 402,406 individuals: Evidence from the UK Biobank cohort. *Eur Heart J*. 2020; 41:1479–1486.

12. Wiggins DL, Strasburger JF, Gotteiner NL, Cuneo B, Wakai RT. Magnetophysiologic and echocardiographic comparison of blocked atrial bigeminy and 2:1 atrioventricular block in the fetus. *Heart Rhythm*. 2013; 10(8):1192–1198.

13. Ge H, Li X, Liu H, Jiang H. Predictors of pharmacological therapy of ectopic atrial tachycardia in children. *Pediatr Cardiol.* 2017 February; 38(2):289–295. doi: 10.1007/s00246-016-1511-7. Epub 2016 November 24.

14. Bradley DJ, Fischbach PS, Law IH, Serwer GA, Dick M. The clinical course of multifocal atrial tachycardia in infants and children. *J Am Coll Cardiol.* 2001 August; 38(2):401–408. doi: 10.1016/s0735-1097(01)01390-0

15. Khongphatthanayothin A, Chotivitayatarakorn P, Lertsupcharoen P, Muangmingsuk S, Thisyakorn C. Atrial tachycardia from enhanced automaticity in children: Diagnosis and initial management. *J Med Assoc Thai.* 2001 September; 84(9):1321–1328.

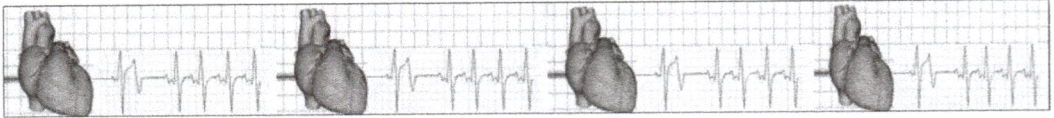

Case 14 Sick Sinus Syndrome

Rein Kolk and Kristel Köbas

CLINICAL CASE

A 5-year-old boy was examined in the Children's Clinic with a view to pacemaker implantation. During the Holter ECG examination, sinus pauses and junctional rhythm were observed; hence, the advice of an electrophysiologist was requested.

Patient Name:		ID#:	
Address:		Age: 5 years DOB:	Sex: Male
Pacemaker:	None	Weight: Height:	
Supervising Physician:		Referring Physician or Facility:	
Indications:			
Medications:			

HEART RATE		VENTRICULAR ECTOPY		HEART RATE VARIABILITY	
Minimum HR-4 Intervals:	40 bpm at 10:45	VE Total:	0	SDNN-24 Hour:	94
Maximum HR-4 Intervals:	190 bpm at 23:26	V-Pair Total:	0	SDANN Index:	83
Average HR-24 Hours:	105 bpm	V-Run Total:	0	SDNN Index:	45
Minimum HR-Hourly:	83 bpm at 1:00	Longest V-Run:	N/A	rMSSD:	32
Maximum HR-Hourly:	127 bpm at 17:00	Maximum HR V-Run:	N/A	pNN50:	11
Analyzed Beats:	150073	Minimum HR V-Run:	N/A	Spectral Power-24 Hour:	1767.3
Analyzed Minutes:	1429	VE's per 1000/per Hour:	0.00/0.00	Min Spectral Power Hour:	1297.6
ECG Monitoring Period:	26 hours 13 minute	Ventricular R on T:	N/A	Max Spectral Power Hour:	2480.9

ST SEGMENT ANALYSIS		SUPRAVENTRICULAR ECTOPY		PAUSES	
Total ST Minutes CH1:	0	SVE Total:	0	Pauses in Excess of 2.50 sec:	8
Total ST Minutes CH2:	0	SVE Pair Total:	0	Max Pause:	4.05 sec at 10:44
Total ST Minutes CH3:	1184	SV-Run Total:	0	QT	
Max Abs. ST Depression:	-4.3 at 21:02@CH 3	Longest SV-Run:	N/A	Max QT:	439 ms (Ch. 1)
Max Abs. ST Elevation:	N/A	Maximum HR SV-Run:	N/A	Max QTc:	453 ms
Max ST Episode:	405 Minutes at 0:16	SVE's per 1000/per hour:	0.00/0.00	Time of Max QT:	at 15:45. HR 90 bpm.
Max HR In ST Episode:	165	Total Aberrant Beats/Runs:	0/0	IdioV	1
		Atrial Fib/Flutter:	0.0%		

Figure 14.1 The summary page shows a minimum heart rate of 40 bpm and 8 pauses of more than 2.5 seconds. The longest pause was 4.1 seconds. No PVCs or PACs were detected.

DOI: 10.1201/9781003545040-14

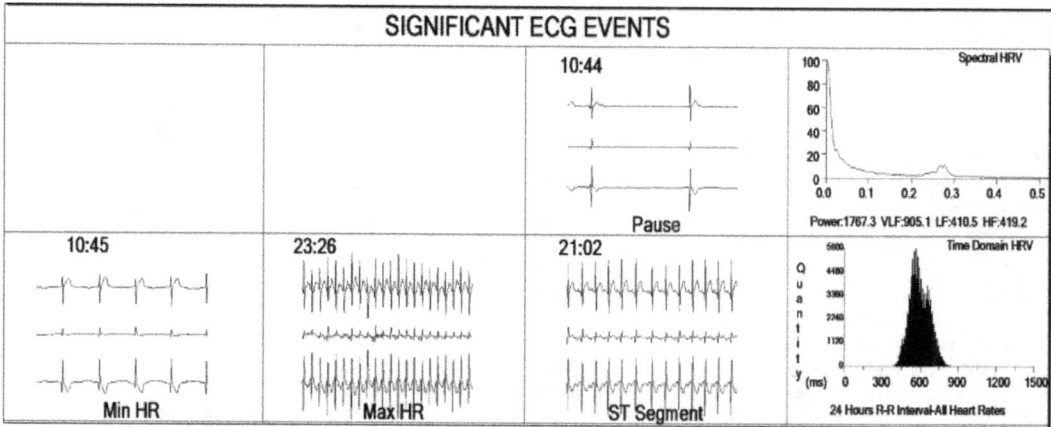

Figure 14.2 Significant ECG events from the 24 hours recording a minimum heart rate of 40 bpm, a maximum pause of 4.1 seconds, a maximum heart rate of 190 bpm, and a ST segment depression of 4.3 mm, HRV SDNN of 94.

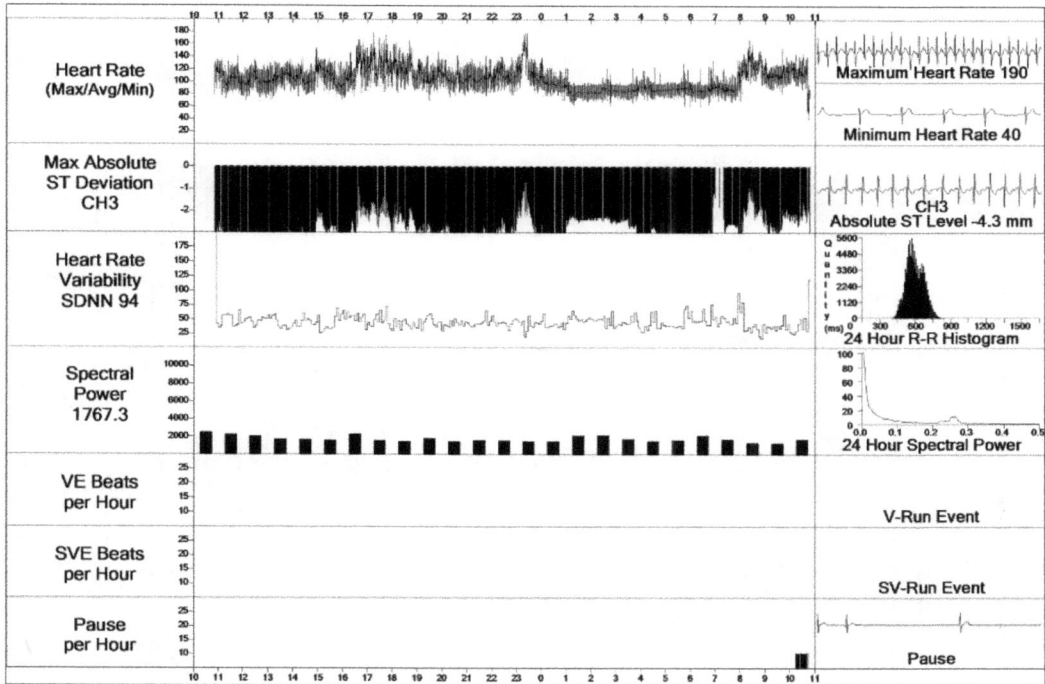

Figure 14.3 Significant ECG events from the 24 hours recording: heart rate, ST deviation, HRV, PVCs, PACs and pauses.

Time	Total Beats	Avg HR	Min HR	Max HR	SDNN	Spectral Power	Absolute ST CH 1		Absolute ST CH 2		Absolute ST CH 3		VE	pair	run	SVE	sin	pair	run	Pause > 2.5 sec	SV-Bi	SV-Tri	V-Big	V-Tri	IdiV
10:49	1039	116	78	133	77	2480.9	0	+3.3	0	-0.1	2	-3.6	0 0 0			0 0 0 0				0	0	0	0	0	0
11:00	6220	104	70	139	60	2239.5	0	+3.5	0	-0.3	14	-4.0	0 0 0			0 0 0 0				0	0	0	0	0	0
12:00	6090	102	72	132	58	2054.6	0	+3.6	0	-0.3	8	-4.1	0 0 0			0 0 0 0				0	0	0	0	0	0
13:00	6435	107	68	129	49	1716.7	0	+3.7	0	-0.4	38	-4.1	0 0 0			0 0 0 0				0	0	0	0	0	0
14:00	6316	106	76	152	59	1682.6	0	+3.7	0	-0.4	53	-4.1	0 0 0			0 0 0 0				0	0	0	0	0	0
15:00	6483	108	72	144	70	1592.5	0	+3.2	0	-0.4	42	-3.7	0 0 0			0 0 0 0				0	0	0	0	0	0
16:00	6943	117	74	163	80	2360.9	0	+3.4	0	-0.4	60	-3.9	0 0 0			0 0 0 0				0	0	0	0	0	0
17:00	7529	127	87	173	57	1564.7	0	+2.5	0	-0.3	60	-3.0	0 0 0			0 0 0 0				0	0	0	0	0	0
18:00	7246	122	84	164	59	1485.5	0	+2.6	0	-0.5	59	-3.2	0 0 0			0 0 0 0				0	0	0	0	0	0
19:00	6595	110	77	141	55	1798.9	0	+3.1	0	-0.4	60	-3.6	0 0 0			0 0 0 0				0	0	0	0	0	0
20:00	6313	105	76	140	55	1485.0	0	+4.1	0	-0.4	60	-4.1	0 0 0			0 0 0 0				0	0	0	0	0	0
21:00	6333	106	81	131	49	1625.9	0	+4.0	0	-0.3	57	-4.3	0 0 0			0 0 0 0				0	0	0	0	0	0
22:00	6550	110	80	139	49	1568.3	0	+3.4	0	-0.3	53	-3.9	0 0 0			0 0 0 0				0	0	0	0	0	0
23:00	7423	124	82	190	76	1464.6	0	+3.3	0	-0.2	58	-3.7	0 0 0			0 0 0 0				0	0	0	0	0	0
0:00	5906	99	71	139	53	1481.0	0	+3.8	0	-0.2	60	-4.3	0 0 0			0 0 0 0				0	0	0	0	0	0
1:00	5017	83	64	112	57	2145.3	0	+2.5	0	-0.1	60	-2.7	0 0 0			0 0 0 0				0	0	0	0	0	0
2:00	5161	86	67	114	52	2178.7	0	+2.3	0	-0.1	60	-2.6	0 0 0			0 0 0 0				0	0	0	0	0	0
3:00	5205	86	65	115	50	1784.5	0	+3.2	0	-0.1	60	-3.4	0 0 0			0 0 0 0				0	0	0	0	0	0
4:00	5360	89	60	125	48	1531.6	0	+3.6	0	0.0	60	-3.8	0 0 0			0 0 0 0				0	0	0	0	0	0
5:00	5375	89	61	127	50	1614.5	0	+3.2	0	0.0	60	-3.4	0 0 0			0 0 0 0				0	0	0	0	0	0
6:00	5267	88	60	129	57	2155.3	0	+3.2	0	0.0	42	-3.5	0 0 0			0 0 0 0				0	0	0	0	0	0
7:00	5489	91	63	143	69	1727.8	0	+3.4	0	0.0	53	-3.5	0 0 0			0 0 0 0				0	0	0	0	0	0
8:00	7543	127	72	165	51	1316.8	0	+3.2	0	-0.2	42	-3.3	0 0 0			0 0 0 0				0	0	0	0	0	0
9:00	6769	113	82	150	43	1297.6	0	+3.3	0	-0.1	55	-3.6	0 0 0			0 0 0 0				0	0	0	0	0	0
10:00	5466	112	40	156	49	1716.7	0	+3.0	0	-0.3	0	-3.6	0 0 0			0 0 0 0				8	0	0	0	0	1
Totals	150073	105	40	190	94	1767.3	0	+4.1	0	-0.5	1184	-4.3	0 0 0			0 0 0 0				8	0	0	0	0	1

Figure 14.4 Summary table with the heart rate, HRV, ST segment modifications, PVCs, PACs and pauses. The 8 pauses with a duration of > 2.5 seconds were detected at the end of monitoring at 10:00.

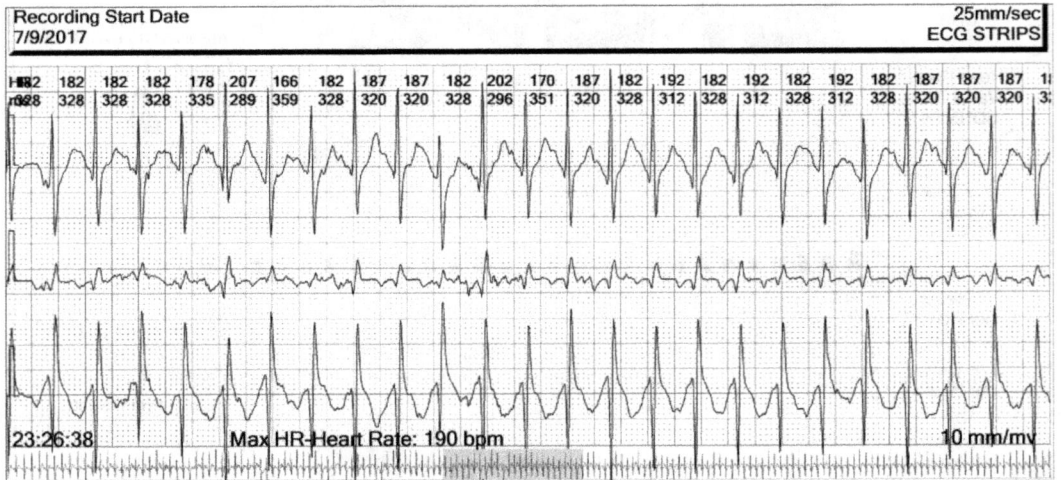

Figure 14.5 Maximum heart rate recorded during monitoring. Sinus rhythm 190 bpm.

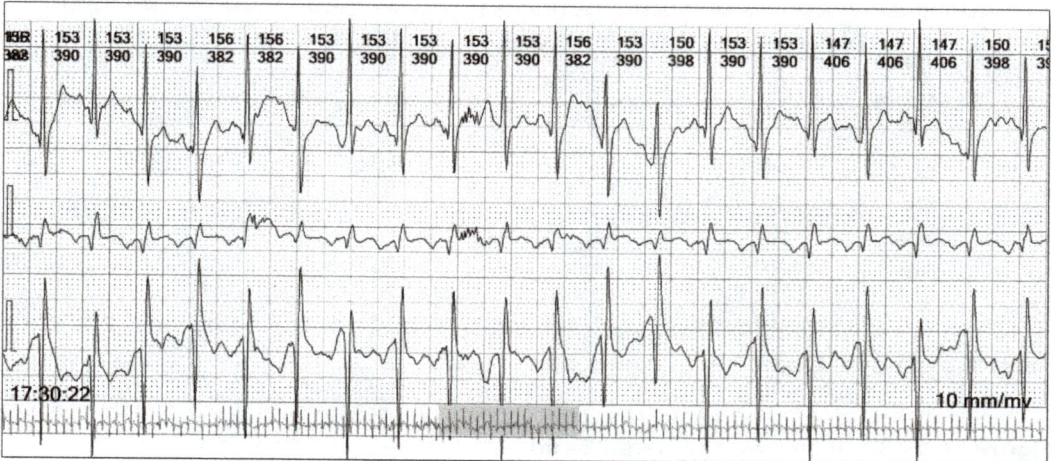

Figure 14.6 Sinus rhythm 153 bpm.

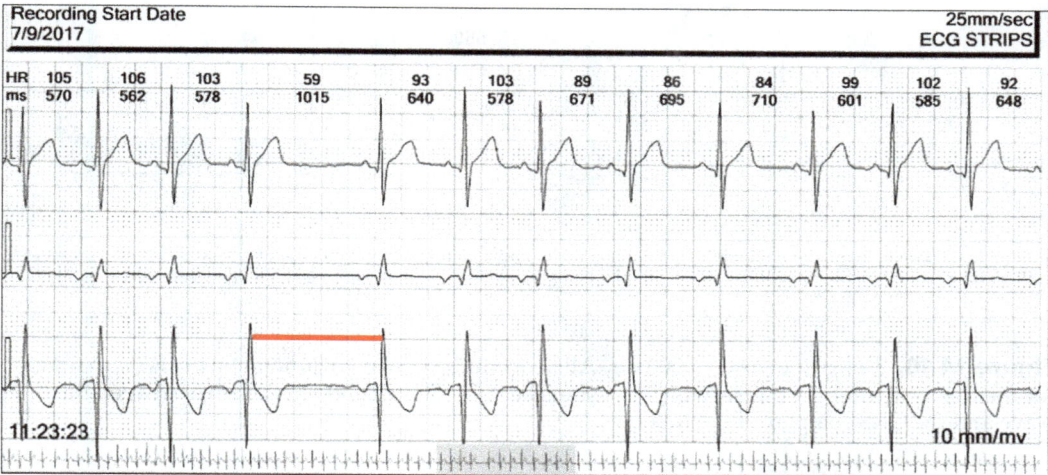

Figure 14.7 Non-significant sinus pause of 1015 ms.

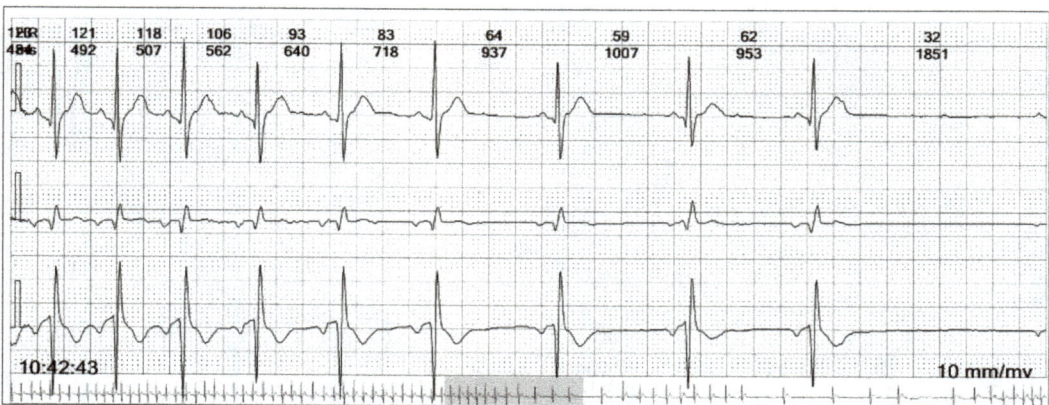

Figure 14.8 Longer sinus pause of 1851 ms.

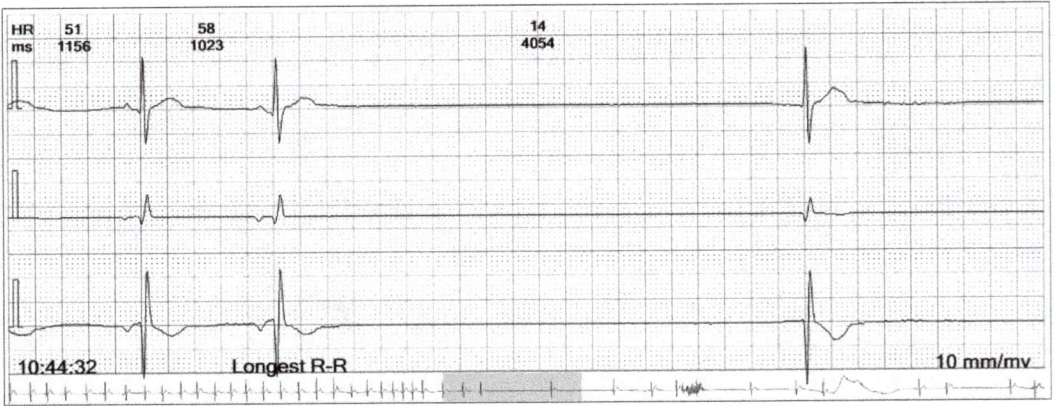

Figure 14.9 Significant sinus pause of 4054 ms.

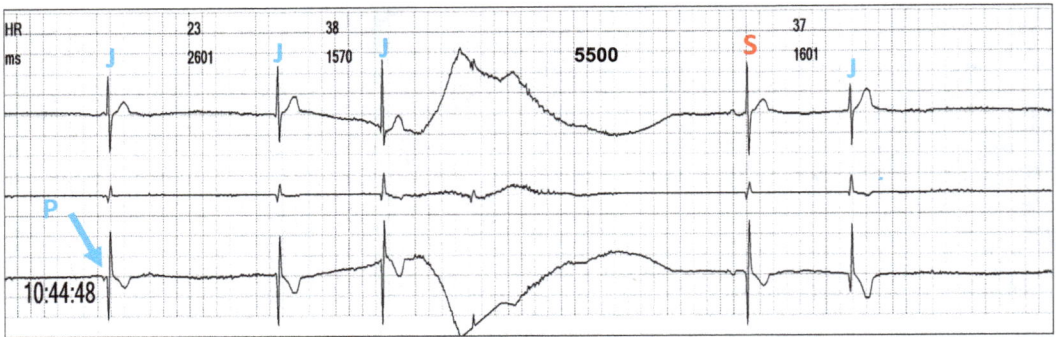

Figure 14.10 Longest pause of 5500 ms. All beats in the image are junctional beats (J), except for the first beat after the pause, which is a sinus beat (S). There is no relationship between the P wave and the QRS complex of the first beat.

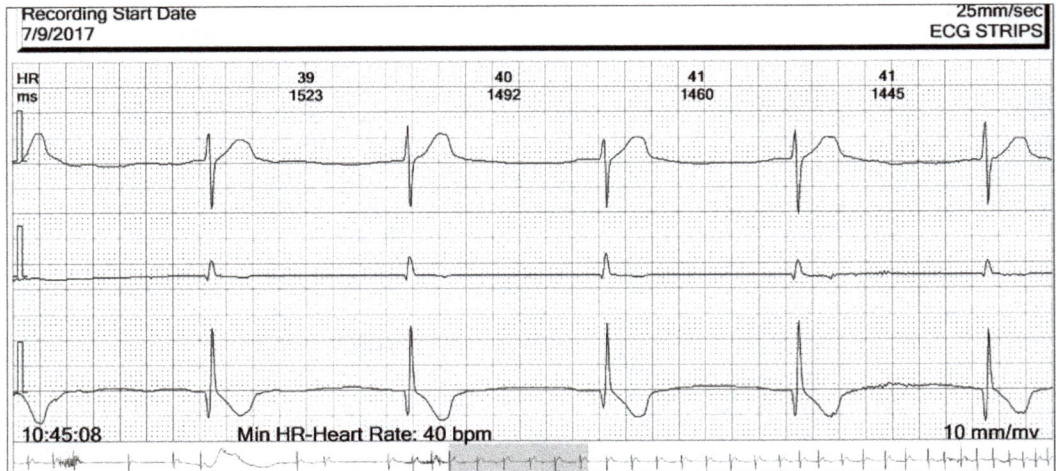

Figure 14.11 Junctional rhythm 40 bpm.

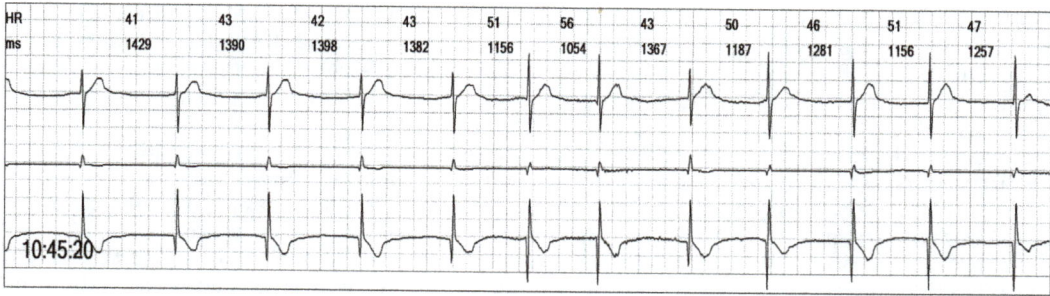

Figure 14.12 Junctional rhythm 45 bpm, different paper speed.

HOLTER SUMMARY

Accelerated idioventricular rhythm was detected during Holter monitoring with a heart rate lower than the sinus rate. The arrhythmia had wide QRS complexes, suggesting a ventricular origin and the P waves were dissociated from the QRS complexes.

DISCUSSION

Sinus node dysfunction manifests when the atrial rate is inadequate to meet physiological cardiac output, leading to clinical symptoms and a diagnosis of sick sinus syndrome. In pediatric patients, sinus node dysfunction, whether symptomatic or asymptomatic, is very rare and typically associated with elevated vagal tone or structural heart disease. Pauses of up to 24 seconds have been documented in children experiencing breath-holding spells.

Sick sinus syndrome includes the following manifestations:

1. Sinus bradycardia. The sinus node generates slow rate beats.

2. Sinus arrest. Sinus node makes a pause and then continues its activity.

3. Sinoatrial exit block is very rare in children. Conduction from the sinus node to the atria is delayed or blocked, resulting in pauses or missed beats.

4. Chronotropic incompetence. It is the main manifestation of sinus node disease in children with congenital heart disease. The heart rate is normal at rest but fails to rise sufficiently with physical exertion.

5. Tachycardia–bradycardia syndrome. The heart rate exhibits irregular fluctuations between slow and rapid impulses, frequently accompanied by prolonged pauses between beats.

Congenital forms of sinus node dysfunction have been documented in pediatric populations, related to several ion channels, ion channel regulatory subunits, and structural proteins.

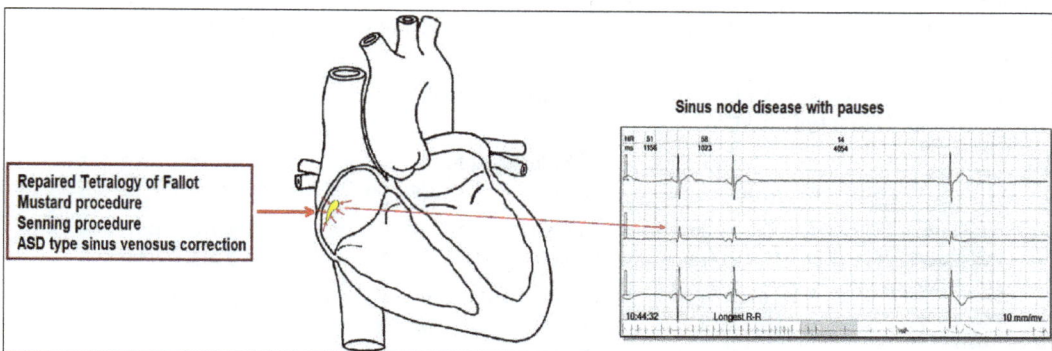

Figure 14.13 If surgery on the right atrium damages the sinus node, sick sinus syndrome can result, possibly manifesting as sinus pauses.

Sick sinus syndrome in children is often due to scar-like damage of the sinus node, especially in heart surgery on the upper chambers when the superior right atrium is affected: atrial septal defect correction for type sinus venosus, transposition of great vessels (after Mustard or Senning operations), Tetralogy of Fallot. Furthermore, injury of the arterial supply to sinus node can be incriminated for sinus dysfunction.

Sinus node dysfunction is commonly reported as a secondary phenomenon in children. In premature newborns, it is prevalent as a reaction to apnea. Prolonged sinus pauses without any escape rhythm is also observed in newborns and young children after reflex asystolic syncope. In older children, it may indicate increased vagal tone, sometimes followed by syncope.

No threshold exists for the duration of sinus pauses in an asymptomatic children, and the ACC/AHA/NASPE guidelines for pacemaker implantation in children with sinus pauses or bradycardia rely exclusively on the presence of symptomatology. Pacemaker implantation is the definitive treatment in the case of symptoms. If the atrioventricular conduction is normal and the sinus node is the sole affected structure, atrial pacing would be enough. In case of AV block, a double chamber pacemaker is preferred.

BIBLIOGRAPHY

1. Beder SD, Gillette PC, Garson AJ, Porter CB, McNamara DG. Symptomatic sick sinus syndrome in children and adolescents as the only manifestation of cardiac abnormality or associated with unoperated congenital heart disease. *Am J Cardiol.* 1983;51:1133–1136.

2. Marcus B, Gillette PC, Garson A Jr. Electrophysiologic evaluation of sinus node dysfunction in postoperative children and young adults utilizing combined autonomic blockade. *Clin Cardiol.* 1991 January;14(1):33–40. doi: 10.1002/clc.4960140108. PMID: 2019029.

3. Dahlqvist JA, Wiklund U, Karlsson M, Hanséus K, Strömvall-Larsson E, Nygren A, Eliasson H, Rydberg A. Sinus node dysfunction in patients with Fontan circulation: Could heart rate variability be a predictor for pacemaker implantation? *Pediatr Cardiol.* 2019 April;40(4):685–693. doi: 10.1007/s00246-019-02092-5. Epub 2019 March 27. PMID: 30918992; PMCID: PMC6451711.

4. Ector H, Bourgois J, Verlinden M, Hermans L, Vanden Eynde E, Fagard R, De Geest H. Bradycardia, ventricular pauses, syncope, and sports. *Lancet.* 1984;2:591–594.

5. Nagashima M, Matsushima M, Ogawa A, Ohsuga A, Kaneko T, Yazaki T, Okajima M. Cardiac arrhythmias in healthy children revealed by 24-hour ambulatory ECG monitoring. *Pediatr Cardiol.* 1987;8:103–108.

6. Gregoratos G, Abrams J, Epstein AE, et al. and Committee. ACC/AHA/NASPE guideline update for implantation of cardiac pacemakers and antiarrhythmia devices: Summary article. A report of the American College of Cardiology/American Heart Association Task Force on Practice Guidelines (ACC/AHA/NASPE Committee to Update the 1998 Pacemaker Guidelines). *J Cardiovasc Electrophys.* 2002;13:1183–1199.

7. Molgaard H, Sorensen KE, Bjerregaard P. Minimal heart rates and longest pauses in healthy adult subjects on two occasions eight years apart. *Eur Heart J.* 1989;10:758–764.

8. Kelly AM, Porter CJ, McGoon MD, Espinosa RE, Osborn MJ, Hayes DL. Breath-holding spells associated with significant bradycardia: Successful treatment with permanent pacemaker implantation. *Pediatrics.* 2001;108:698–702.

9. Mairesse GH, Marchand B. Prolonged asymptomatic sinus pause indicated by implantable loop recording. *Heart.* 2003;89:244.

10. Madan N, Levine M, Pourmoghadam K, Sokoloski M. Severe sinus bradycardia in a patient with Rett syndrome: A new cause for a pause? *Pediatr Cardiol.* 2004;25:53–55.

11. Anderson JB, Benson DW. Genetics of sick sinus syndrome. *Card Electrophysiol Clin.* 2010 Dec 1;2(4):499–507. doi: 10.1016/j.ccep.2010.09.001. PMID: 21499520; PMCID: PMC3076695.

12. Semelka M, Gera J, Usman S. Sick sinus syndrome: A review. *Am Fam Physician.* 2013 May 15;87(10):691–696. PMID: 23939447.

13. Tseng JJ, Lin MC. Congenital sick sinus syndrome: Prenatal diagnosis and postnatal follow-up. *Taiwan J Obstet Gynecol.* 2017 Aug.;56(4):573–575. doi: 10.1016/j.tjog.2016.09.011. PMID: 28805625.

14. Zheng M, Erhardt S, Cao Y, Wang J. Emerging signaling regulation of sinoatrial node dysfunction. *Curr Cardiol Rep.* 2023 Jul.;25(7):621–630. doi: 10.1007/s11886-023-01885-8. Epub 2023 May 25. PMID: 37227579; PMCID: PMC11418806.

15. Bakalli A, Jashari I, Krasniqi X, Spahiu L. A case of successfully implanted dual chamber pacemaker in a young patient with dextrocardia and sick sinus syndrome. *Clin Med Insights Case Rep.* 2021 Jul. 2;14:11795476211017733. doi: 10.1177/11795476211017733. PMID: 34276232; PMCID: PMC8255552.

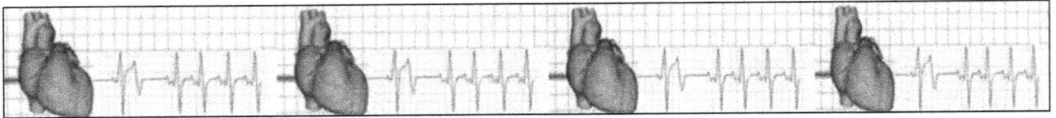

Case 15 Multifocal Premature Ventricular Contractions in a Complex CHD Patient

Cristina Filip and Maria-Evelyn Kecskes

CLINICAL HISTORY

A 9-year-old patient who underwent surgery during the first year of life for pulmonary atresia with ventricular septal defect and major aorto-pulmonary collateral suffered complications from a ruptured right ventricular pseudoaneurysm and presented at her annual check-up. During the echocardiography she presents multiple premature ventricular contractions(PVCs) and an ECG with multifocal PVCs (left bundle branch block(LBBB) and right bundle branch block(RBBB) like morphology). The findings prompted a 24 hour continuous ECG monitoring and introduction of beta blocker therapy with Metoprolol. She has a long-standing right ventricular dysfunction, large ventricular septal defect(VSD), right ventricle-pulmonary artery(RV-PA) conduit and occlusion of the left pulmonary branch; there is no history of syncope.

Concluzie

Ritm cardiac		
Total bătăi	90 219	(0% paced)
HR max / min	**129 / 58 bpm**	
Media HR	**Ø 82 bpm**	
HR Max / Min Sinus	129 / 58 bpm	
Media HR (Treaz/Adormit)	84 / 79 bpm	
Index circadian	1.06	
Tahicardie / Bradicardie	- % / 87 %	

Pauze		
RR Max	**1 520 ms**	
Pauze (>2000ms)	0	

Fibrilaţie atrială / Flutter atrial		
Total AF	-	
AF HR Max	0 bpm	
Cel mai lung AF	-	

Bradicardie		
Cea mai mică	Ø 72 bpm	05:23:16
Cea mai mare	Ø 72 bpm	05:23:16

ST		
St ridicare max	-	
ST depresurizare max	-	

Ectopie ventriculară		
V Total	24296	(27%)
V / Ora Max	2 300	pe oră
Episoade Tahicardie V		-
Cea mai rapidă Tahicardie V		-
V Cea mai lungă secvenţă	Ø 114 bpm	1 sec
Triplete / Execută	35	Σ 105 bătăi
Cuplete	663	Σ 1326 bătăi
Bigeminism	5852	Σ 16993 bătăi
Trigeminism	3885	Σ 11145 bătăi

Ectopie supraventriculară		
S Tot	101	(< 1%)
Episoade Tahicardie SV		-
Cea mai rapidă Tahicardie SV		-
S Cea mai lungă secvenţă		-
Triplete / Execută	0	Σ 0 bătăi
Cuplete	0	Σ 0 bătăi

Figure 15.1   The Holter summary reveals a heart rate between 58 and 129 bpm and a high number of PVCs: 27%/24 hours.

DOI: 10.1201/9781003545040-15

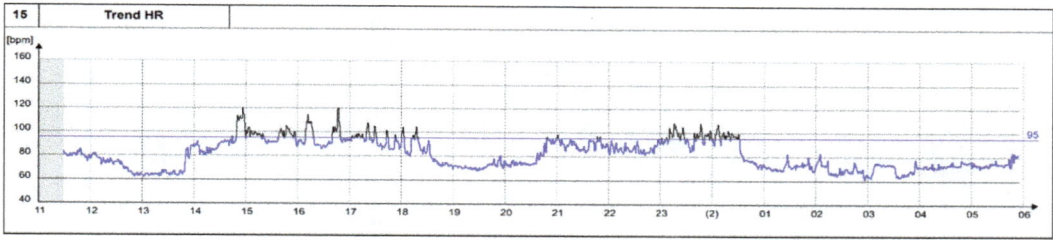

Figure 15.2   The Heart rate Chart shows the mean heart rate during the 24 hours monitoring.

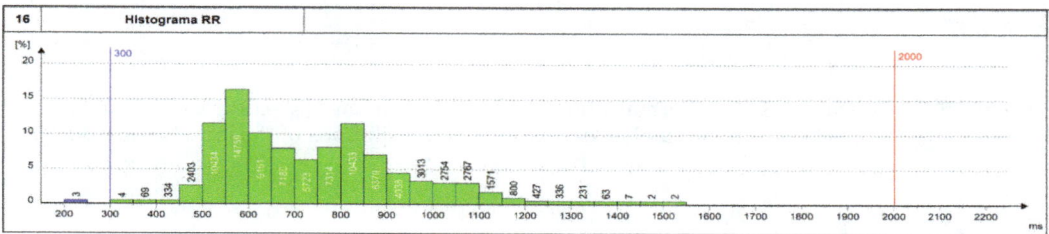

Figure 15.3   RR histogram shows 3categories of values: with blue short RR intervals, with light green normal RR intervals and with red long RR intervals.

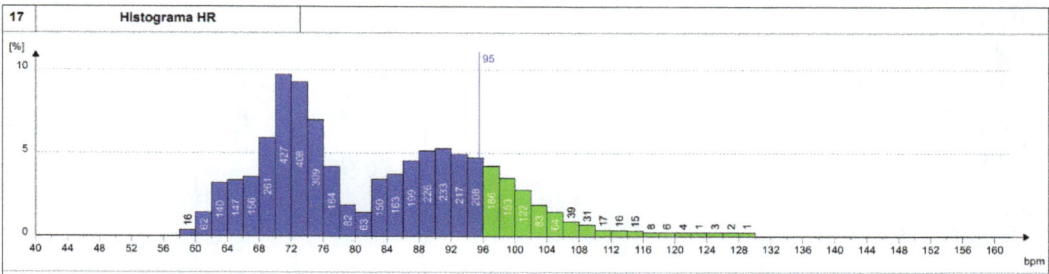

Figure 15.4   The HR Histogram shows the heart rates during the 24 hours monitoring. By establishing a minimum threshold of 58 bpm and a maximum threshold of 129 bpm, two distinct groups of values can be identified and distinguished using two different colors: blue for lower rates, light green for higher rates.

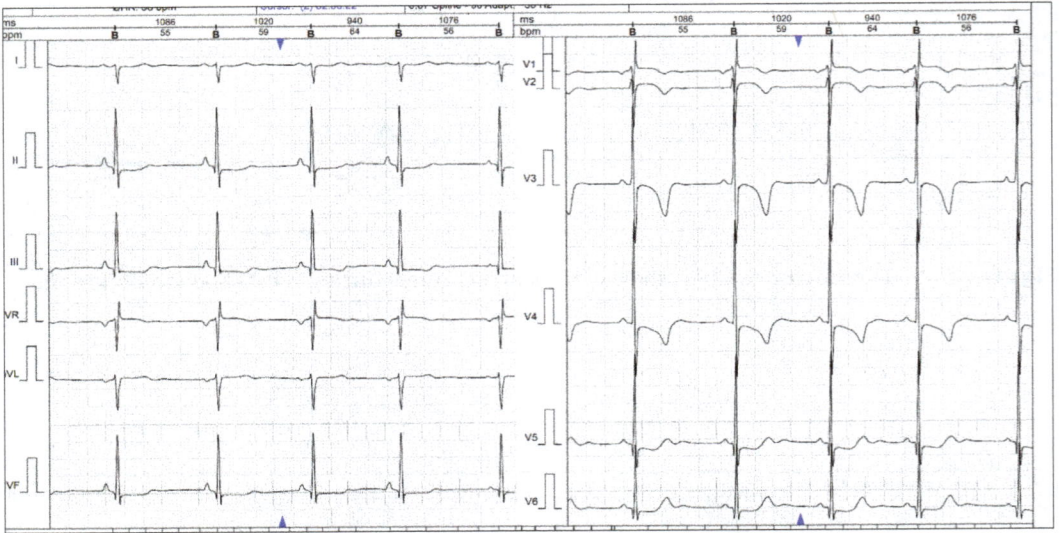

Figure 15.5 This image shows normal sinus rhythm with narrow QRS complexes, heart rate 58 bpm. Negative T waves in precordial leads are due to modifications of the left ventricle due to VSD.

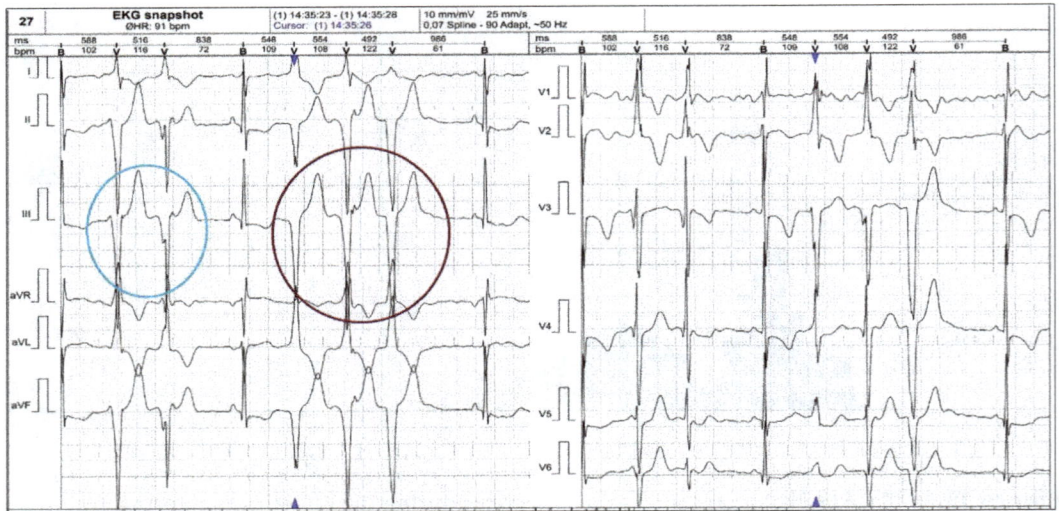

Figure 15.6 This image shows PVCs with atypical right bundle branch block pattern (Couplets – blue, Triplets – red).

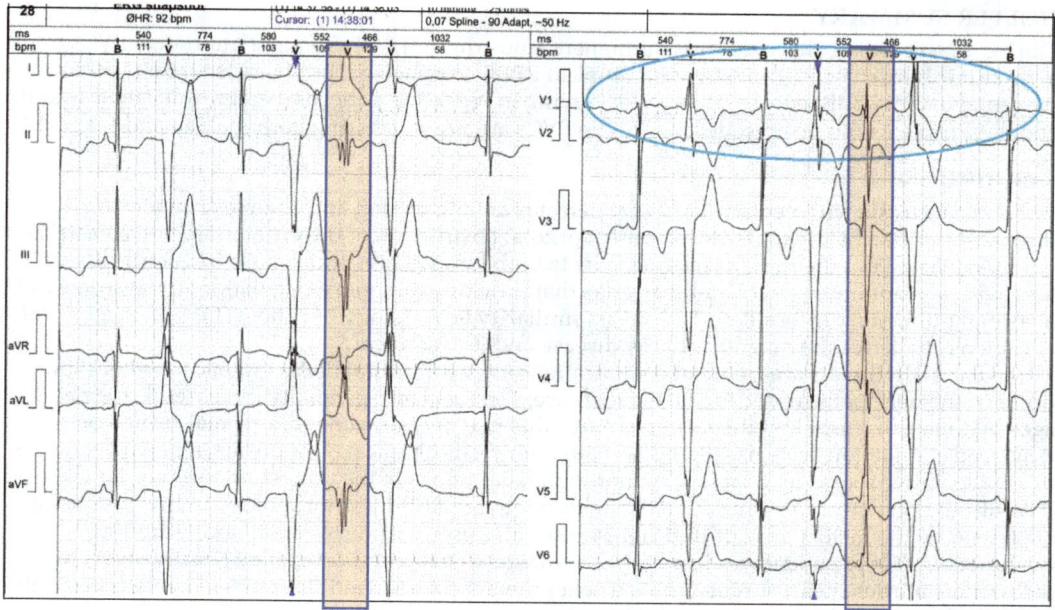

Figure 15.7 This image shows PVCs and fusion beats marked with a red square.

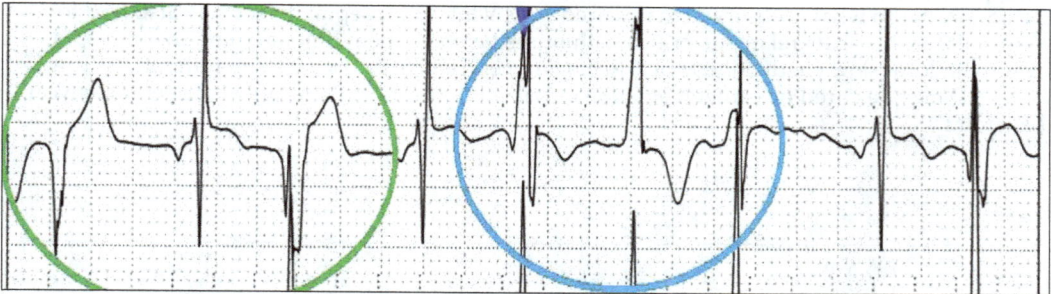

Figure 15.8 This image shows PVCs of two different morphologies in leads V1 (LBBB like – green, RBBB like – blue) organized in repeating patterns of bigeminy and couplet.

HOLTER SUMMARY

During the recording she maintains permanent sinus rhythm with frequent multifocal PVCs (high arrhythmic burden ~ 27%), mostly with atypical RBBB morphology, but there is also a significant percentage with LBBB like morphology, occurring in repeating patterns: bigeminy/trigeminy and couplets/triplets with no episodes of VT. The PVCs are present during both the day and the night.

DISCUSSION

Pulmonary atresia with ventricular septal defect is an uncommon and complex congenital heart disease described by the underdevelopment or total obstruction of the pulmonary valve, restricting blood flow from the right heart chambers to both lungs. This syndrome is frequently associated with aortopulmonary collateral arteries that provide pulmonary circulation in the absence of a normal pulmonary artery flow. Despite its similarity to Tetralogy of Fallot (TOF), its anatomical variations challenge the diagnosis of the disease and its treatment.

Cardiac arrhythmias are frequent complications after congenital heart surgery whether they occur in the perioperative setting or at a distance. The incidence generally increases as the patient ages, with multifactorial predisposing features that may include congenitally malformed or displaced conduction systems, altered hemodynamics, mechanical or hypoxic stress, and residual or postoperative sequelae. That is why thorough follow-up is of the utmost importance for these patients, the polymorphic aspect of PVCs with frequent LBBB-like morphology in this case being explained by the history of ruptured right ventricular pseudoaneurysm and long-standing dysfunction. As the patient was in a high-risk category (structural congenital heart disease, high arrhythmic burden, heart surgery), beta blocker therapy was started (Metoprolol being commonly used). If there is no therapeutic or suboptimal answer to beta-blocker therapy an antiarrhythmic agent can be used (Amiodarone being the preferred agent in case of systolic disfunction). Catheter ablation can be used in selected cases.

The reported incidence of ventricular tachycardia in children with pulmonary atresia and ventricular septal defect is lower than that of TOF. Although this malformation is not as complex as the TOF, surgery results in a compromised muscular tissue between the pulmonary and tricuspid valves, which could serve as a slowly conducting critical isthmus for ventricular tachycardia, similar to what is observed in repaired TOF. Ventricular septal defect may also lead to ventricular tachycardia related to critical isthmuses between the pulmonary and the tricuspid valve with local slow conduction zones. Reentrant ventricular tachycardias in pulmonary atresia with VSD may be cured by catheter ablation of critical parts of the reentrant ventricular tachycardia circuit.

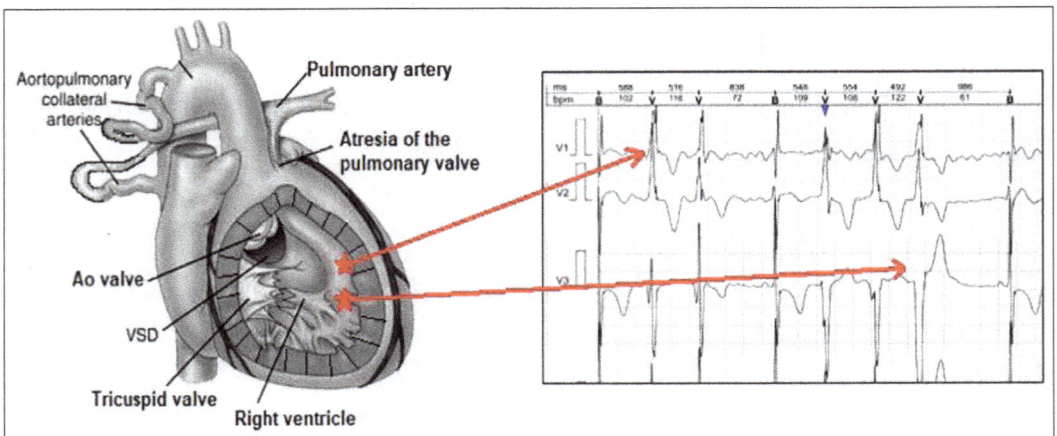

Figure 15.9 In pulmonary atresia with ventricular septal defect a diseased right and left ventricle may lead to multiple abnormal foci of automatism. The ECG printout shows PVCs with an RBBB-like morphology.

BIBLIOGRAPHY

1. Silvetti MS, Colonna D, Gabbarini F, Porcedda G, Rimini A, D'Onofrio A, Leoni L. New guidelines of pediatric cardiac implantable electronic devices: What is changing in clinical practice? *J Cardiovasc Dev Dis.* 2024;11:99.

2. Khairy P, Balaji S. Cardiac arrhythmias in congenital heart diseases. *Indian Pacing Electrophysiol J.* 2009 Nov 1;9(6):299–317. PMID: 19898654; PMCID: PMC2766579.

3. Cohle SD, et al. Sudden death due to ventricular septal defect. *Pediatr Dev Pathol.* 1999;2:32.

4. Nollert G, et al. Long-term survival in patients with repair of tetralogy of Fallot: 36-year follow-up of 490 survivors of the first year after surgical repair. *J Am Coll Cardiol.* 1997;30:1374.

5. Gillette PC, et al. Sudden cardiac death in the pediatric population. *Circulation.* 1992;85(1 Suppl):I64.

6. Zeppenfeld K, et al. Catheter ablation of ventricular tachycardia after repair of congenital heart disease: Electroanatomic identification of the critical right ventricular isthmus. *Circulation.* 2007;116:2241.

7. Anderson RH, Ho SY. The disposition of the conduction tissues in congenitally malformed hearts with reference to their embryological development. *J Perinat Med.* 1991;19(Suppl 1):201–206.

8. Brugada J, Blom N, Sarquella-Brugada G, Blomstrom-Lundqvist C, Deanfield J, Janousek J, European Heart Rhythm Association; Association for European Paediatric and Congenital Cardiology, et al. Pharmacological and nonpharmacological therapy for arrhythmias in the pediatric population: EHRA and AEPC-Arrhythmia Working Group joint consensus statement. *Europace.* 2013; 15:1337–1382.

9. Khairy P. Ventricular arrhythmias and sudden cardiac death in adults with congenital heart disease. *Heart.* 2016;102:1703–1709.

10. Priori SG, Blomström-Lundqvist C, Mazzanti A, Blom N, Borggrefe M, Camm J et al. ESC Guidelines for the management of patients with ventricular arrhythmias and the prevention of sudden cardiac death. *Europace.* 2015;17:1601–1687.

11. Backer CL, Tsao S, Deal B, Mavroudis C. Maze procedure in single ventricle patients. *Semin Thorac Cardiovasc Surg Pediatr Card Surg Annu.* 2008;11:44–48.

12. Khairy P, Landzberg MJ, Gatzoulis MA, Lucron H, Lambert J, Marcon F et al. Value of programmed ventricular stimulation after tetralogy of Fallot repair: a multicenter study. *Circulation.* 2004;109:1994–2000.

13. Teuwen CP, Ramdjan TTTK, Götte M, Brundel BJJM, Evertz R, Vriend JWJ et al. Non-sustained ventricular tachycardia in patients with congenital heart disease: an important sign? *Int J Cardiol.* 2016;206:158–163.

14. Bessière F, Waldmann V, Combes N, Metton O, Dib N, Mondésert B, O'Leary E, De Witt E, Carreon CK, Sanders SP, Moore JP, Triedman J, Khairy P. Ventricular Arrhythmias in Adults with Congenital Heart Disease, Part II: JACC State-of-the-Art Review. *J Am Coll Cardiol.* 2023 Sep 12;82(11):1121–1130. doi: 10.1016/j.jacc.2023.06.036. PMID: 37673513.

15. Ntiloudi D, Rammos S, Karakosta M, Kalesi A, Kasinos N, Giannakoulas G. Arrhythmias in patients with congenital heart disease: An ongoing morbidity. *J Clin Med.* 2023 Nov 10;12(22):7020. doi: 10.3390/jcm12227020. PMID: 38002634; PMCID: PMC10672721.

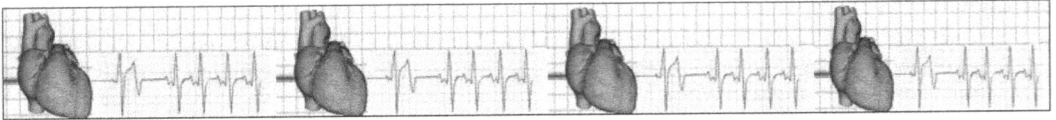

Case 16 Congenital Junctional Ectopic Tachycardia

Marie Bartos

CLINICAL CASE

A 2-year-old child was diagnosed with congenital junctional ectopic tachycardia shortly after birth. The boy presented no symptoms and underwent routine Holter monitoring. His usual heart rate was 130 bpm. Following his most recent Holter monitoring, the Sotalol dosage increased to reduce the arrhythmia burden. His last Holter is presented below.

Allmän	
Slag	192506
Normalslag	192504 (100,00%)
Ventrikelslag	2 (0,00%)
SVES	0 (-)
PM-slag	0 (0,00%)
BBB (Grenblock)	0 (0,00%)
Artefakter%	0,01%

Hjärtfrekvenser	
Min. HR	112 @ 00:45:56
Max. HR	159 @ 13:41:18
Medel HF	134
Medel HF Dag	137
Medel HF Natt	130
Paus	0
Längsta Paus	--- @ ---

Händelser	
V extraslag	2 (-)
Kopplade VES	Mono: 0 Poly: 0
VES i bigemini	0
Triplet (3 VES i rad)	0
Ideoventrikulär rytm	0
VT < 30 sek	0
VT > 30 sek	0
Längsta V	--- (definieras som längd) med --- @ ---
AV Block I	0
AV Block II typ 1	0
AV Block II typ 2	0
AV Block III	0

PSVT	0
Bradykardi	0
Längsta bradykardi	--- (definieras som HF) med --- @ ---

Figure 16.1 The summary page shows a mean heart rate of 134 bpm, suggesting an arrhythmia with high rate during monitoring. The number of PVCs is low during the entire Holter period.

DOI: 10.1201/9781003545040-16

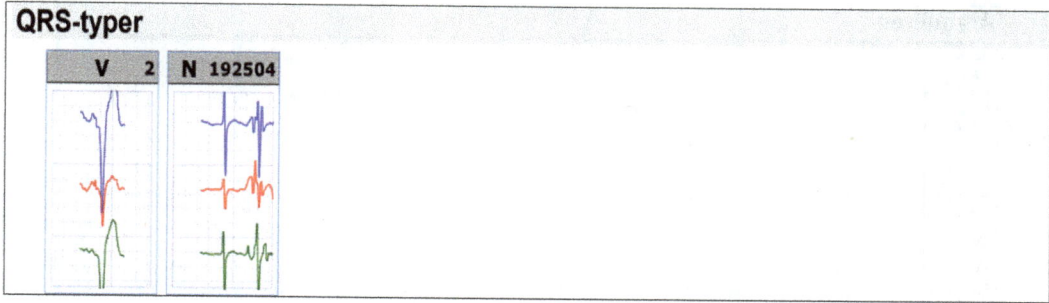

Figure 16.2 This figure displays the templates used by the software for beat classification: there were 2 PVCs and 192,504 regular beats. This number is excessively elevated, indicating a rapid arrhythmia.

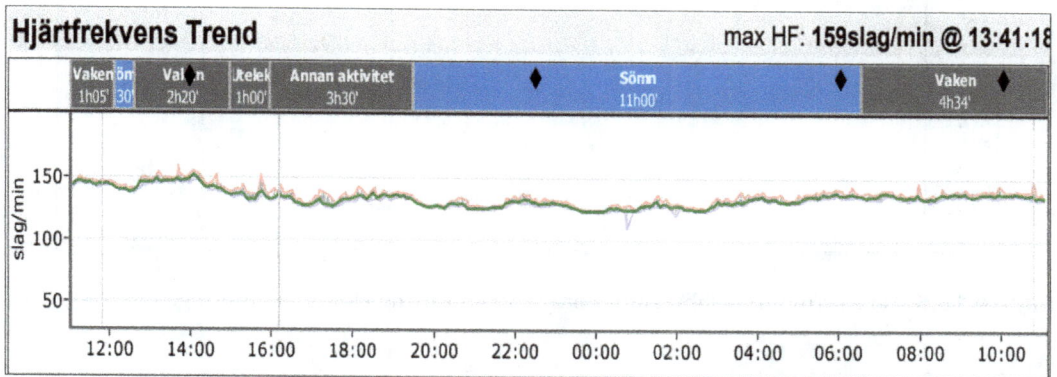

Figure 16.3 The heart rate histogram shows increased rate from 11:00 to 11:00 the next day, suggesting a fast arrhythmia during the monitoring period.

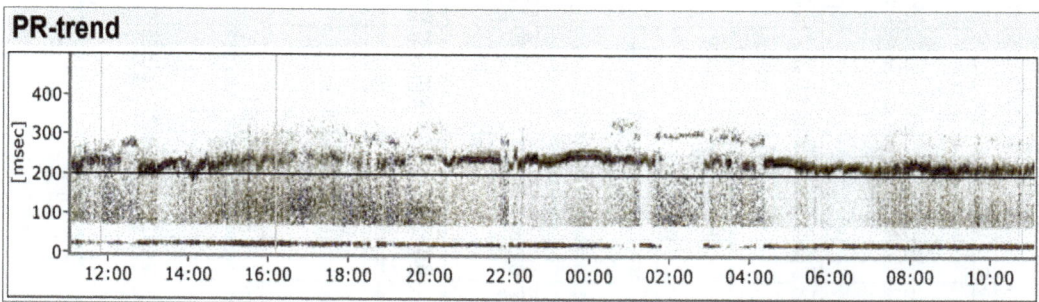

Figure 16.4 This PR trend from 11:00 to 11:00 the next day.

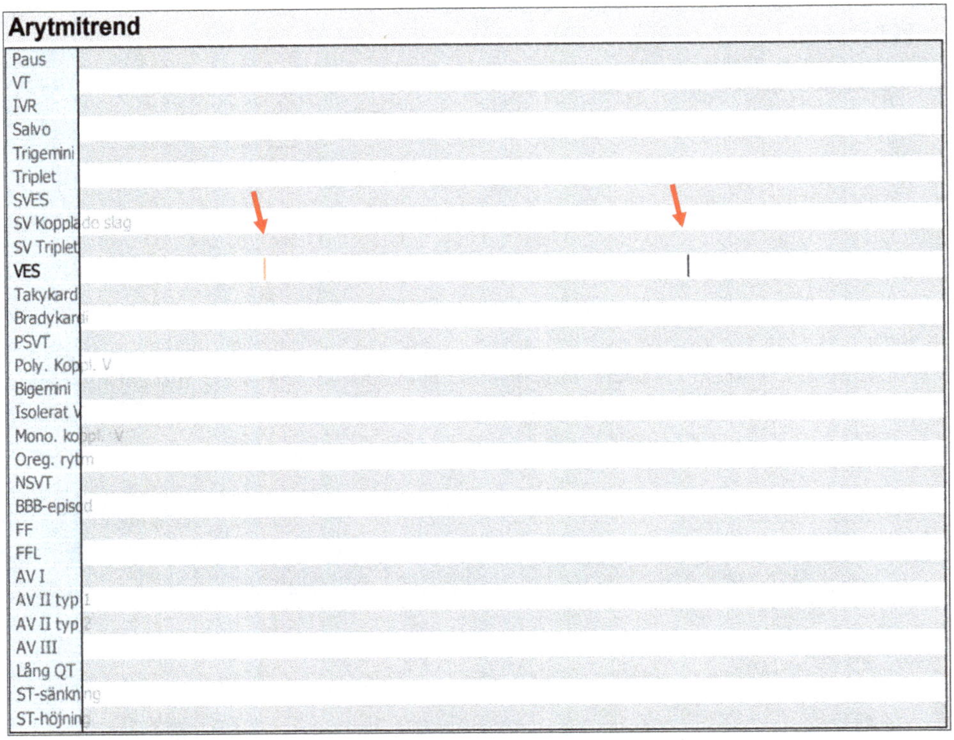

Arytmitrend

Paus
VT
IVR
Salvo
Trigemini
Triplet
SVES
SV Kopplade slag
SV Triplet
VES
Takykard
Bradykard
PSVT
Poly. Koppl. V
Bigemini
Isolerat V
Mono. koppl. V
Oreg. rytm
NSVT
BBB-episod
FF
FFL
AV I
AV II typ 1
AV II typ 2
AV III
Lång QT
ST-sänkning
ST-höjning

Figure 16.5 The arrhythmia table shows only 2 PVCs during Holter monitoring.

Händelser, sammanfattning   max HR: **159b/min @ 13:41:18**

Tid	Min HF	Medel HF	Max HF	VES	N - SVES	total N	total V	Giltighet [%]	Totalt antal slag
Fullständig reg.	112	134	159	2	192504	192504	2	100	192506
Natt	112	130	144	1	89405	89405	1	100	89406
Dag	125	137	159	1	103099	103099	1	100	103100
11:04	140	145	149		7959	7959		100	7959
12:00	136	142	149		8504	8504		100	8504
13:00	144	147	159		8829	8829		100	8829
14:00	135	143	154		8603	8603		100	8603
15:00	129	135	149		8102	8102		100	8102
16:00	125	131	142	1	7879	7879	1	100	7880
17:00	125	130	138		7786	7786		100	7786
18:00	130	135	142		8081	8081		100	8081
19:00	125	131	139		7887	7887		100	7887
20:00	124	127	133		7644	7644		100	7644
21:00	123	127	135		7602	7602		100	7602
22:00	127	130	137		7826	7826		100	7826
23:00	122	126	132		7556	7556		100	7556
00:00	112	124	129		7466	7466		100	7466
01:00	121	128	136		7671	7671		100	7671
02:00	122	126	134		7545	7545		100	7545
03:00	128	131	140	1	7888	7888	1	100	7889
04:00	129	133	139		7950	7950		100	7950
05:00	129	135	141		8128	8128		100	8128
06:00	133	136	144		8167	8167		100	8167
07:00	132	136	145		8180	8180		100	8180
08:00	131	136	142		8137	8137		100	8137
09:00	134	137	144		8231	8231		100	8231
10:00	132	137	146		8216	8216		100	8216
11:00	133	135	138		667	667		100	667

Figure 16.6 The table shows minimum heart rate, medium and maximum rate as well as the PVC burden, which is 2 PVCs/24 hours.

130

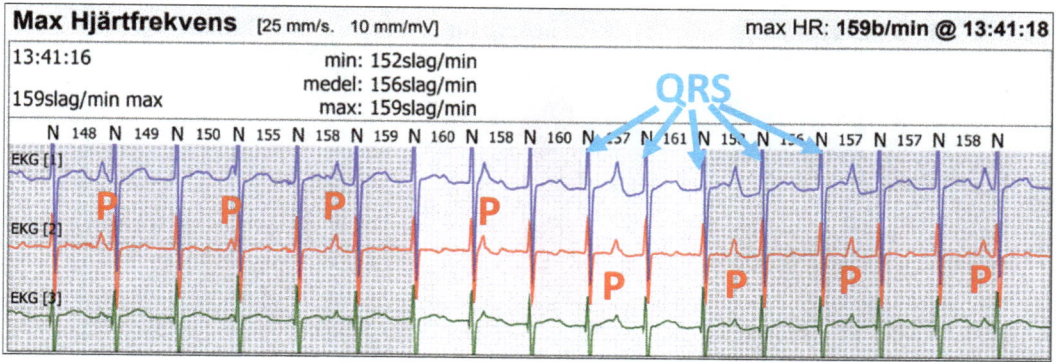

Figure 16.7 The highest rate during monitoring was 159 bpm. The ventricular rate is high (159 bpm); however, the atrial rate is low (77 bpm), suggesting a junctional ectopic tachycardia with a dissociated low rate sinus rhythm. The PP interval is also irregular.

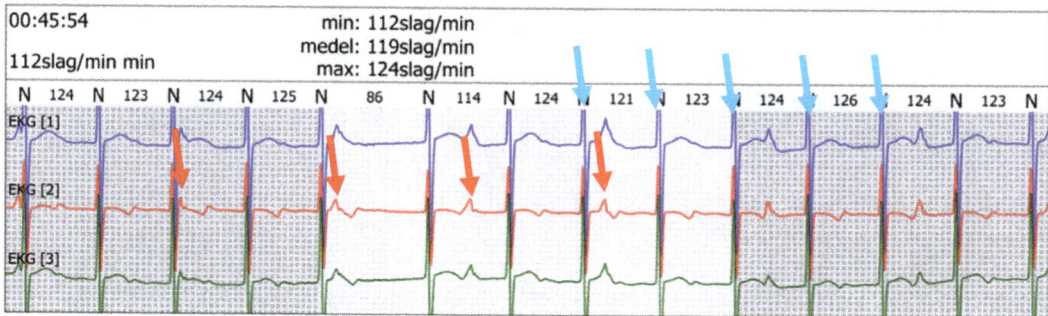

Figure 16.8 The lowest rate was 112 bpm at 00:45, during a junctional ectopic tachycardia while asleep (blue arrows) with dissociated atrial rhythm (red arrows) at 64 bpm.

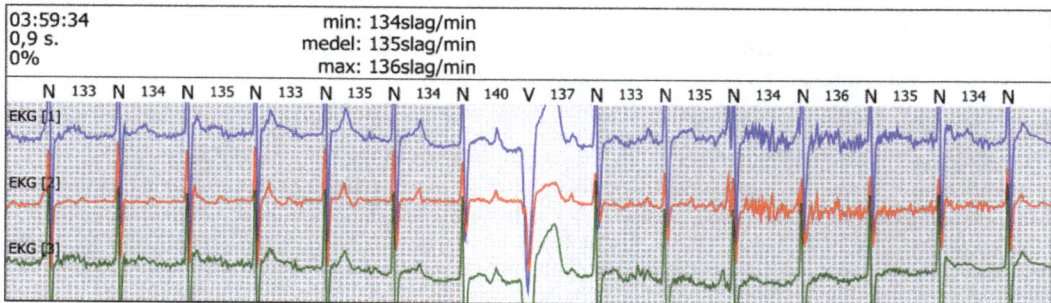

Figure 16.9 One of the 2 premature ventricular contractions.

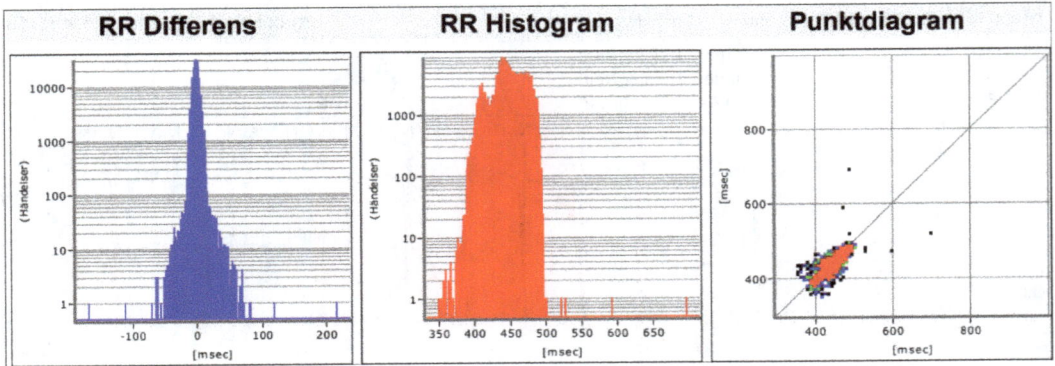

Figure 16.10 Heart rate variability charts with Poincaré graph.

HRV Statistik				validitet 100,0%
SDNN-i	SDANN-i	Circadian Index	TINN	HRV Index
4,3ms	21,1ms	1,06	101,6	6,2

	SDNN	rMSSD	pNN50
totalt	21,6	5,1	0,02
medel	4,3	5,0	0,02
median	3,8	4,6	0,00

Figure 16.11 Heart rate variability indices: SDNN index (mean of the standard deviations of all the NN intervals for each 5 min. segment of a 24 h HRV recording), SDANN index (mean of Standard Deviation of all the average NN intervals for each 5 min. segment of a 24 h HRV recording), TINN (Baseline width of the RR interval histogram).

HOLTER SUMMARY

Junctional ectopic tachycardia with atrioventricular dissociation was detected during monitoring. Junctional tachycardia was observed throughout the whole 24-hour monitoring period. Sinus node dysfunction was suggested due to irregular low-rate P waves.

DISCUSSION

The sinoatrial node is the natural cardiac pacemaker located in the upper right atrium. The atrioventricular node is a separate cardiac pacemaker located in the inferior-posterior right atrium. Junctional rhythm emerges when the electrical impulse in the heart originates from the atrioventricular node rather than the sinoatrial node. In typical circumstances, subsidiary pacemakers are inhibited by the faster impulses originating from superior sources like sinus rhythm. In JET, increased automaticity is considered the principal cause of arrhythmia. Additional processes were also involved, including triggered activity, calcium overload, and enhanced local inflammation. JET occurring after surgery and post-ablation may share an identical etiology, since RF treatments in the vicinity of Koch's triangle can induce localized micro-hemorrhages and coagulation necrosis, similar to those generated after surgical procedures or electrocauterization. Zahn et al. and Thibault et al. show, through experimental investigations, that the introduction of ice or warm water to the area of Koch's triangle near its anterior point provoked an active junctional rhythm. from the SA node.

Congenital junctional ectopic tachycardia was first described in 1975 by Professor Philippe Coumel (1935–2004). It is thought to be a congenital arrhythmia as it was noted in newborns and

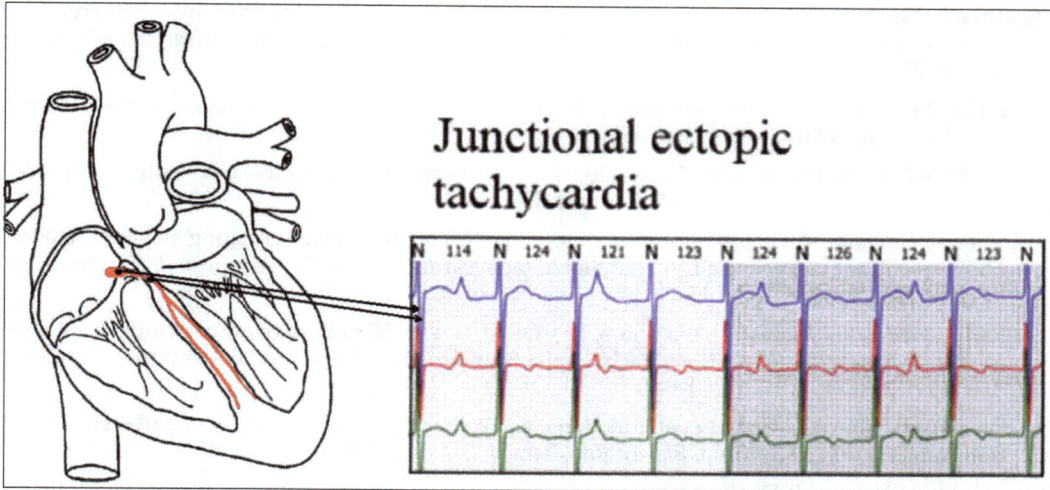

Figure 16.12 In junctional ectopic tachycardia, the arrhythmia originates from the AV node or His bundle; the QRS complexes and P waves are dissociated.

infants <6 months of age. Junctional ectopic tachycardia is often seen as an autonomic condition arising from the distal atrioventricular node or His bundle. In cases with 1:1 retrograde conduction through the fast pathway, the JET has characteristics similar to those of typical atrioventricular nodal re-entrant tachycardia.

ECG features of junctional ectopic tachycardia rhythm are: increased rate over 100 bpm, narrow QRS complexes, and no relationship between P waves and the QRS complexes. The ventricular rate usual range is 150 to 350 bpm. JET should be differentiated from typical atrioventricular node reentrant tachycardia, especially in case of retrograde 1:1 conduction to the atrium.

The electrophysiological diagnosis of JET is made based on the presence of a His bundle potential preceding ventricular depolarization, with an HV interval in normal range.

JET is a severe arrhythmia that can induce tachycardia-induced cardiomyopathy with low ejection fraction and increased risk of sudden cardiac death. This type of arrhythmia is usually resistant to antiarrhythmic drugs, and Amiodarone is frequently used to decrease the heart rate and ultimately stop the arrhythmia. The starting dose is 500 mg/m² for 1 week, continued with a maintenance dose of 250 mg/m². When Amiodarone is not effective, Sotalol can be used as an alternative. Electrical cardioversion is not effective in this type of tachycardia as the mechanism is ectopic. Catheter ablation remains an alternative to conventional antiarrhythmic drugs; however, it has a risk of damage of the conduction system with subsequent AV block.

In the case of antenatal tachycardia detected during fetal echocardiography, the treatment is made with Amiodarone or Sotalol, given to the mother in order to reduce the heart rate of the fetus.

BIBLIOGRAPHY

1. Padanilam BJ, Manfredi JA, Steinberg LA, Olson JA, Fogel RI, Prystowsky EN. Differentiating junctional tachycardia and atrioventricular node re-entry tachycardia based on response to atrial extrastimulus pacing. *J Am Coll Cardiol*, 2008; 52: 1711–1717.

2. Alasti M, Mirzaee S, Machado C, et al. Junctional ectopic tachycardia (JET). *J Arrhythm*, 2020; 36: 837–844.

3. Dar T, Turagam MK, Yarlagadda B, et al. Outcomes of junctional ectopic tachycardia ablation in adult population—A multicenter experience. *J Interv Card Electrophysiol*, 2021; 61: 19–27.

4. Liu CF, Ip JE, Markowitz SM, Lerman BB. Junctional tachycardia. *Zipes and Jalife's Cardiac Electrophysiology, From Cell to Bedside* (8th ed.), Elsevier 2022, pp. 853–860.

5. Tokuda M, Yamane T, Matsuo S, et al. Paradoxical responses to pacing maneuvers differentiating atrioventricular node reentrant tachycardia and junctional tachycardia. *Heart Vessels,* 2016; 31: 256–260.

6. Refaat MM, Scheinman M, Badhwar N. Narrow complex tachycardia: What is the mechanism? *Card Electrophysiol Clin,* 2016; 8: 67–69.

7. Di Biase L, Gianni C, Bagliani G, Padeletti L. Arrhythmias involving the atrioventricular junction. *Card Electrophysiol Clin,* 2017 Sep; 9(3): 435–452.

8. Chen H, Shehata M, Cingolani E, Chugh SS, Chen M, Wang X. Differentiating atrioventricular nodal re-entrant tachycardia from junctional tachycardia: Conflicting responses? *Circ Arrhythm Electrophysiol,* 2015; 8: 232–235.

9. Fan R, Tardos JG, Almasry I, Barbera S, Rashba EJ, Iwai S. Novel use of atrial overdrive pacing to rapidly differentiate junctional tachycardia from atrioventricular nodal reentrant tachycardia. *Heart Rhythm,* 2011; 8: 840–844.

10. Cismaru G, Simu G, Puiu M et al. Junctional ectopic tachycardia as an AVNRT catheter ablation complication in children. *Biomed Res Therapy,* 2023; 10(2): 5545–5549.

11. Sarubbi B, Vergara P, D'Alto M, Calabro R. Congenital junctional ectopic tachycardia: presentation and outcome. *Indian Pacing Electrophysiol J,* 2003; 3(3): 143–147. PMID: 16943912; PMCID: PMC1502046.

12. Coumel P, Fidelle JE, Attuel P, et al. Tachycardies focales hisiennes congenitales: etude cooperative de sept cas. *Arch Mal Coeur,* 1976; 69: 899–903.

13. Villazon E, Fouron JC, Fournier A, et al. Prenatal diagnosis of junctional ectopic tachycardia. *Pediatr Cardiol,* 2001; 22: 160–162.

14. Sarubbi B, Musto B, Ducceschi V, et al. Congenital junctional ectopic tachycardia in children and adolescents: A 20 year experience based study. *Heart,* 2002; 88: 188–190.

15. Garson W, Gillette PC. Junctional ectopic tachycardia in children: Electrocardiography, electrophysiology and pharmacological response. *Am J Cardiol,* 1979; 44: 298–302.

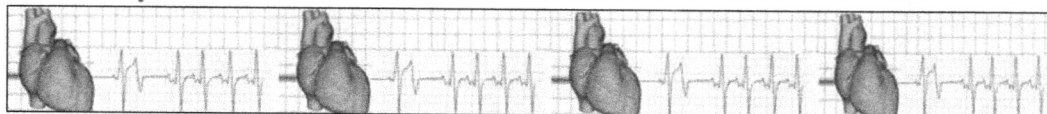

Case 17 Low Atrial Rhythm in a Newborn

Simona Cainap, Diana Jecan Toader and Roxana Rusu

CLINICAL CASE

A dystrophic premature had borderline QT interval at birth and low atrial rhythm. At 7 months of age a Holter ECG confirmed persistence of the low atrial rhythm with normal QT intervals. No congenital heart disease or anomaly of the systemic venous connection was detected in echocardiography. The Holter images are presented below.

Ritm cardiac		
Total bătăi	155 516	(0% paced)
HR max / min	**174 / 86 bpm**	
Media HR	**Ø 119 bpm**	
HR Max / Min Sinus	174 / 86 bpm	
Media HR (Treaz/Adormit)	124 / 113 bpm	
Index circadian	1,10	
Tahicardie / Bradicardie	- % / 12 %	

Pauze	
RR Max	**898 ms**
Pauze (>2000ms)	0

Fibrilaţie atrială / Flutter atrial	
Total AF	-
AF HR Max	0 bpm
Cel mai lung AF	-

Bradicardie		
Cea mai mică	Ø 99 bpm	22 sec
Cea mai mare	Ø 104 bpm	00:04:12

ST	
St ridicare max	-
ST depresurizare max	-

Ectopie ventriculară		
V Total	0	(< 1%)
V / Ora Max	0	pe oră
Episoade Tahicardie V	-	
Cea mai rapidă Tahicardie V	-	
V Cea mai lungă secvenţă	-	
Triplete / Execută	0 Σ 0 bătăi	
Cuplete	0 Σ 0 bătăi	
Bigeminism	0 Σ 0 bătăi	
Trigeminism	0 Σ 0 bătăi	

Ectopie supraventriculară		
S Tot	0	(< 1%)
Episoade Tahicardie SV	-	
Cea mai rapidă Tahicardie SV	-	
S Cea mai lungă secvenţă	-	
Triplete / Execută	0 Σ 0 bătăi	
Cuplete	0 Σ 0 bătăi	

Figure 17.1 The summary page shows a maximum heart rate of 174 bpm and a minimum rate of 86 bpm. The PVC and PAC burden are 0.

DOI: 10.1201/9781003545040-17

135

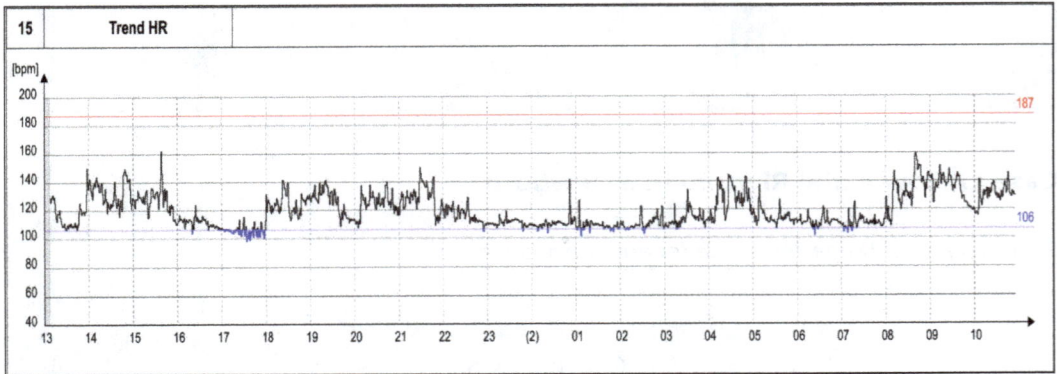

Figure 17.2   The heart rate trend shows the mean rate over 24 hours of monitoring.

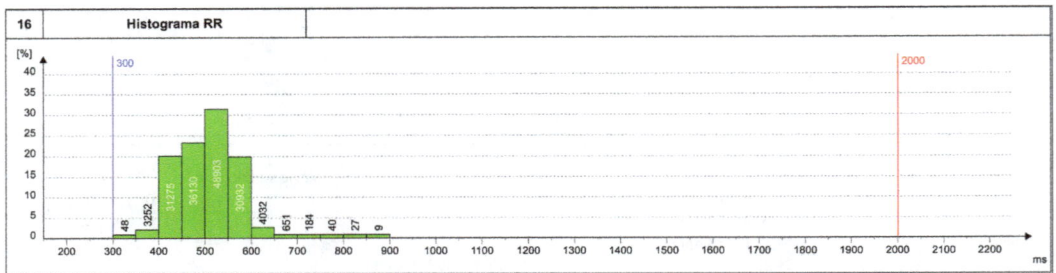

Figure 17.3   The RR histogram shows cycle length between 400 and 600 ms corresponding to normal sinus rhythm 100 to150 bpm. It never falls below 300 ms or increases above 800 ms.

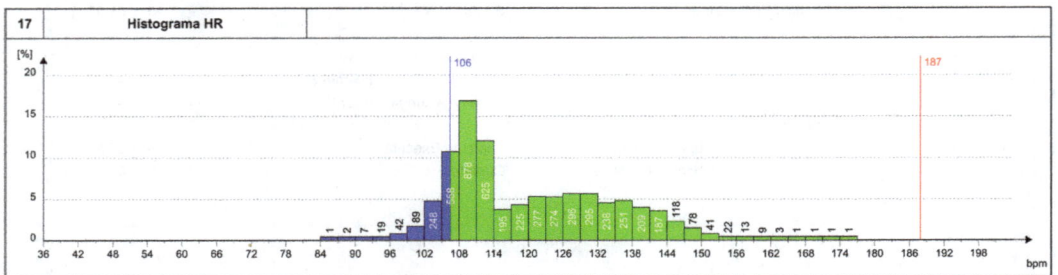

Figure 17.4   The HR histogram shows heart rates during 24 hours period of monitoring. Blue color shows rates down to 86 bpm.

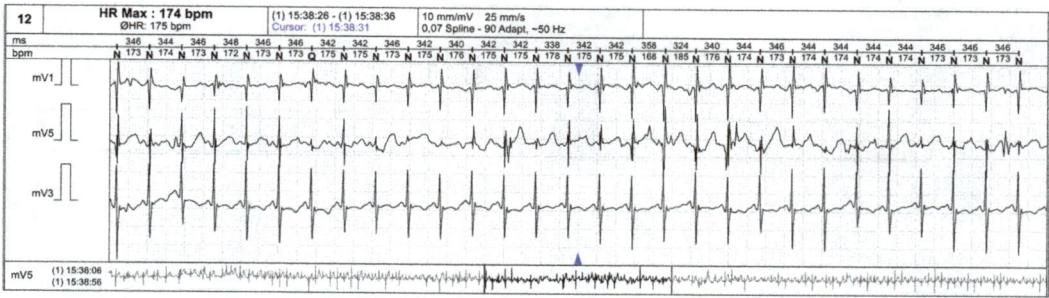

Figure 17.5 The tracing shows the maximum heart recorded which is 174 bpm during sinus rhythm.

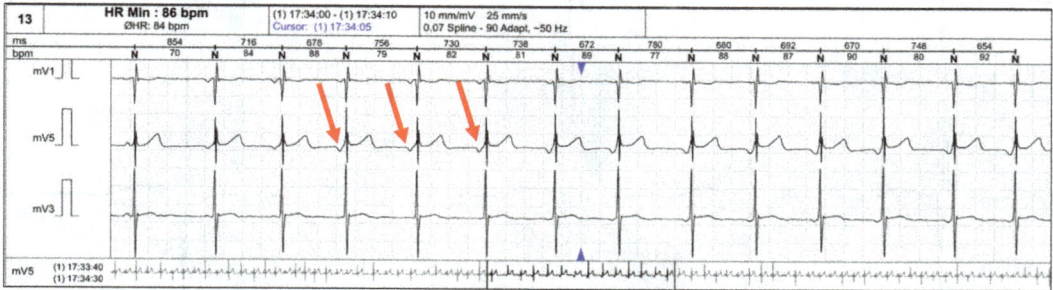

Figure 17.6 The tracing shows the minimum heart rate of 86 bpm during low atrial rhythm.

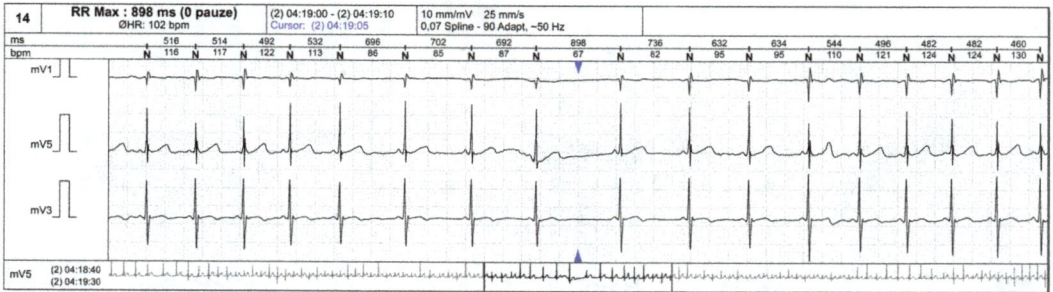

Figure 17.7 The tracing shows the maximum RR interval which is 898 ms, during sinus rhythm and respiratory arrhythmia, which is normal for a newborn.

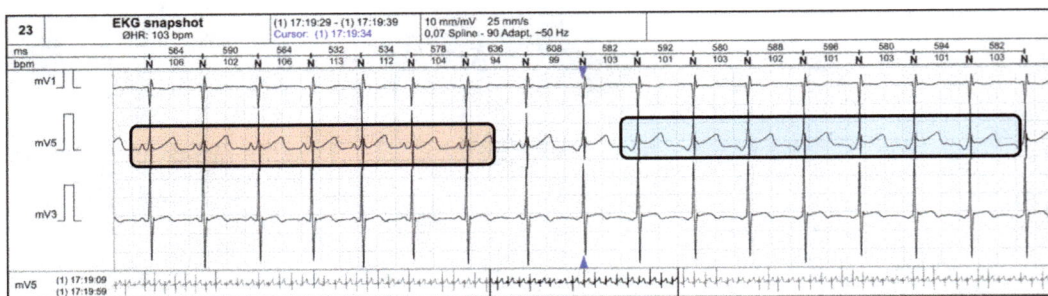

Figure 17.8 The tracing shows sinus rhythm with a rate of 113 bpm alternating with low atrial rhythm with a rate of 103 bpm.

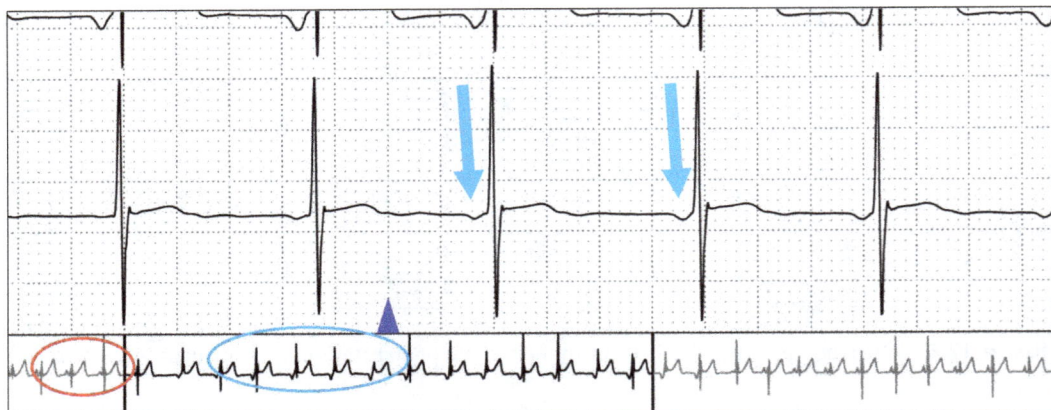

Figure 17.9 The tracing is a zoom of Figure 17.8 showing low atrial rhythm with negative P wave on channel 2 (mV5).

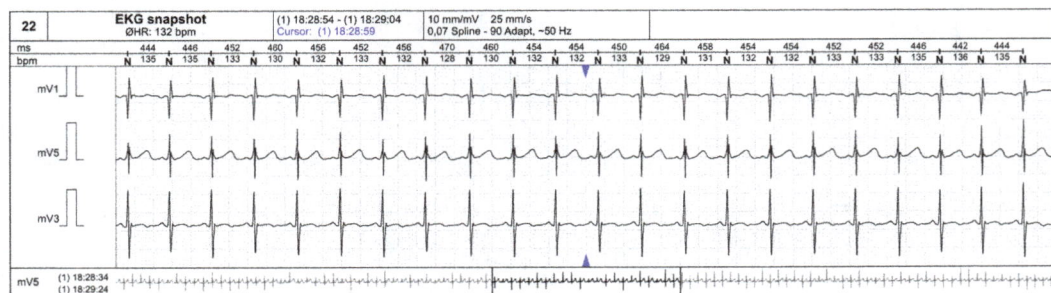

Figure 17.10 The tracing shows sinus rhythm with a rate of 132 bpm.

HOLTER SUMMARY

During 24 hours of Holter monitoring, there was sinus rhythm alternating with low atrial rhythm. There was no PAC or PVC. Low atrial rhythm manifested at a rate lower than that of sinus rhythm.

DISCUSSION

Low atrial rhythm is characterized by P waves preceding each QRS complex, with P wave inversion in leads II, III and avF, and normal or shorter PR interval.

It has been shown that the origin of this rhythm is the inferior right or left atrium, the AV node or the ostium of the coronary sinus. When pacing the ostium of the coronary sinus the obtained rhythm resembles that of low atrial rhythm, with negative P waves in inferior leads. The coronary sinus is the cardiac venous system that starts at the ostium situated in the right atrium and terminates at the origin of the great cardiac vein. The coronary sinus is an anatomical structure of particular interest to electrophysiologists, as it is a potential source of atrial arrhythmias.

Since the 1970s, the arrhythmogenic potential of the thoracic veins has been acknowledged in general. The pulmonary veins, the superior vena cava, and the coronary sinus are potential sources of atrial arrhythmias or ectopic rhythms.

Scherf et al. observed that the electrocardiogram of the low atrial rhythm exhibited a deeply inverted P wave in leads II and III, accompanied by a normal or slightly shortened PR interval. The focus of origin of this rhythm was located in the upper part of the A-V node.

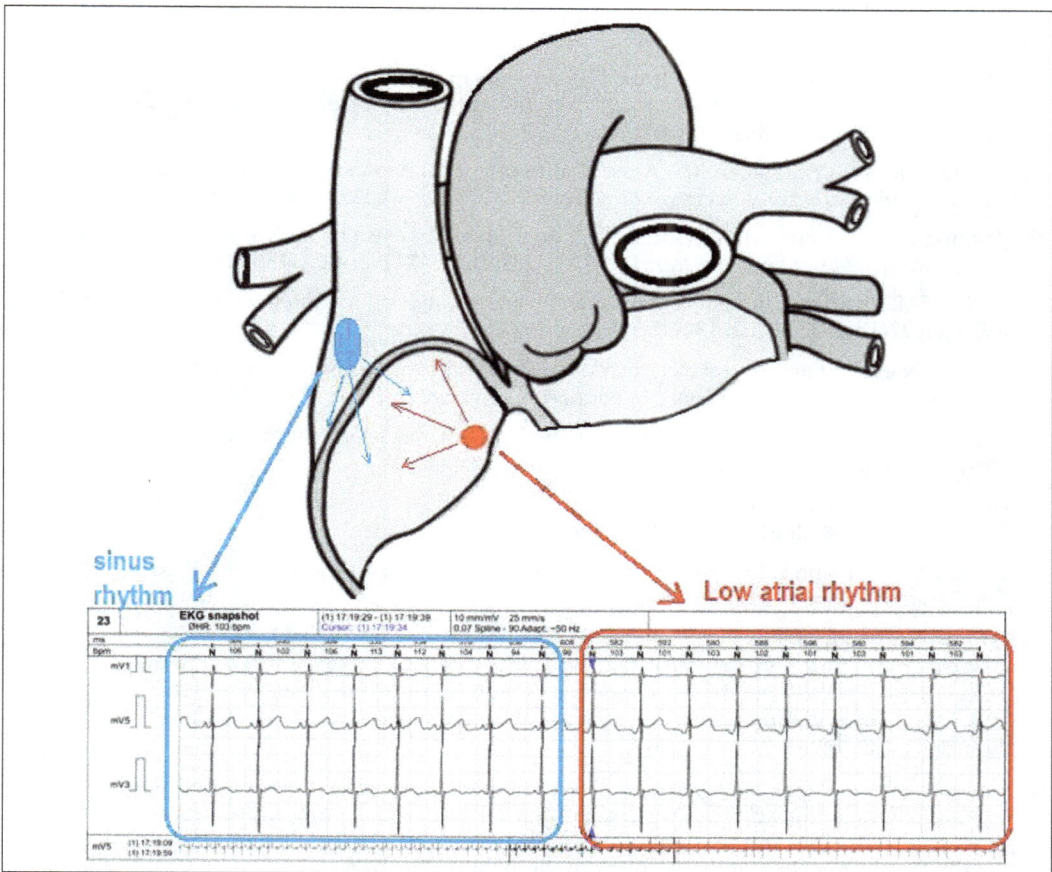

Figure 17.11 In sinus rhythm, the activation of the right atrium occurs in a superior to inferior direction, from the top to the bottom of the atrium, resulting in a positive P wave in leads II, III, and aVF. During low atrial rhythm, atrial activation occurs in an inferior-to-superior direction, resulting in a negative P wave in leads II, III, and aVF.

Hancock et al. further defined low atrial rhythm by claiming that the P wave with left axis deviation was the result of a pacemaker localized in the coronary sinus region or the A-V node and was either persistent from embryonic life when the left superior vena cava was present, or assumed the pacemaking function when the S-A node was completely anatomically absent, as in a sinus venosus type atrial septal defect.

Furure et al. studied low atrial rhythm in patients with congenital heart diseases and anomalous venous systemic connection. Low atrial rhythm was present in two-thirds of patients with absent inferior vena cava, and one-third of patients with persistent left superior vena cava. In patients without anomalies of the systemic venous connection, low atrial rhythm was present in 15% of patients with atrial septal defect, and in 14% of patients with ventricular septal defect. The presence of low atrial rhythm should alert physicians to venous return abnormalities, which complicate the right heart through cardiac catheterization. This procedure is typically performed through an inferior approach using the common femoral vein and inferior cava.

In the embryonic heart, the pacemakers are symmetrically located at the junction between common cardinal veins with the right and left horns of the sinus venosus. Patten described the development of the sinoatrial node from the right cardinal vein pacemaker and the atrioventricular node from the left cardinal vein pacemaker. The left superior vena cava develops from the left cardinal vein. In case of PLSVC left-sided pacemaker of the heart may persist, without its normal involution, functioning as an abnormal pacemaker at the level of the coronary sinus ostium. Absent inferior vena cava can also be associated with an abnormal persistence of the left cardinal vein pacemaker which leads to a low atrial rhythm.

BIBLIOGRAPHY

1. Moorman AF, Lamers WH. Current developments in cardiovascular embryology. II. Development of the conduction system and its significance for understanding congenital heart defects. *Ned Tijdschr Geneeskd.* 1992 Dec. 19;136(51):2509–2516.

2. Van der Horst RL, Gotsman MS. Abnormalities of atrial depolarization in infradiaphragmatic interruption of inferior vena cava. *Br Heart J.* 1972 Mar.;34(3):295–300. doi:10.1136/hrt.34.3.295

3. Thomas Jr HM, Spicer MJ, Nelson WP. Evaluation of P wave axis in distinguishing anatomical site of atrial septal defect. *Br Heart J.* 1973 Jul.;35(7):738–742. doi:10.1136/hrt.35.7.738

4. Patten BM. The development of the sinoventricular conduction system. *Med Bull (Ann Arbor).* 1956 Jan;22(1):1–21. PMID: 13291603.

5. Mifflin, N et al. "Paradoxical electrocardiographic rhythm during peripherally inserted central catheter insertion from persistent left superior vena cava." *J Assoc Vasc Access.* 2017;22:15–18.

6. Freedom RM, Schaffer MS, Rowe RD. Anomalous low insertion of right superior vena cava. *Br Heart J.* 1982 Dec.;48(6):601–603. doi:10.1136/hrt.48.6.601

7. Freedom RM, Ellison RC. Coronary sinus rhythm in the polysplenia syndrome. *Chest.* 1973 Jun;63(6):952–958. doi:10.1378/chest.63.6.952. PMID: 4711867.

8. Bellakehal M, Laine Y. Rythme du sinus coronaire [Coronary sinus rhythm]. *Rev Prat.* 2024 Sep;74(7):773. French. PMID: 39412024.

9. Giraud G, Latour H, Puech P. L'electrocardiographie du sinus coronaire. II. Etude électrocardiographique endocavitaire des dysrythmies du sinus coronaire chez l'homme [Electrocardiography of the coronary sinus. II. Endocavitary electrocardiographic study of dysrhythmias of the coronary sinus in man]. *Arch Mal Coeur Vaiss.* 1954 Dec;47(12):1008–1025. French. PMID: 14362676.

10. Giraud G, Latour H, Puech P, Roujon J. Rythmes de substitution d'origine coronarienne et nodale au cours d'une déficience sinusale; analyse électrocardiographique oesophagienne et endocavitaire [Substitute rhythms of coronary and nodal origin during a sinus deficiency; esophageal and endocavitary electrocardiographic analysis]. *Arch Mal Coeur Vaiss.* 1957 Aug;50(8):735–747. French. PMID: 13479172.

11. Wu J, Stork TL, Perron AD, Brady WJ. The athlete's electrocardiogram. *Am J Emerg Med.* 2006 Jan.;24(1):77–86. doi:10.1016/j.ajem.2005.04.009

12. Eliska O, Eliskova M. Morphology of the region of the coronary sinus in respect to coronary sinus rhythm. *Int J Cardiol.* 1990 Nov.;29(2):141–153. doi: 10.1016/0167-5273(90)90216-r. PMID: 2269534.

13. Sealy WC, Seaber AV. Cardiac rhythm following exclusion of the sinoatrial node and most of the right atrium from the remainder of the heart. *J Thorac Cardiovasc Surg.* 1979 Mar.;77(3):436–447. PMID: 762987.

14. Eckardt L. Automaticity in the coronary sinus. *J Cardiovasc Electrophysiol.* 2002;13:288–289. doi:10.1046/j.1540-8167.2002.00288.x

15. von Ludinghausen M. Clinical anatomy of cardiac veins, Vv. cardiacae. *Surg Radiol Anat.* 1987;9(2): 159–168. doi:10.1007/BF02086601

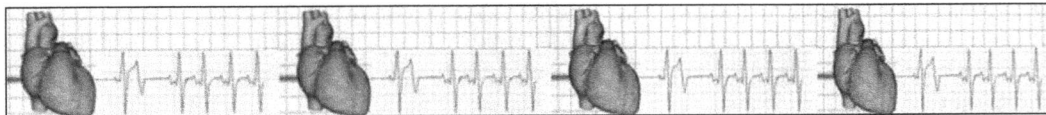

Case 18 PVCs in a 15-Year-Old Athlete

Ioana Ciuca

CLINICAL CASE

A 15-year-old female athlete, competing in the 3000 m and 5000 m running probes, was discovered to have premature ventricular contractions (PVCs) during a routine sports medicine evaluation. She participates in five training sessions per week, each lasting one hour. The Holter ECG recorded 27,000 PVCs. Treatment with vitamin D increased the blood levels from 20 to 42 ng/ml; thereafter, in conjunction with Flecainide 2x50 mg/day, the frequency of ExV decreased to 10,000 PVC/24 hours.

Concluzie

Ritm cardiac		
Total bătăi	111 454	(0% paced)
HR max / min	**161 / 49 bpm**	
Media HR	**Ø 77 bpm**	
HR Max / Min Sinus	150 / 49 bpm	
Media HR (Treaz/Adormit)	83 / 68 bpm	
Index circadian	1.22	
Tahicardie / Bradicardie	6 % / < 1 %	

Pauze		
RR Max	**1 714 ms**	
Pauze (>2000ms)	**0**	

Fibrilație atrială / Flutter atrial		
Total AF	5	(< 1%)
AF HR Max	133 bpm	
Cel mai lung AF	Ø 113 bpm	00:03:01

Bradicardie		
Cea mai mică	Ø 52 bpm	18 sec
Cea mai mare	Ø 53 bpm	00:01:24

ST		
St ridicare max	0,45 mV	mV1
ST depresurizare max	-	

Ectopie ventriculară		
V Total	27532	(25%)
V / Ora Max	2 464	pe oră
Episoade Tahicardie V		29 Σ 00:01:09
Cea mai rapidă Tahicardie V	Ø 161 bpm	1 sec
V Cea mai lungă secvență	Ø 136 bpm	2 sec
Triplete / Execută		474 Σ 1493 bătăi
Cuplete		1173 Σ 2346 bătăi
Bigeminism		4255 Σ 13947 bătăi
Trigeminism		3454 Σ 9011 bătăi

Ectopie supraventriculară		
S Tot	0	(< 1%)
Episoade Tahicardie SV		-
Cea mai rapidă Tahicardie SV		-
S Cea mai lungă secvență		-
Triplete / Execută		0 Σ 0 bătăi
Cuplete		0 Σ 0 bătăi

Figure 18.1 The image displays the summary of the Holter recording: maximum heart rate of 161 bpm, lowest rate of 49 bpm, PVC burden of 25% and absence of premature atrial contractions.

DOI: 10.1201/9781003545040-18

7	Ectopii						Run-uri V sunt compuse din mai puțin de 5 bătăi. Run-uri S sunt compuse din mai puțin de 20 bătăi.															
Interval		TOTAL	act.	HR[bpm]			Bătăi V							Modele V / Bătăi S							Modele S	Pauza	Buton
De la	Dur.	Bătăi	[%]	Min	Media	Max	Σ Individu	Bi	Tri	Cvadr	Cupl	Tripl	Ruleaza	Σ Individu	Bi	Tri	Cvadr	Cupl	Tripl	Ruleaza			
(1) 15:57	00:02	214	40.00	92	101	111	103	0	20	11	1	7	3	1	0	0	0	0	0	0	0	0	0
(1) 16:00	01:00	5792	27.00	74	97	160	2314	28	422	226	168	177	46	3	0	0	0	0	0	0	0	0	0
(1) 17:00	01:00	4937	4.00	70	82	95	1495	27	244	293	243	26	10	0	0	0	0	0	0	0	0	0	0
(1) 18:00	01:00	4514	5.00	65	75	90	1258	48	233	178	211	20	1	0	0	0	0	0	0	0	0	0	0
(1) 19:00	01:00	4269	3.00	61	71	95	1011	68	153	84	191	4	1	0	0	0	0	0	0	0	0	0	0
(1) 20:00	01:00	4259	3.00	60	71	88	801	123	115	87	122	1	0	0	0	0	0	0	0	0	0	0	0
(1) 21:00	01:00	4551	12.00	58	76	92	918	163	38	134	151	8	4	0	0	0	0	0	0	0	0	0	0
(1) 22:00	01:00	4882	17.00	66	81	104	886	157	6	90	186	12	0	0	0	0	0	0	0	0	0	0	0
(1) 23:00	01:00	4686	18.00	63	78	99	784	211	6	108	138	4	2	0	0	0	0	0	0	0	0	0	0
(2) 00:00	01:00	4238	9.00	56	71	91	482	185	51	25	68	1	1	0	0	0	0	0	0	0	0	0	0
(2) 01:00	01:00	4167	6.00	53	69	90	457	240	24	27	53	3	0	0	0	0	0	0	0	0	0	0	0
(2) 02:00	01:00	3764	3.00	56	63	85	228	142	11	5	24	2	0	0	0	0	0	0	0	0	0	0	0
(2) 03:00	01:00	3865	3.00	55	64	88	369	120	56	10	48	8	0	0	0	0	0	0	0	0	0	0	0
(2) 04:00	01:00	3639	3.00	52	61	86	143	33	34	2	20	2	0	0	0	0	0	0	0	0	0	0	0
(2) 05:00	01:00	3784	3.00	50	63	90	271	89	45	13	25	9	0	0	0	0	0	0	0	0	0	0	0
(2) 06:00	01:00	3699	4.00	49	62	97	253	113	23	18	24	7	1	0	0	0	0	0	0	0	0	0	0
(2) 07:00	01:00	3861	4.00	51	64	93	375	119	27	29	56	12	3	0	0	0	0	0	0	0	0	0	0
(2) 08:00	01:00	4351	6.00	53	73	110	962	60	246	54	210	34	8	1	0	0	0	0	0	0	0	0	0
(2) 09:00	01:00	5618	26.00	74	94	156	1971	36	325	311	180	122	46	10	0	0	0	0	0	0	0	0	0
(2) 10:00	01:00	5187	18.00	70	86	129	1610	41	243	237	195	63	25	4	0	0	0	0	0	0	0	0	0
(2) 11:00	01:00	5331	22.00	71	89	161	1948	39	347	254	127	118	40	13	0	0	0	0	0	0	0	0	0
(2) 12:00	01:00	5469	18.00	75	91	160	1939	30	294	290	190	133	45	3	0	0	0	0	0	0	0	0	0
(2) 13:00	01:00	5485	25.00	65	91	157	2053	24	333	311	160	132	44	17	0	0	0	0	0	0	0	0	0
(2) 14:00	01:00	5570	19.00	73	93	146	2437	6	501	375	103	160	53	11	0	0	0	0	0	0	0	0	0
(2) 15:00	00:58	5322	18.00	78	91	143	2464	2	458	282	83	108	70	8	0	0	0	0	0	0	0	0	0
Σ adormit	09:00	36724	7.00	49	68	104	3873	1290	256	298	586	48	4	0	0	0	0	0	0	0	0	0	0
Σ treaz	15:00	74730	14.00	51	83	161	23659	814	3999	3156	2391	1125	399	71	0	0	0	0	0	0	0	0	0
TOTAL	24:00	111454	12.00	49	77	161	27532	2104	4255	3454	2977	1173	403	71	0	0	0	0	0	0	0	0	0

Figure 18.2 The table illustrates the distribution of PVCs during sleep and waking periods. The majority of PVCs occurred during waking hours: 23,659 compared to 3,873 during sleeping hours. The column in red shows the PVD distribution during the daytime and night time hours , starting from 15:57 to 15:00 the next day.

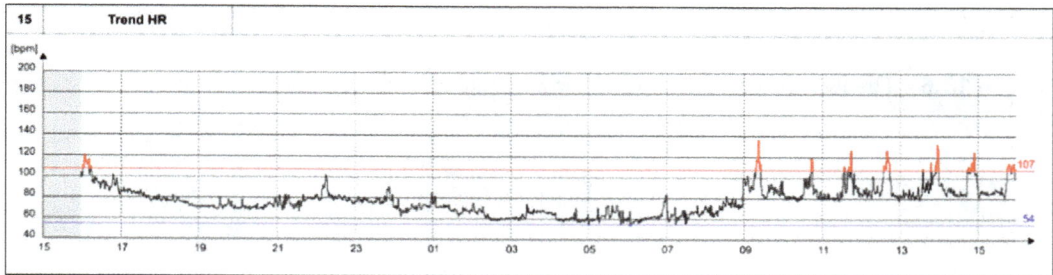

Figure 18.3 The histogram shows the HR curve with mean rates between 54 and 107 bpm. The red color on the curve indicates rates over 107 bpm.

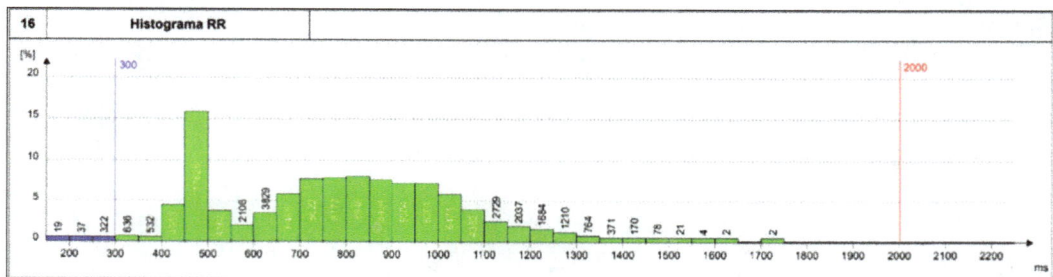

Figure 18.4 The RR histogram shows intervals between 300 and 2000 ms marked with green color and intervals below 300 ms marked with blue color.

143

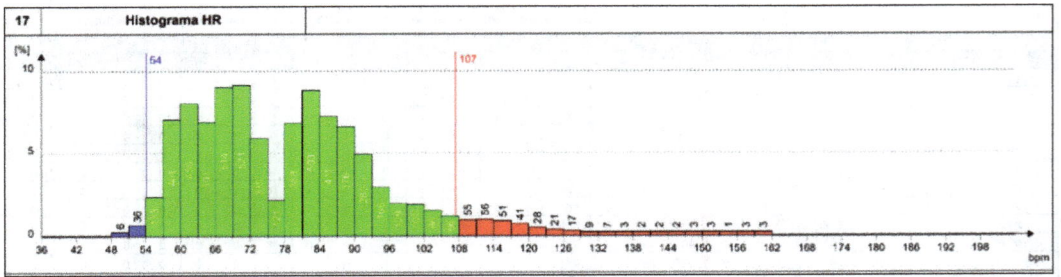

Figure 18.5 The HR histogram shows rates above 107 bpm marked with red color, rates between 54 and 107 bpm marked with green color and rates below 54 bpm marked with blue color.

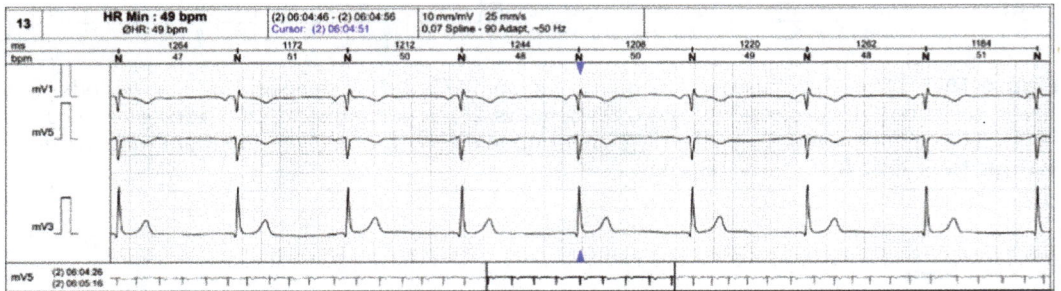

Figure 18.6 The ECG recording shows the lowest rate of 49 bpm observed during sinus rhythm.

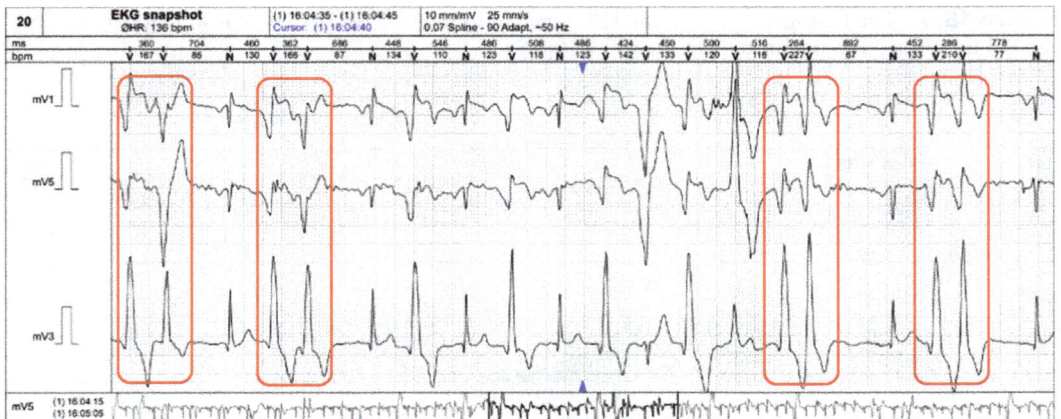

Figure 18.7 The ECG recording shows and increased rate of 136 bpm and frequent PVCs with couplets marked with a red square (2 consecutive PVCs).

144

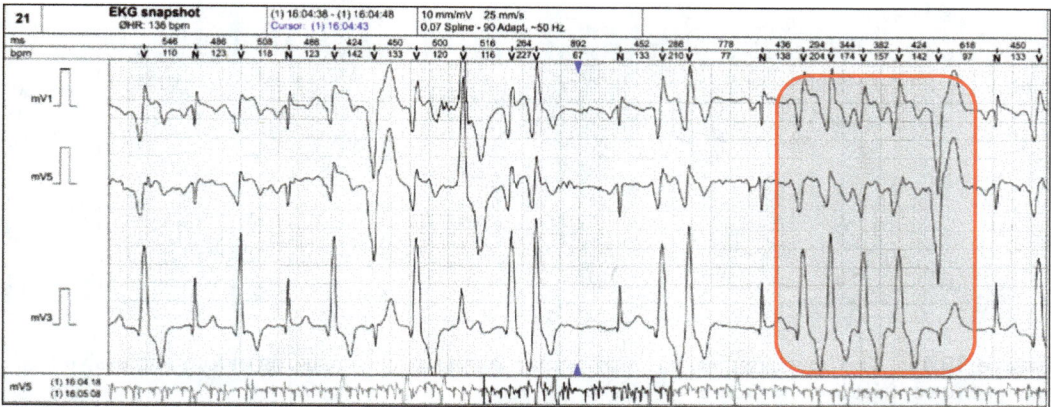

Figure 18.8 The ECG recording shows frequent PVCs with couplets and a ventricular salvo of 5 consecutive beats (marked with a red square).

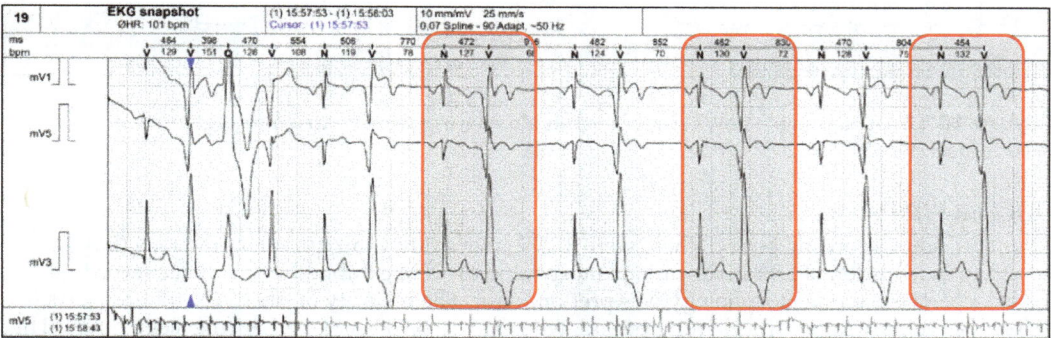

Figure 18.9 The image shows ventricular bigeminy, every second beat being a PVC.

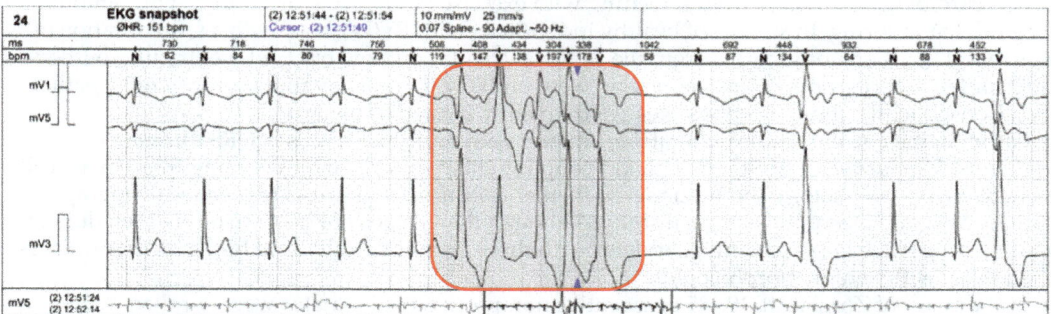

Figure 18.10 The image shows a ventricular salvo, made of 5 consecutive PVCs.

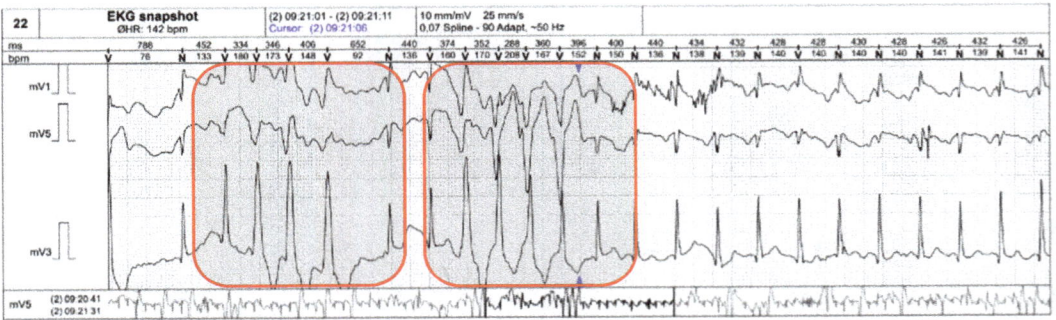

Figure 18.11 The image depicts two ventricular salvoes, each consisting of four successive premature ventricular contractions (PVCs).

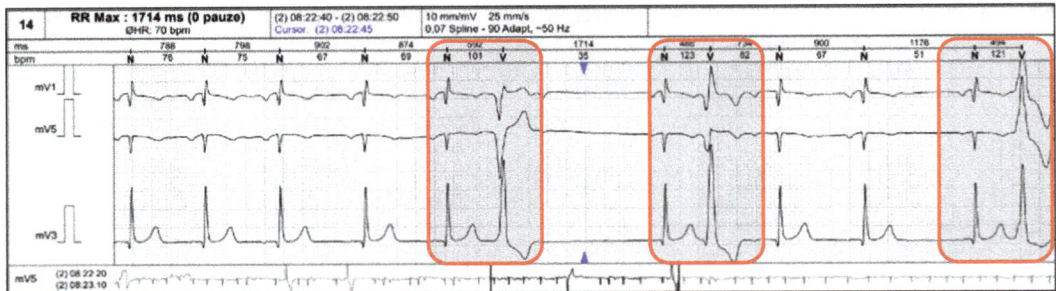

Figure 18.12 The image shows sinus rhythm alternating with ventricular bigeminy, every second beat being a PVC.

HOLTER SUMMARY

Over a 24-hour recording period, there were 27,532 premature ventricular contractions (PVCs), resulting in a burden of 25%. Four unique morphologies were exhibited by the three recording leads; nevertheless, one morphology was predominant. The majority of the PVCs, totaling 23,000, were observed during the awakening period, whereas just 3,000 occurred during sleep hours. The maximum measured rate was 161 bpm, while the minimum rate was 49 bpm. No premature atrial contractions were present.

DISCUSSION

The athletic preparticipation evaluation approach recommended by the European Society of Cardiology includes medical history, physical examination, and resting ECG. In 2016 EHRA and EAPC published a consensus statement on preparticipation evaluation.

Characterization of benign PVC morphology derives from large cohorts of athletes referred to sports cardiology experts or from screening with exercise ECG testing or 12- to 24-hour ambulatory ECG monitoring. In studies of healthy individuals with PVCs, those with a QRS duration of less than 140 ms and originating from the right ventricular outflow tract, left ventricular outflow tract, or left anterior or posterior fascicular, were unlikely to have any underlying cardiac pathology. Consequently, those morphologies are frequently labeled as benign.

Based on the current medical literature, athletes with multifocal PVCs, a QRS duration of >140 ms, high burden on Holter ECG, short coupling interval or variable coupling interval as well as nonbenign morphology should undergo further testing such as stress test, echocardipgraphy, cardiac MRI and elecrophysiological study. Although these types of PVCs are rarely seen during routine preparticipation screening, athletes with these findings might be at higher arrhythmic risk than those with benign morphologies.

In the study of Zorzi et al. 10,985 consecutive non-professional athletes were enrolled, with a median age of 15 years undergoing evaluation for sports participation. Of those individuals, 9% had abnormal findings, 4% being detected on medical, examination or 12 lead ECG, however,

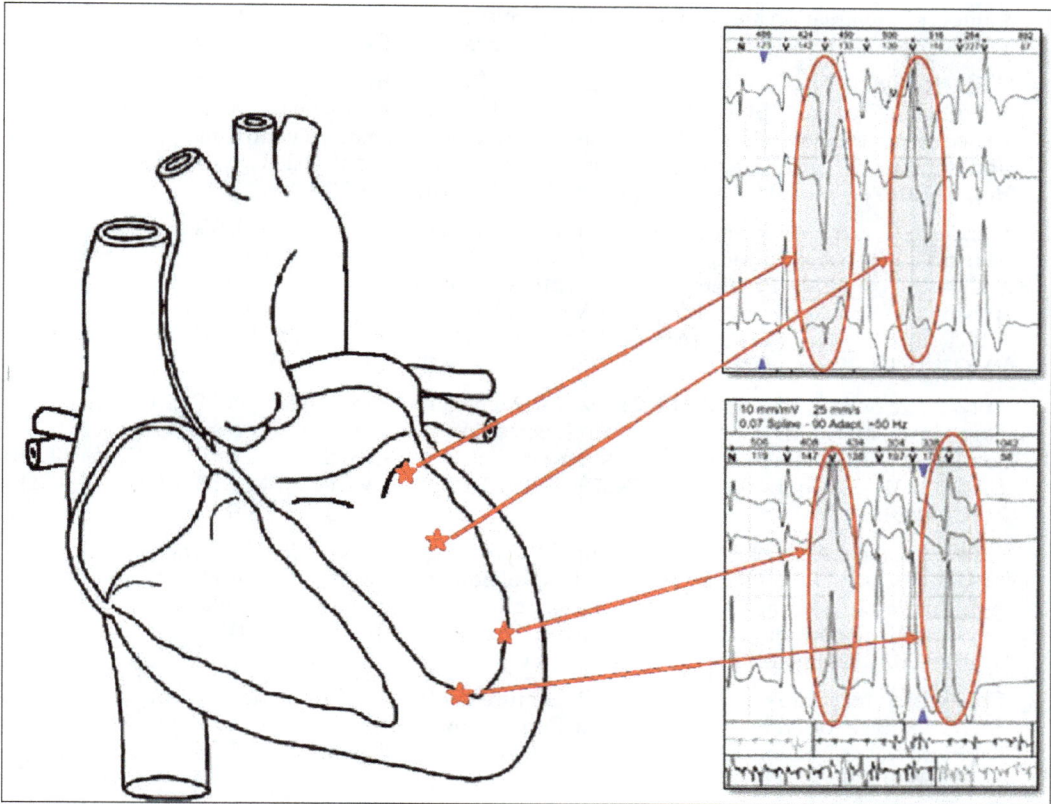

Figure 18.13 The figure shows 4 types of premature ventricular contractions from different foci inside the right and left ventricle. The morphology in the 3 ECG leads differs between the 4 PVCs.

5% were detected only during stress test. Abnormal findings were ventricular arrhythmias such as premature ventricular beats, couplets triplets and non-sustained ventricular tachycardia, which was present in 14% of cases. Subsequent examinations in athletes with stress-test induced ventricular arrhythmias included a 24-hour Holter ECG monitoring and echocardiography. In those with complex ventricular arrhythmias, Cardiac Magnetic Resonance(CMR) was performed. Overall, 0.5% of all athletes showed modifications at risk of developing sudden cardiac death and were stopped from participating in competitive sports.

Therapeutic decisions for athletes with PVCs might be difficult. It is advisable for every patient to adopt lifestyle modifications, including the avoidance of stimulants, specific supplements after long hours of training, and overtraining, a nutritious diet and sleep hygiene. Athletes with nonbenign PVC morphologies should be evaluated for treatment following an extensive arrhythmologic evaluation. Individuals with a significant PVC load, regardless of benign or malign PVC morphologies, may require treatment. Although PVC morphology and classification are more suggestive of the risk for cardiomyopathy or sudden cardiac death than the PVC load itself, a high PVC burden can still be detrimental by provoking symptoms, impairing athletic performance, and potentially leading to PVC-induced cardiomyopathy.

BIBLIOGRAPHY

1. Gomez SE, Hwang CE, Kim DS, Froelicher VF, Wheeler MT, Perez MV. Premature ventricular contractions (PVCs) in young athletes. *Prog Cardiovasc Dis*. 2022 Sep–Oct;74:80–88. doi: 10.1016/j.pcad.2022.10.011. Epub 2022 Oct 26. PMID: 36309100.

2. Klewer J, Springer J, Morshedzadeh J. Premature ventricular contractions (PVCs): A narrative review. *Am J Med*. 2022 Nov;135(11):1300–1305. doi: 10.1016/j.amjmed.2022.07.004. Epub 2022 Jul 27. PMID: 35907515.

3. Lampert R. Evaluation and management of arrhythmia in the athletic patient. *Prog Cardiovasc Dis.* 2012 Mar–Apr;54(5):423–431. doi: 10.1016/j.pcad.2012.01.002. PMID: 22386293.

4. Basile P, Soldato N, Pedio E, Siena P, Carella MC, Dentamaro I, Khan Y, Baggiano A, Mushtaq S, Forleo C, Ciccone MM, Pontone G, Guaricci AI. Cardiac magnetic resonance reveals concealed structural heart disease in patients with frequent premature ventricular contractions and normal echocardiography: A systematic review. *Int J Cardiol.* 2024 Oct 1;412:132306. doi: 10.1016/j.ijcard.2024.132306. Epub 2024 Jun 29. PMID: 38950789.

5. Crescenzi C, Zorzi A, Vessella T, Martino A, Panattoni G, Cipriani A, De Lazzari M, Perazzolo Marra M, Fusco A, Sciarra L, Sperandii F, Guerra E, Tranchita E, Fossati C, Pigozzi F, Sarto P, Calò L, Corrado D. Predictors of Left Ventricular Scar Using Cardiac Magnetic Resonance in Athletes With Apparently Idiopathic Ventricular Arrhythmias. *J Am Heart Assoc.* 2021 Jan 5;10(1):e018206. doi: 10.1161/JAHA.120.018206. Epub 2020 Dec 31. PMID: 33381977; PMCID: PMC7955495.

6. Zorzi A, Vessella T, De Lazzari M, Cipriani A, Menegon V, Sarto G, Spagnol R, Merlo L, Pegoraro C, Marra MP, Corrado D, Sarto P. Screening young athletes for diseases at risk of sudden cardiac death: role of stress testing for ventricular arrhythmias. *Eur J Prev Cardiol.* 2020 Feb;27(3):311–320. doi: 10.1177/2047487319890973. Epub 2019 Dec 2. PMID: 31791144; PMCID: PMC7008549.

7. Papanastasiou CA, Bazmpani MA, Kampaktsis PN, Zegkos T, Gossios T, Parcharidou D, Kokkinidis DG, Tziatzios I, Economou FI, Nikolaidou C, Kamperidis V, Tsapas A, Ziakas A, Efthimiadis G, Karamitsos TD. Cardiac magnetic resonance for ventricular arrhythmias: a systematic review and meta-analysis. *Heart.* 2024 Aug 26;110(18):1113–1123. doi: 10.1136/heartjnl-2024-324182. PMID: 39084706.

8. Chukwurah MI, Chung EH. Incidental Premature Ventricular Contractions in Young Athletes: Shape and Size (of Premature Ventricular Contractions burden) Matter. *Circ Arrhythm Electrophysiol.* 2024 Oct;17(10):e013345. doi: 10.1161/CIRCEP.124.013345. Epub 2024 Sep 20. PMID: 39301716.

9. Gomez SE, Perez MV, Wheeler MT, Hadley D, Hwang CE, Kussman A, Kim DS, Froelicher V. Classification of premature ventricular contractions in athletes during routine preparticipation exams. *Circ Arrhythm Electrophysiol.* 2024 Sep;17(9):e012835. doi: 10.1161/CIRCEP.124.012835. Epub 2024 Aug 28. PMID: 39193774; PMCID: PMC11452187.

10. Delise P, Lanari E, Sitta N, Centa M, Allocca G, Biffi A. Influence of training on the number and complexity of frequent VPBs in healthy athletes. *J Cardiovasc Med (Hagerstown).* 2011 Mar;12(3):157–161. doi: 10.2459/JCM.0b013e32834102ea. PMID: 21139509.

11. D'Ascenzi F, Zorzi A, Alvino F, Bonifazi M, Mondillo S, Corrado D. L'extrasistolia ventricolare nel giovane atleta: inquadramento e percorso diagnostico [Premature ventricular beats in young athletes: interpretation and diagnostic pathway]. *G Ital Cardiol (Rome).* 2019 Apr;20(4):229–241. Italian. doi: 10.1714/3126.31076. PMID: 30920550.

12. Crescenzi C, Panattoni G, Stazi A, Martino A, Sgueglia M, De Ruvo E, Calò L. Ventricular arrhythmias and risk stratification of cardiac sudden death in athletes. *Minerva Cardioangiol.* 2020 Apr;68(2):110–122. doi: 10.23736/S0026-4725.20.05178-6. PMID: 32429629.

13. Valeri Y, Compagnucci P, Volpato G, Luciani L, Crepaldi E, Maiorino F, Parisi Q, Cipolletta L, Campanelli F, D'Angelo L, Gaggiotti G, Gasperetti A, Giovagnoni A, Curcio A, Dello Russo A, Casella M. Idiopathic premature ventricular contraction catheter ablation, sedentary population vs. athlete's populations: Outcomes and resumption of sports activity. *J Clin Med.* 2024 Mar 24;13(7):1871. doi: 10.3390/jcm13071871. PMID: 38610635; PMCID: PMC11012949.

14. Lawless CE, Briner W. Palpitations in athletes. *Sports Med.* 2008;38(8):687–702. doi: 10.2165/00007256-200838080-00006. PMID: 18620468.

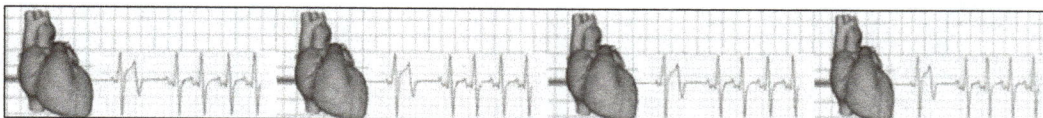

Case 19 Asymptomatic Complete AV Block

Maria Ilina

CLINICAL CASE

A 5-year-old female patient was evaluated in the Cardiology Department for bradycardia. She was diagnosed with AV block by a pediatrician and then referred to the pediatric cardiologist. She was asymptomatic. An ECG revealed third-degree AV block; hence, a Holter ECG was requested.

3 Lead Holter Report

(5 years)   Gender: Female

Analyzed Length: 1 day 2 hr 20 min 57 sec, 2.2% artifact
Analyzed by: . Thu 22 Feb 2024

Beats

Beats	Total		Normal		Ventricular		Supraventricular		Paced	
Count	95,718	95,690	>99%		0	0%	0	0%	0	0%
Max/Hour		4,341	Wed 14, 08:00		0		0		0	

Heart Rates

Heart Rates (1 min avg)	Rate (bpm)	Time
Max	106	Wed 14, 10:20
Min	46	Wed 14, 02:20
Mean	62	
Mean HR (Day)	65	07:00:00 - 23:00:00
Mean HR (Night)	54	23:00:00 - 07:00:00

Rate Dependent Events

Rate Dependent Events	Count	Most Severe Rate (bpm)	Longest (beats / secs)
Pause	0	-	
Dropped Beat		-	-
Bradycardia	15	43 : Wed 14, 02:08	10 beats : Wed 14, 02:33
Tachycardia	0		

Ventricular Arrhythmias

Ventricular Beats : 0 (0%)   Max/Hour : 0   Max/Minute: 0   Average/Hour : 0

Event	Event Count	V Beat Count	% V Beats	% Total Beats	Per 1000	Max Rate (bpm)	Longest (beats / cycles)
VT	0	0	0%	0%	0		
V-Run/AIVR	0	0	0%	0%	0		
IVR	0	0	0%	0%	0		
Triplet	0	0	0%	0%	0	-	-
Couplet	0	0	0%	0%	0	-	-
Bigeminy	0	0	0%	0%	-		-
Trigeminy	0	0	0%	0%	-		-
Single VE Events	0	0	0%	0%	0	-	-

Supraventricular Arrhythmias

Supraventricular Beats : 0 (0%)   Max/Hour : 0   Max/Minute: 0   Average/Hour : 0

Event	Event Count	SV Beat Count	% SV Beats	% Total Beats	Per 1000	Max Rate (bpm)	Longest (beats)
SVT	0	0	0%	0%	0		
SVE Run	0	0	0%	0%	0		
SVE Couplet	0	0	0%	0%	0	-	-
Single SVE Events	0	0	0%	0%	0	-	-

Figure 19.1   The summary page shows demographical data: age and gender, the minimum heart rate of 46 and the maximum heart rate of 106 bpm. No PVCs or PACs were detected during monitoring. There were no significant pauses.

DOI: 10.1201/9781003545040-19

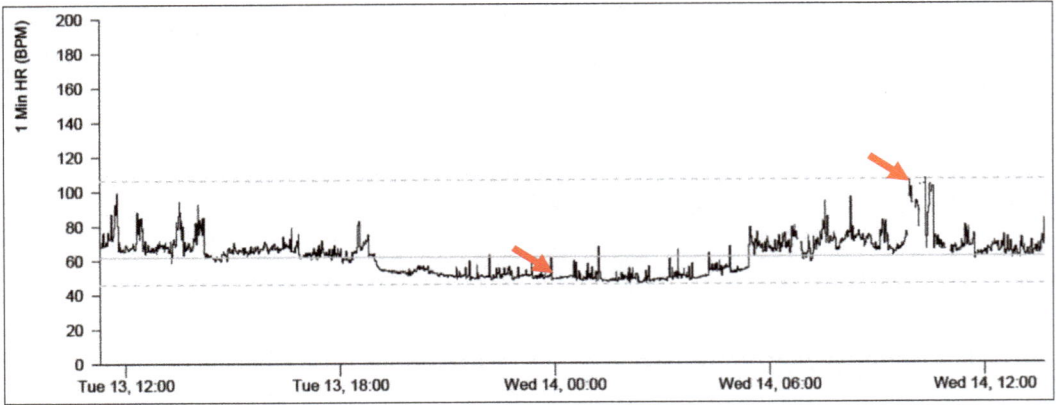

Figure 19.2 Heart rate trend shows a minimum rate of 46 bpm and a maximum of 106 bpm during physical activity.

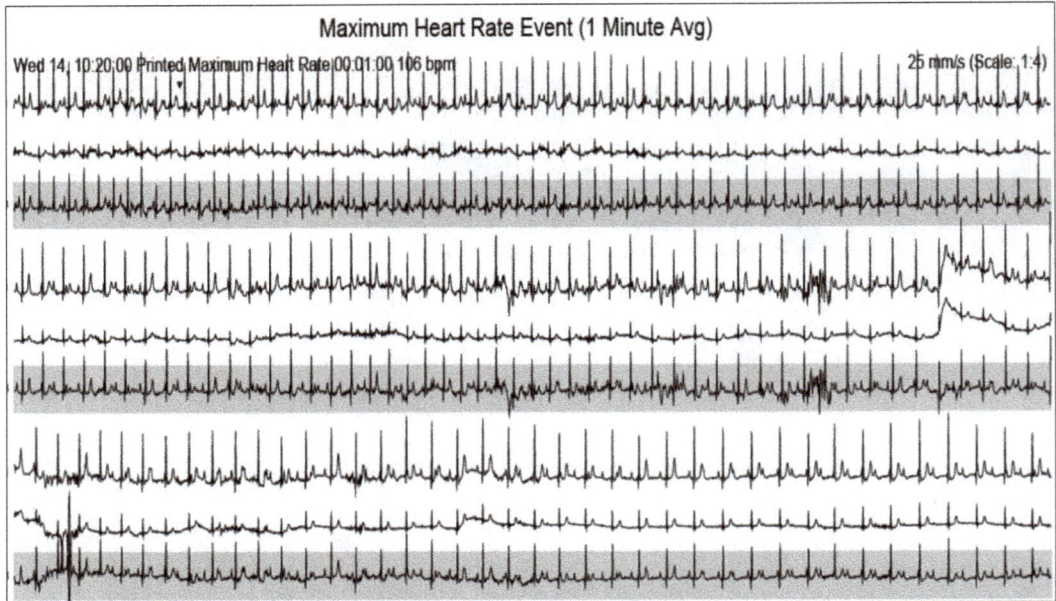

Figure 19.3 The maximum recorded rate was 106 bpm and the inferior part of the image clearly shows dissociated P waves and QRS complexes.

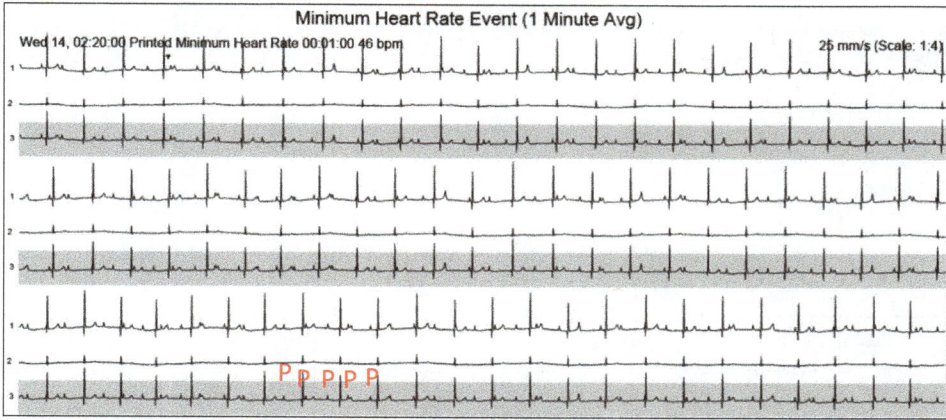

Figure 19.4 The image shows the lowest rate during monitoring with P waves being completely dissociated from the QRS complexes.

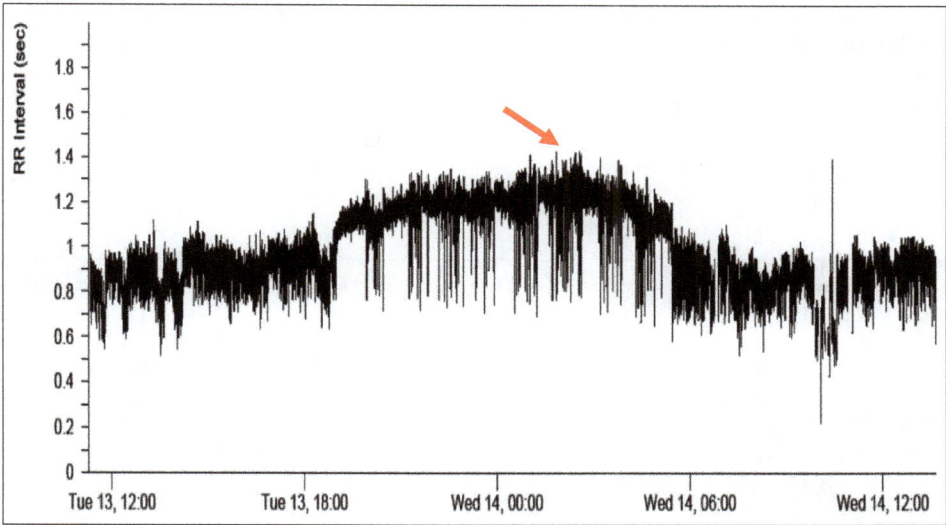

Figure 19.5 RR histogram shows the lowest rates during sleep with values >1500 ms.

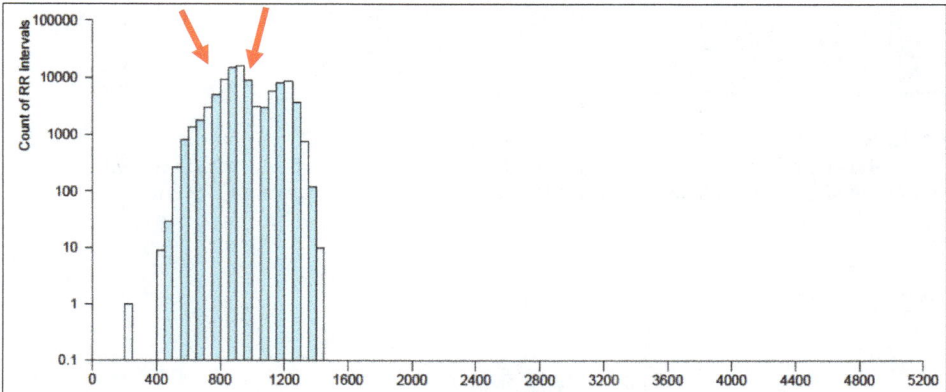

Figure 19.6 The count of RR intervals indicates that the majority of the RR values ranged from 900 to 1000 ms.

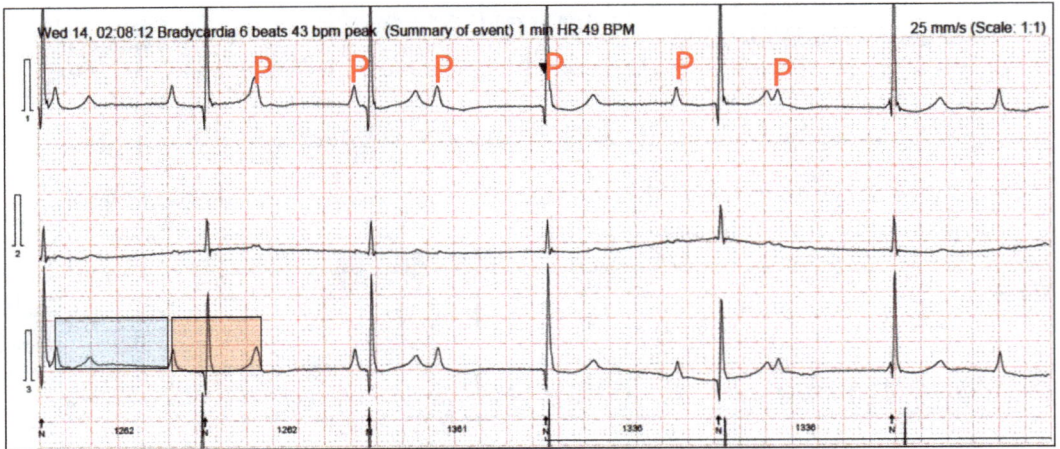

Figure 19.7 The image shows complete AV block (P waves are dissociated from QRS complexes). Ventriculophasic arrhythmia can be observed on the strip: the PP intervals that include the QRS complex (red square) are of shorter duration than the PP intervals that do not have a QRS complex (blue square).

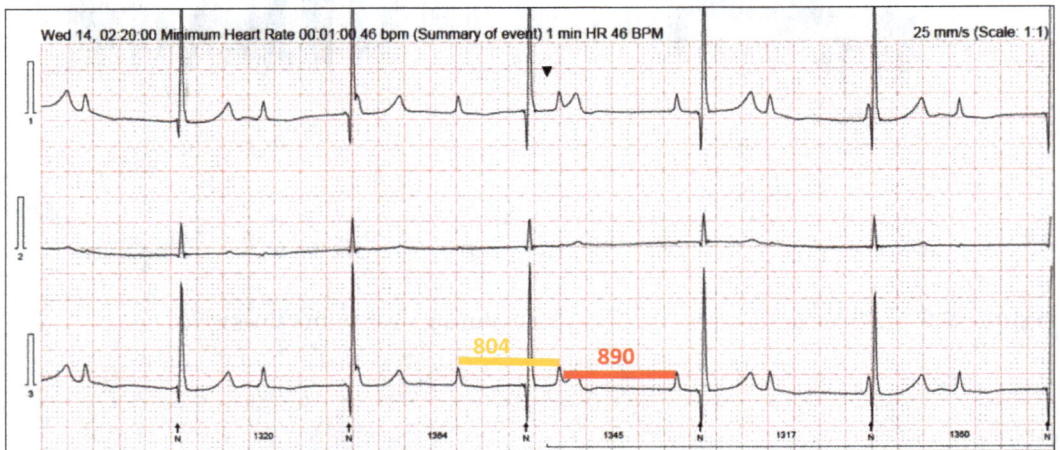

Figure 19.8 Complete AV block: P waves are dissociated from QRS complexes. Ventriculophasic arrhythmia is demonstrated by the PP intervals that include the QRS complex (804 ms) are of shorter duration than the PP intervals that do not have a QRS complex (890 ms).

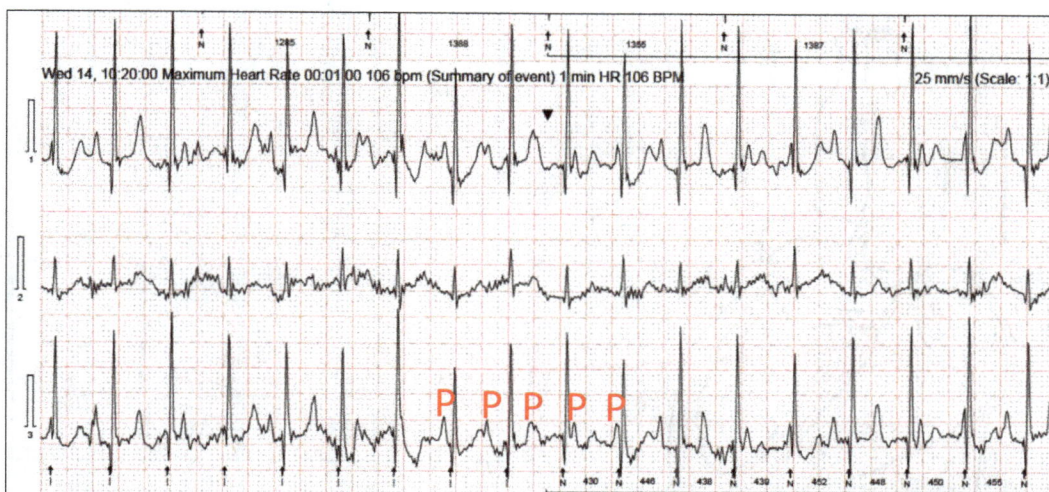

Figure 19.9 Complete AV block during physical activity. Both the atrial and ventricular rates increase, demonstrating the supra-Hisian origin of the block. There is no relationship between P waves and QRS complexes.

HOLTER SUMMARY

The monitoring revealed complete AV block with a minimum rate of 46 bpm, and a maximum rate of 106 bpm during physical activity. No pause has been identified. The patient was asymptomatic during Holter monitoring.

DISCUSSION

Atrioventricular block is a rare disorder in children. It may manifest in children with structurally normal hearts or in association with congenital heart disease. All symptomatic, irreversible complete AV blocks necessitate the insertion of a permanent pacemaker. In the case of an asymptomatic complete AV block, the decision is based on other high-risk predictors.

Ventriculophasic arrhythmia is a non-respiratory sinus arrhythmia, seen in children with complete AV block. Typically, it is seen as PP intervals that include the QRS complex of shorter duration compared to the PP intervals that do not contain a QRS complex. Thus, sinus cycle length is reduced when a QRS complex occurs between 2 P waves. Ventriculophasic arrhythmia is defined as a shortening of > 3% in the PP interval if the QRS complex occurs within the 60% of the anticipated PP interval. It is a phenomenon more frequently seen in women (81%) than in men (37%).

The suggested mechanisms for ventriculophasic arrhythmia comprise: (a) modifications in baroreceptor output due to stroke volume from ventricular contraction within a PP interval; (b) distension of the right atrium and sinus node during ventricular contraction that enhances sinus node automaticity; and (c) variations in sinus rate caused by modifications in sinus node blood supply in response to ventricular contraction.

In 1955, Rosenbaum and Lepeschkin postulated a positive and negative chronotropic mechanism to clarify the ventriculophasic arrhythmia: The positive chronotropic effect causes an accelerated sinus nodal discharge of a P wave after a QRS, leading to a reduction of the PP interval that includes the QRS. The negative chronotropic effect leads to an extension of the subsequent PP interval without a preceding QRS complex. The increase in arterial blood pressure during ventricular systole activates arterial baroreceptors, resulting in a reflex reduction of sinus node firing due to heightened vagal tone, hence extending the PP interval in the absence of a QRS complex.

It has been shown that ventriculophasic sinus arrhythmia is absent in recipient atria after orthotopic cardiac transplant. This is in spite of the intact autonomic innervation of the recipient atria. This could be explained by the absence of pulsatile blood flow to the sinus node.

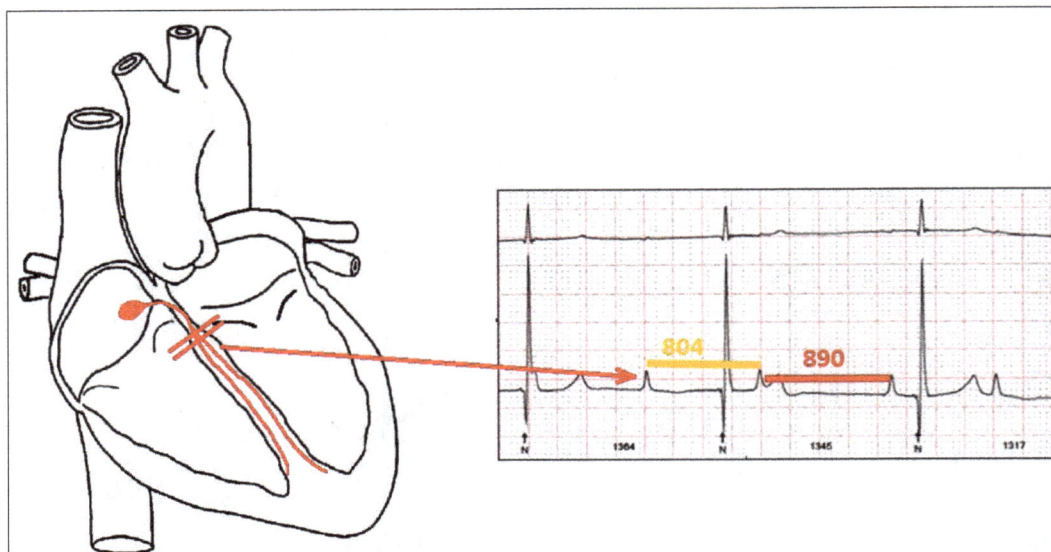

Figure 19.10 Complete AV block: P waves are dissociated from the QRS complexes. Ventriculophasic arrhythmia can be seen: PP interval of 804 ms is shorter than PP interval of 890 ms.

BIBLIOGRAPHY

1. Rosenbaum MB, Lepeschkin E. The effect of ventricular systole on auricular rhythm in auriculoventricular block. *Circulation*. 1955; 11: 240–261.

2. Liu T, Shehata M, Wang X. Paradoxical ventriculophasic sinus arrhythmia during 2:1 atrioventricular block. *J Cardiol Cases*. 2011; 3: e37–e39.

3. Gazes PC, Culler RM, Taber E, Kelly TE. Congenital familial cardiac conduction defects. *Circulation*. 1965; 32: 32–34. doi:10.1161/01.CIR.32.1.32

4. Erlanger J, Blackman JR. Further studies in the physiology of heart block in mammals. Chronic auriculo-ventricular block in the dog. *Heart*. 1910; 1: 177–230.

5. Jaeggi ET, Hamilton RM, Silverman ED, Zamora SA, Hornberger LK. Outcome of children with fetal, neonatal or childhood diagnosis of isolated congenital atrio-ventricular block. *J Am Coll Cardiol*. 2002; 39: 130–137. doi:10.1016/S0735-1097(01)01697-7

6. Shah MJ, Silka MJ, Silva JNA, et al. 2021 PACES expert consensus statement on the indications and management of cardiovascular implantable electronic devices in pediatric patients *Heart Rhythm*. 2021; 18: 1888–1924.

7. Jičínský M, Kubuš P, Pavlíková M, Ložek M, Janoušek J. Natural history of nonsurgical complete atrioventricular block in children and predictors of pacemaker implantation *J Am Coll Cardiol EP*. 2023; 9(8): 1379–1389.

8. Lazzerini PE, Capecchi PL, Laghi-Pasini F. Isolated atrioventricular block of unknown origin in adults and anti-Ro/SSA antibodies: Clinical evidence, putative mechanisms, and therapeutic implications. *Heart Rhythm*. 2015; 12: 449–454. doi:10.1016/j.hrthm.2014.10.031

9. Liberman L, Silver ES, Chai P, Anderson BR. Incidence and characteristics of heart block after heart surgery in pediatric patients: A multicenter study. *J Thorac Cardiovasc Surg*. 2016 doi:10.1016/j.jtcvs.2016.03.081

10. Michaelsson M, Riesenfeld T, Jonzon A. Natural history of congenital complete atrioventricular block. *Pacing Clin Electrophysiol*. 1997; 20: 2098–2101. doi:10.1111/j.1540-8159.1997.tb03636.x

11. Nakashima T, Nagase M, Shibahara T, Ono D, Yamada T, Tanabe G, Suzuki K, Yamaura M, Ido T, Takahashi S, Okura H, Aoyama T. Electrocardiographic features of paradoxical ventriculophasic response. *J Electrocardiol*. 2022 Mar.–Apr.; 71: 67–73. doi:10.1016/j.jelectrocard.2022.02.002. Epub 2022 Feb 12. PMID: 35183045.

12. de Marchena E, Colvin-Adams M, Esnard J, Ridha M, Castellanos A, Myerburg RJ. Ventriculophasic sinus arrhythmia in the orthotopic transplanted heart: Mechanism of disease revisited. *Int J Cardiol*. 2003 Sep.; 91(1): 71–74. doi:10.1016/s0167-5273(02)00597-1. PMID: 12957731.

13. Manne JR. Paradoxical ventriculophasic arrhythmia in a patient with 2:1 atrioventricular block: A rare phenomenon. *Ann Noninvasive Electrocardiol*. 2016 May; 21(3): 325–327. doi:10.1111/anec.12340. Epub 2016 Jan. 29. PMID: 26824225; PMCID: PMC6931667.

14. Parsonnet AE, Miller R. Heart block: The influence of ventricular systole upon the auricular rhythm in complete and incomplete heart block. *Am Heart J*. 1944; 27: 676–687.

15. Alboni P, Holz A, Brignole M. Vagally mediated atrioventricular block: Pathophysiology and diagnosis. *Heart*. 2013 Jul.; 99(13): 904–908. doi:10.1136/heartjnl-2012-303220. Epub 2013 Jan. 2. PMID: 23286970.

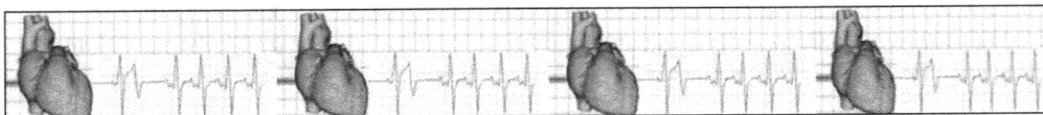

Case 20 High Burden PVCs in a 7-Year-Old Football Player

Cismaru Gabriel, Bogdan Caloian, Horatiu Comsa, Diana Irimie, Florina Fringu, Raluca Tomoaia, and Dana Pop

CLINICAL CASE

A 7-year-old male football player with no symptoms was found with abnormal rhythm during medical consultation. He practiced 4 times per week, 1.5 hours of football per session. The sports doctor found PVCs on the 12-lead ECG, with an RVOT morphology and asked for a Holter ECG. Echocardiography was normal, with a non-dilated left ventricle and an ejection fraction of 60%. The right ventricle and RVOT were also normal. Lab tests were within normal limits, except for vitamin D which had a level of 22 ng/ml, lower than the limit of > 30 ng/ml. Even though he was asymptomatic, the pediatric cardiologist started treatment with Propranolol 10 mg twice/day. The following Holter monitoring was performed after the patient took his daily dose of Propranolol.

The average heart rate was 72 bpm. The minimum heart rate was 50 bpm at 22:50. The maximum heart rate was 116 bpm at 18:20.

Ventricular results:
There were a total of 23385 (23.42%) beats. These comprised 23385 (100%) single beats, there were 1004 (51.52%) bigeminy events.

Supraventricular results:
There were a total of 8 (0.01%) beats. These comprised 4 (50%) single beats, 2 (50%) couplets.

ST episodes:
The maximum ST depression was -0.13 mm at 15:34 in channel CH3. The maximum ST elevation was 3.37 mm at 18:57 in channel CH1.

Rhythm results:
There were 0 pause intervals defined greater than 2400 ms.
Atrial Fibrillation was detected in 0.00% (0 h 00 min) of the total monitoring time.
Atrial flutter was detected in 0.13% (3 h 03 min) of the total monitoring time.

QT results:
The maximum QT interval was 440 ms (51 bpm) at 23:51, the maximum QTc interval was 516 ms (106 bpm) at 07:47.
The minimum QT interval was 336 ms (112 bpm) at 18:20, the minimum QTc interval was 370 ms (69 bpm) at 13:17.

TIME [hh:mm-hh:mm]	TOTAL BEATS	HEART RATE			VENTRICULAR							SUPRAVENTRICULAR							PAUSE	MARKED
		MIN	AVG	MAX	BEATS	SINGLE	CPL	RUN	TCH	BIG	TRIG	BEATS	SINGLE	CPL	RUN	TCH	BIG	TRIG		
17:48-18:00	830	60	77	92	306	306	0	0	0	9	15	0	0	0	0	0	0	0	0	0
18:00-19:00	4710	62	80	116	1712	1712	0	0	0	71	65	2	0	1	0	0	0	0	0	0
19:00-20:00	4769	60	80	93	1756	1756	0	0	0	134	34	0	0	0	0	0	0	0	0	0
20:00-21:00	4216	59	71	90	1081	1081	0	0	0	32	28	2	0	1	0	0	0	0	0	0
21:00-22:00	4343	60	73	92	1112	1112	0	0	0	32	40	0	0	0	0	0	0	0	0	0
22:00-23:00	3705	50	63	83	245	245	0	0	0	5	7	0	0	0	0	0	0	0		
23:00-00:00	3374	50	57	87	24	24	0	0	0	0	0	0	0	0	0	0	0	0		
00:00-01:00	3520	50	59	82	95	95	0	0	0	0	1	0	0	0	0	0	0	0		
01:00-02:00	3650	52	61	89	188	188	0	0	0	0	1	0	0	0	0	0	0	0		
02:00-03:00	3960	54	67	90	409	409	0	0	0	4	3	0	0	0	0	0	0	0		

Figure 20.1   The summary page shows a maximum heart rate of 116 bpm after Propranolol and a minimum rate of 50 bpm. PVC burden is high 23385/24 hours (23.4%).

DOI: 10.1201/9781003545040-20

The maximum ST depression was -0.13 mm at 15:34 in channel CH3. The maximum ST elevation was 3.37 mm at 18:57 in channel CH1.

Rhythm results:
There were 0 pause intervals defined greater than 2400 ms.
Atrial Fibrillation was detected in 0.00% (0 h 00 min) of the total monitoring time.
Atrial flutter was detected in 0.13% (3 h 03 min) of the total monitoring time.

QT results:
The maximum QT interval was 440 ms (51 bpm) at 23:51, the maximum QTc interval was 516 ms (106 bpm) at 07:47.
The minimum QT interval was 336 ms (112 bpm) at 18:20, the minimum QTc interval was 370 ms (69 bpm) at 13:17.

TIME [hh:mm-hh:mm]	TOTAL BEATS	HEART RATE			VENTRICULAR							SUPRAVENTRICULAR							PAUSE	MARKED
		MIN	AVG	MAX	BEATS	SINGLE	CPL	RUN	TCH	BIG	TRIG	BEATS	SINGLE	CPL	RUN	TCH	BIG	TRIG		
17:48-18:00	830	60	77	92	306	306	0	0	0	9	15	0	0	0	0	0	0	0	0	0
18:00-19:00	4710	62	80	116	1712	1712	0	0	0	71	65	2	0	1	0	0	0	0	0	0
19:00-20:00	4769	60	80	93	1756	1756	0	0	0	134	34	0	0	0	0	0	0	0	0	0
20:00-21:00	4216	59	71	90	1081	1081	0	0	0	32	28	2	0	1	0	0	0	0	0	0
21:00-22:00	4343	60	73	92	1112	1112	0	0	0	32	40	0	0	0	0	0	0	0	0	0
22:00-23:00	3705	50	63	83	245	245	0	0	0	5	7	0	0	0	0	0	0	0	0	0
23:00-00:00	3374	50	57	87	24	24	0	0	0	0	0	0	0	0	0	0	0	0	0	0
00:00-01:00	3520	50	59	82	95	95	0	0	0	0	1	0	0	0	0	0	0	0	0	0
01:00-02:00	3650	52	61	89	188	188	0	0	0	0	1	0	0	0	0	0	0	0	0	0
02:00-03:00	3960	54	67	90	409	409	0	0	0	4	3	0	0	0	0	0	0	0	0	0
03:00-04:00	3748	51	63	86	311	311	0	0	0	1	1	0	0	0	0	0	0	0	0	0
04:00-05:00	4122	59	69	90	664	664	0	0	0	7	30	0	0	0	0	0	0	0	0	0
05:00-06:00	4404	62	74	97	861	861	0	0	0	28	34	0	0	0	0	0	0	0	0	0
06:00-07:00	4514	64	76	95	925	925	0	0	0	53	10	0	0	0	0	0	0	0	0	0
07:00-08:00	4581	59	77	113	1182	1182	0	0	0	63	33	1	1	0	0	0	0	0	0	0
08:00-09:00	4477	61	75	97	1260	1260	0	0	0	62	33	1	0	0	0	0	0	0	0	0
09:00-10:00	4659	61	78	100	1699	1699	0	0	0	83	49	1	1	0	0	0	0	0	0	0
10:00-11:00	4498	60	76	96	1609	1609	0	0	0	59	66	0	0	0	0	0	0	0	0	0
11:00-12:00	4631	61	78	104	1523	1523	0	0	0	63	15	1	1	0	0	0	0	0	0	0
12:00-13:00	4344	61	73	94	1211	1211	0	0	0	53	14	0	0	0	0	0	0	0	0	0
13:00-14:00	4265	58	72	94	948	948	0	0	0	50	21	0	0	0	0	0	0	0	0	0
14:00-15:00	4577	60	77	96	1108	1108	0	0	0	55	30	0	0	0	0	0	0	0	0	0
15:00-16:00	4507	64	76	96	1269	1269	0	0	0	64	14	0	0	0	0	0	0	0	0	0
16:00-17:00	4421	60	74	95	1510	1510	0	0	0	56	36	0	0	0	0	0	0	0	0	0
17:00-17:13	1037	66	76	86	377	377	0	0	0	20	6	0	0	0	0	0	0	0	0	0
Awake	69379	58	75	116	20588	20588	0	0	0	959	509	8	4	2	0	0	0	0	0	0
Asleep	30483	50	64	97	2797	2797	0	0	0	45	77	0	0	0	0	0	0	0	0	0
Total	99862	50	72	116	23385	23385	0	0	0	1004	586	8	4	2	0	0	0	0	0	0
Percentage (%)	100				23.42	100	0	0	0	51.52	12.64	0.01	50	50	0	0	0	0	0	0

Figure 20.2 The second part of the summary page shows the distribution of PVCs during 24 hours. There is a higher number of PVCs during the day than during the night.

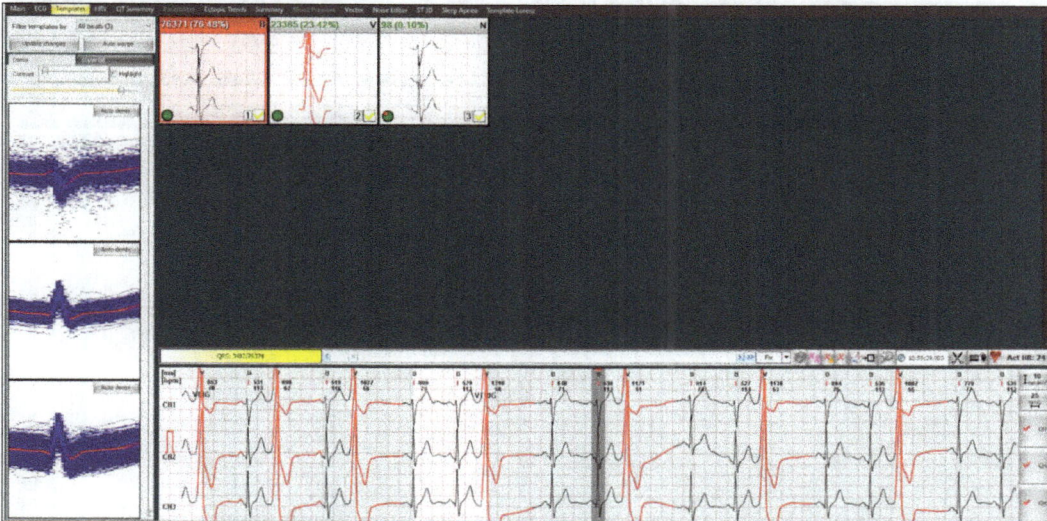

Figure 20.3 The template window shows a sinus beat that is marked with a B. We modified the category and labeled it N (=normal beat).

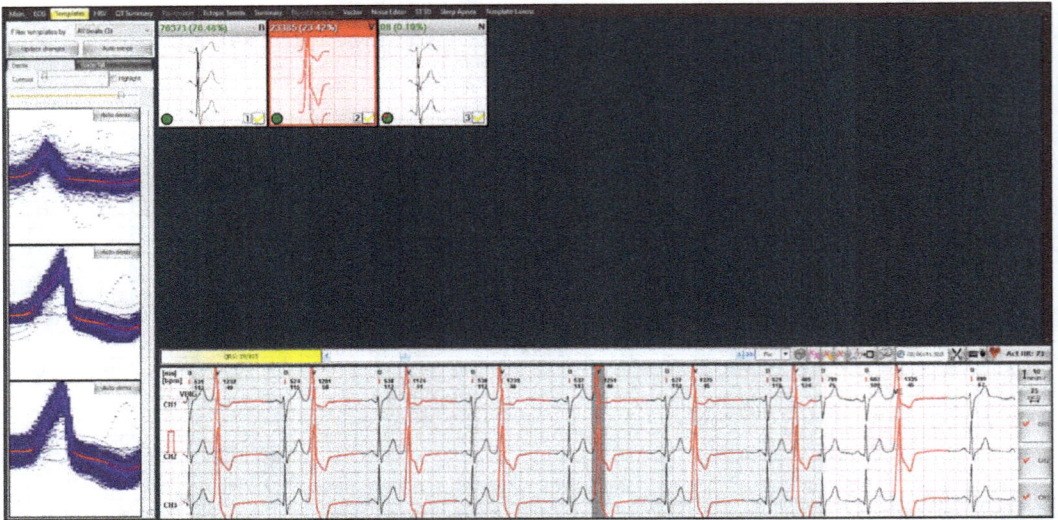

Figure 20.4 The template window shows a premature ventricular contractions, labeled with a V.

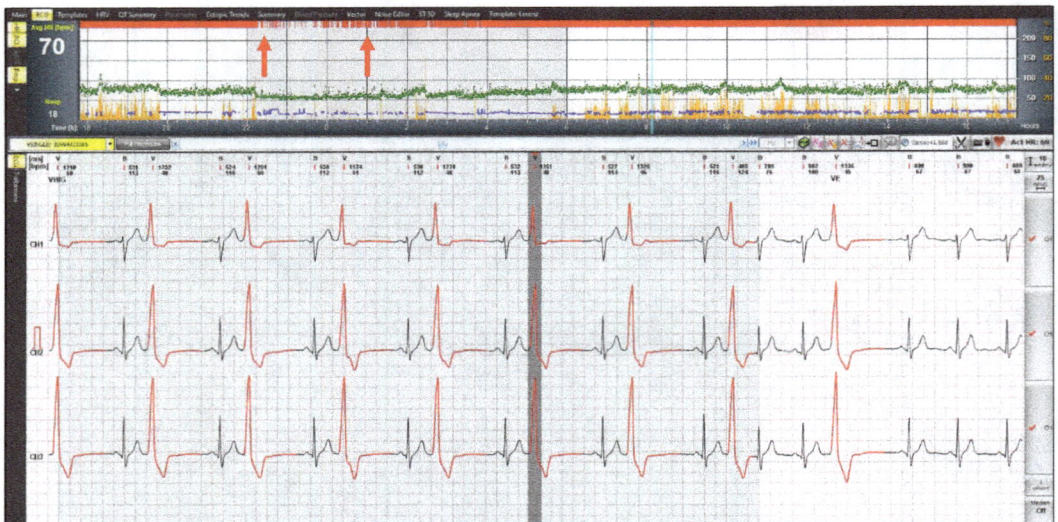

Figure 20.5 The figure shows ventricular bigeminy. Every second beat is a PVC. The upper red line and the arrows show the distribution of PVCs. The lowest number of PVCs were between 22:00 and 01:00.

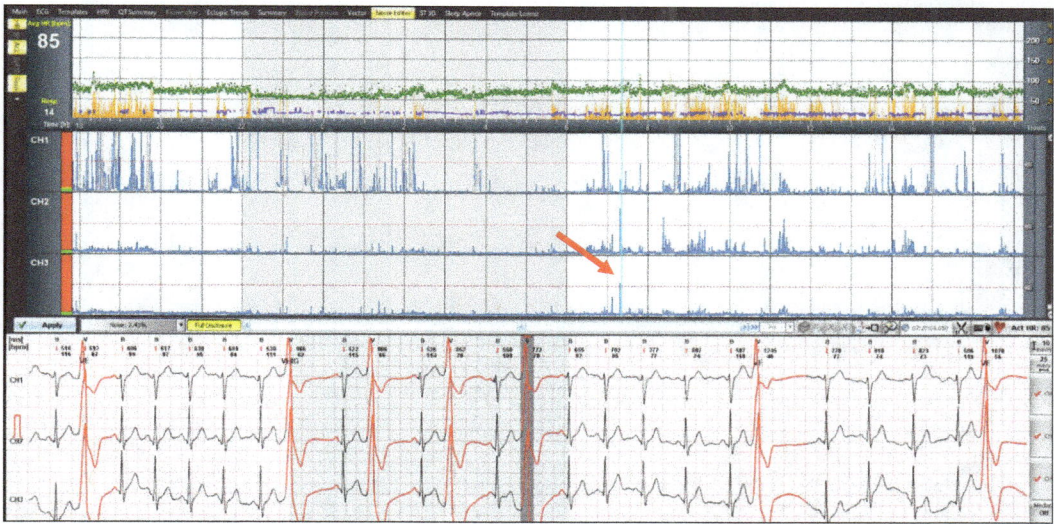

Figure 20.6 The noise window shows periods of recording with high and low electrical noise on channels CH1, CH2 and CH3. The red arrow marks a tracing with an acceptable electrical signal.

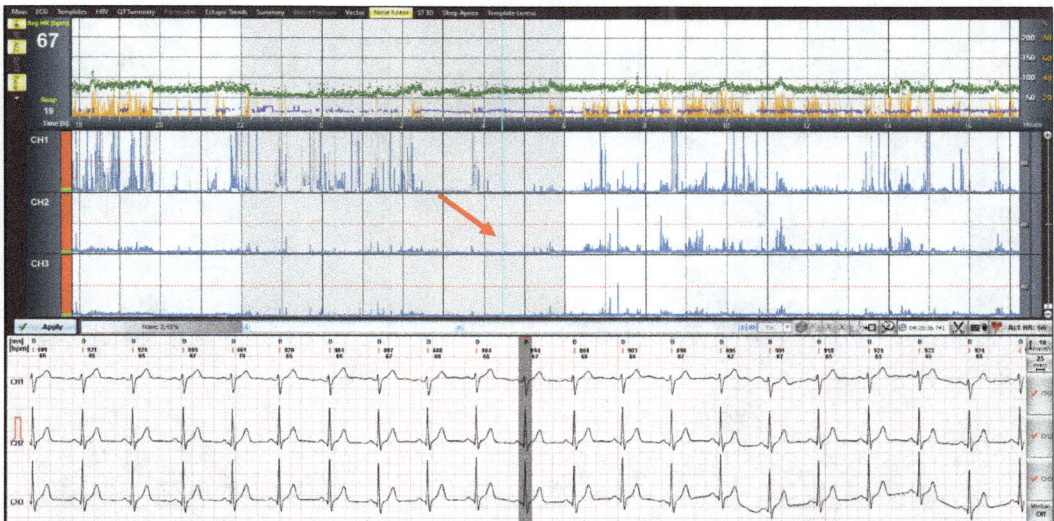

Figure 20.7 The noise window shows periods of recording with high and low electrical noise on channels CH1, CH2 and CH3. The red arrow marks a tracing with good electrical signal.

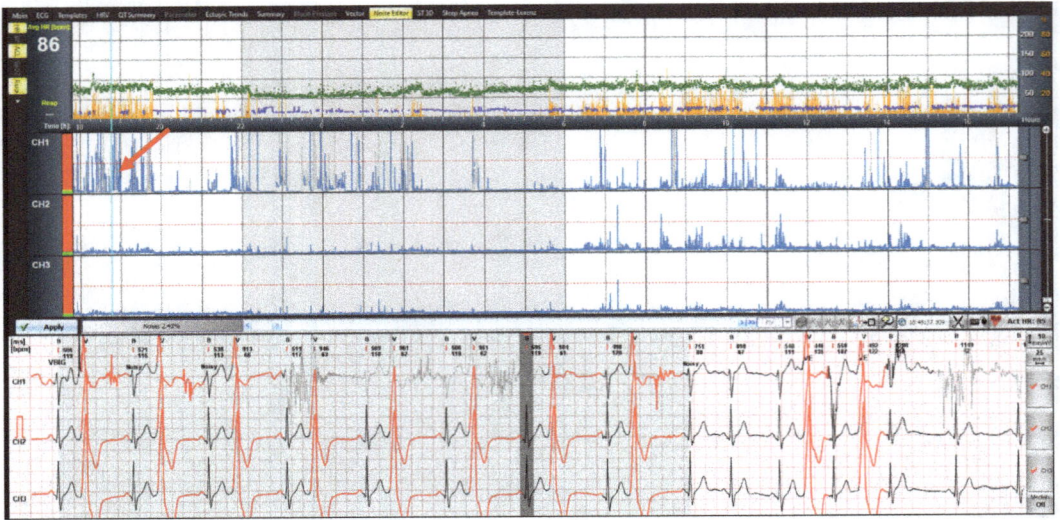

Figure 20.8 The noise window shows periods of recording with high and low electrical noise on channels CH1, CH2 and CH3. The red arrow marks a tracing with a bad signal on channel 1.

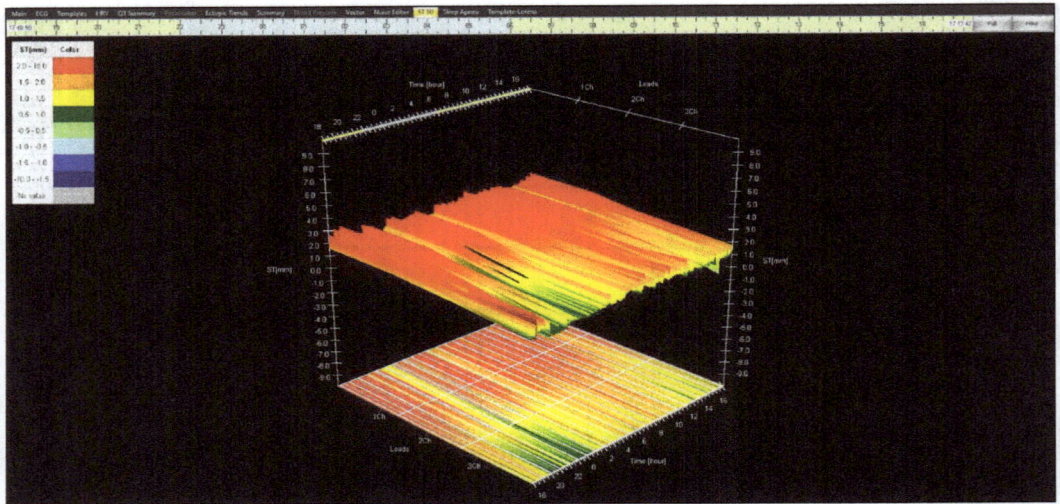

Figure 20.9 The ST segment window shows ST modifications during the recording period. The analysis of the ST segment is unreliable in the presence of numerous PVCs, as they are associated with ST segment alterations not linked to ischemia.

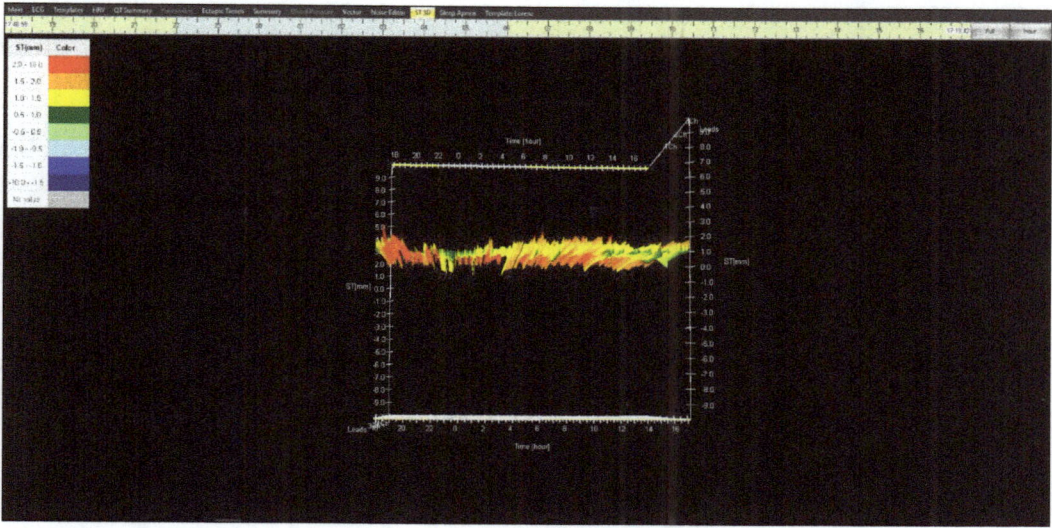

Figure 20.10 The ST segment window: frontal view. The analysis of the ST segment is unreliable in the presence of numerous PVCs, as they are associated with ST segment alterations not linked to ischemia.

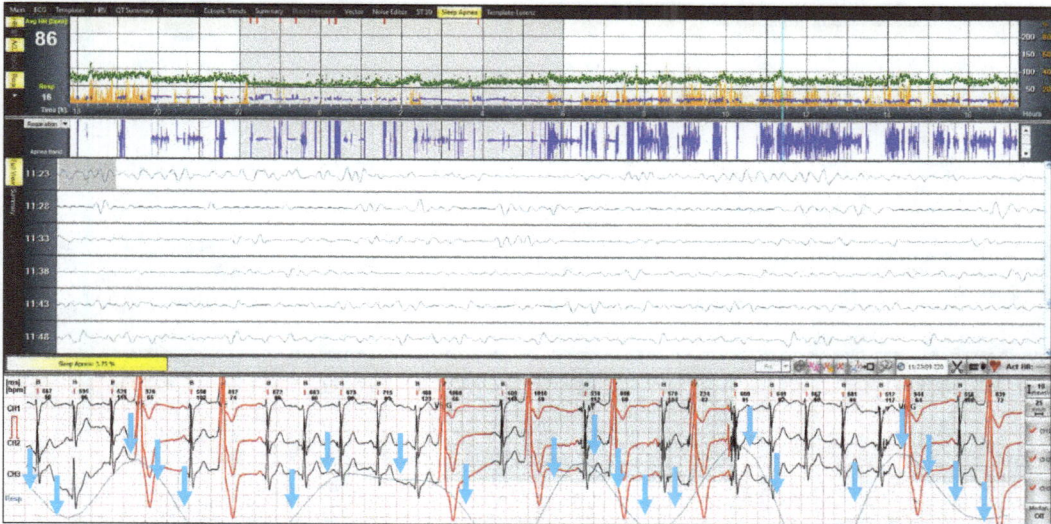

Figure 20.11 Sleep apnea window shows respiratory movements during daytime and nighttime. It is used to detect apnea episodes.

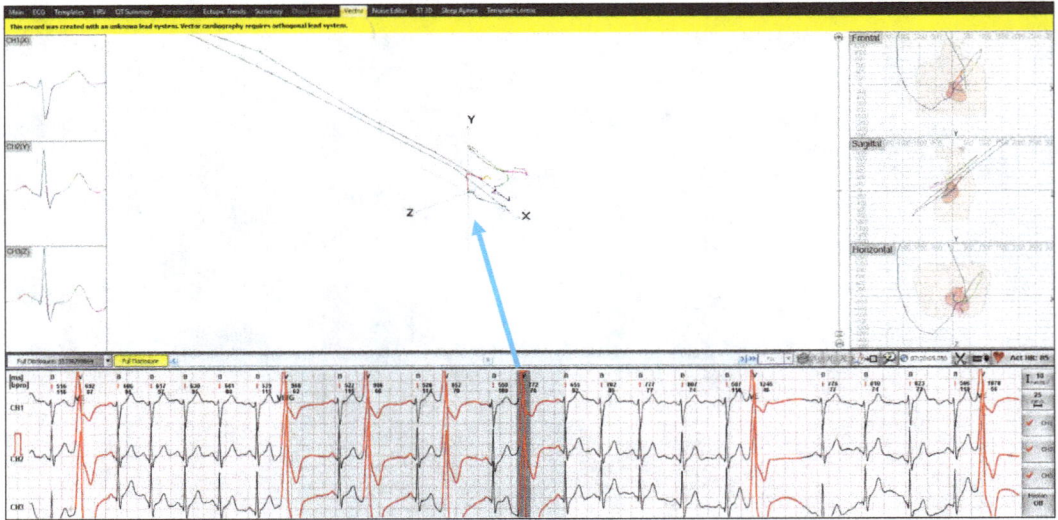

Figure 20.12 Vector window shows the QRS vector in the frontal, sagittal and horizontal plane. In this image the QRS vector is taken for PVCs.

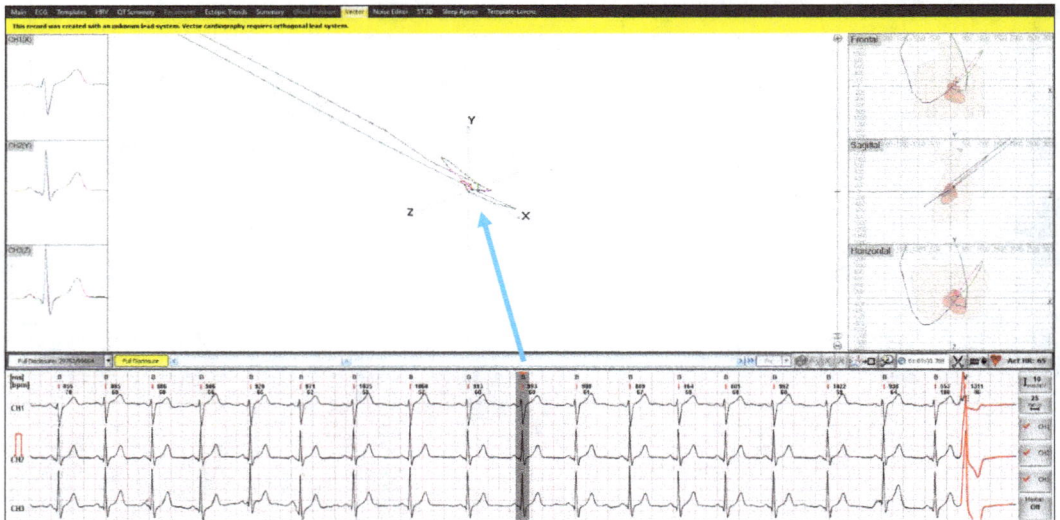

Figure 20.13 Vector window shows the QRS vector in the frontal, sagittal and horizontal plane. In this image the QRS vector is taken for a normal sinus beat.

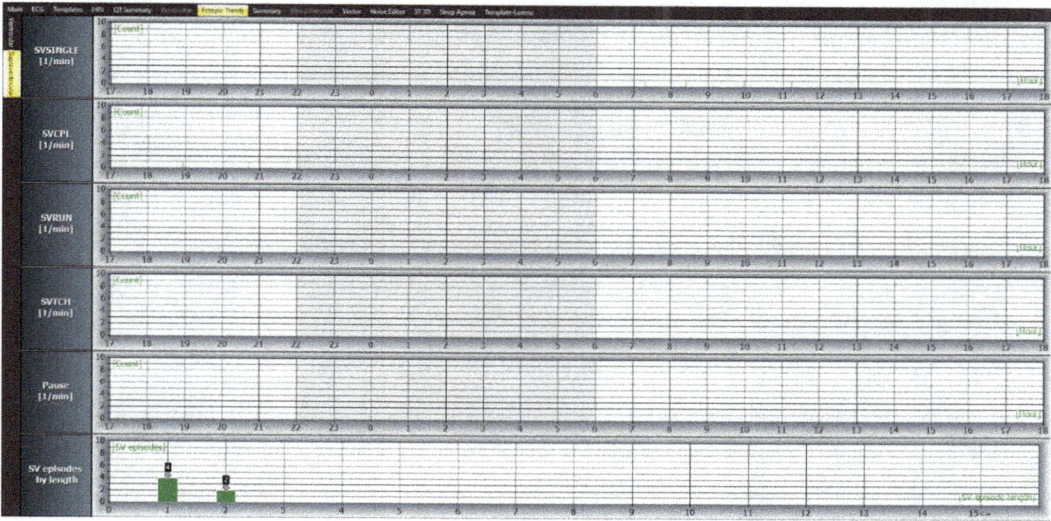

Figure 20.14 Supraventricular ectopic trend with 1 and 2 consecutive beats.

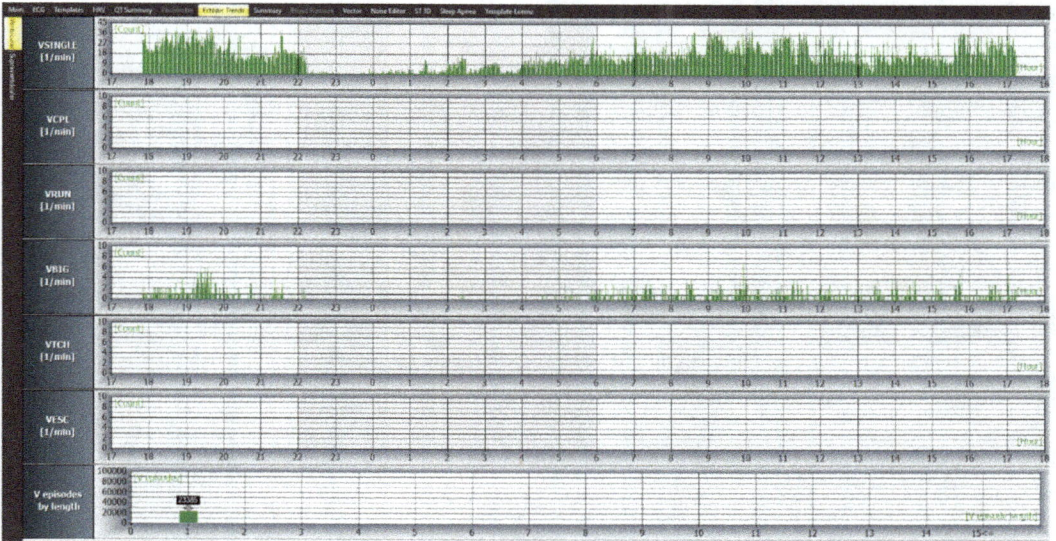

Figure 20.15 Ventricular ectopic trend with singular PVCs and the 24-hour distribution.

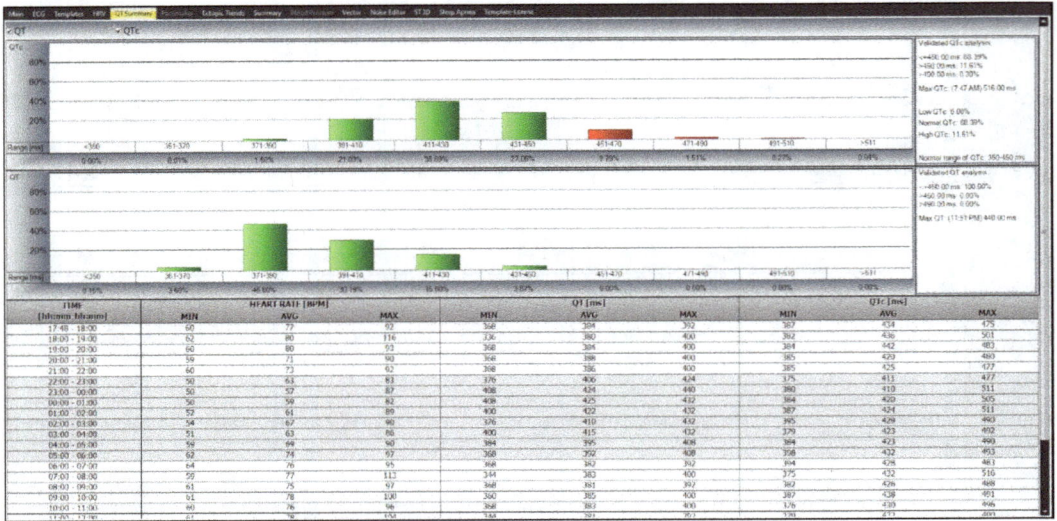

Figure 20.16 QT and QTc intervals. The measurements, however, are unreliable due to PVCs with prolonged QT.

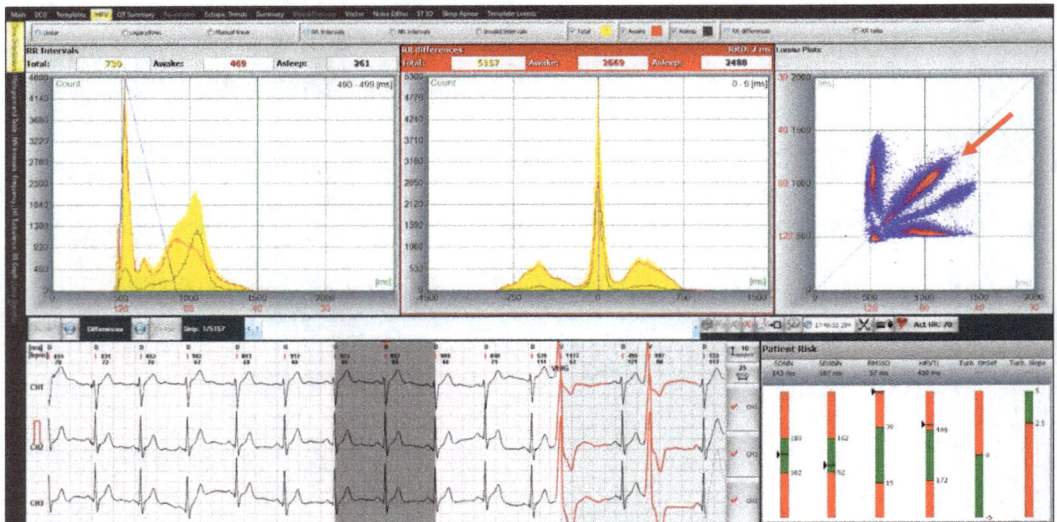

Figure 20.17 Heart rate variability with Lorenz Plots and Poincaré graphs. The red arrow indicates a point situated on the 45° line where the "n" and "n + 1" intervals are equal.

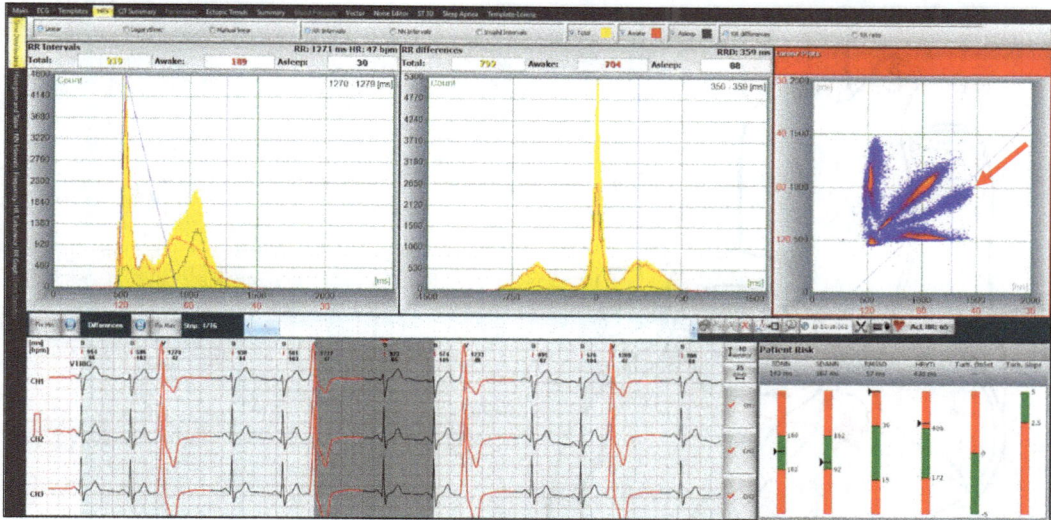

Figure 20.18 Heart rate variability with Lorenz Plots and Poincaré graphs. The red arrow indicates a point situated on the 35° line where the "n" is greater than the "n + 1" interval.

HOLTER SUMMARY

This Holter shows the result of treatment with Propranolol on PVC burden. There were 23385 PVCs /24 hours. The mean heart rate was 72 bpm, with a maximum of 116 and a minimum of 50 bpm. They were present both during the day and during the night; however, the daily burden was higher.

DISCUSSION

Ventricular premature contractions demonstrate significant diurnal variations. Circadian suscepti-bility to ventricular arrhythmias has been associated with multiple triggering pathways, including the autonomic nervous system. A circadian rhythm is a periodic fluctuation of a physiological process occurring throughout a 24-hour cycle. Numerous cardiovascular parameters, such as heart rate, heart rate variability, QT interval, and blood pressure, exhibit a pronounced circadian pattern. The RR interval lengthens at night, indicating a decrease of the heart rate. During nocturnal hours, there is a prolongation of the PR interval, QRS duration, and QT interval. This indicates reduced conduction across the atrioventricular node, His–Purkinje system, and decreased ventricular repolarization. Brugada syndrome and catecholaminergic polymorphic ventricular tachycardia exhibit a diurnal variation, with sudden arrhythmias being particularly prominent at night in Brugada syndrome and in the afternoon in CPVT.

It is documented that under pathological conditions, most ventricular arrhythmias are triggered or exacerbated by sympathetic stimulation or vagal withdrawal, while they are suppressed by increased vagal tone. Impaired vagal tone is associated with ventricular arrhythmias in post-infarction animals, and therapeutic interventions that reduce sympathetic tone, such as beta blockers, or improve vagal tone have been demonstrated to be protective against ventricular arrhythmias. Conversely, parasympathetic dysfunction has been linked to ventricular arrhythmias in patients with heart failure. Vagal nerve stimulation results in a quick reduction in the heart rate. The vagal nerve terminations generate acetylcholine, which attaches to M2 muscarinic receptors of the sinus node myocytes, activating the ACh-activated K+ current and inhibiting the funny current (If) and the L-type Ca2+ current. Conversely, activation of the sympathetic nervous system results in a rapid elevation of heart rate. Sympathetic nerve terminations release noradrenaline, which attaches to β-receptors on the sinus node myocytes, amplifying the If and ICa,L currents.

The exact mechanism through which autonomic system affects idiopathic ventricular arrhyth-mias is not completely understood. Sympathetic stimulation may increase the automaticity in ectopic foci and generate cAMP-mediated triggered activity, consequently inducing idiopathic PVCs.

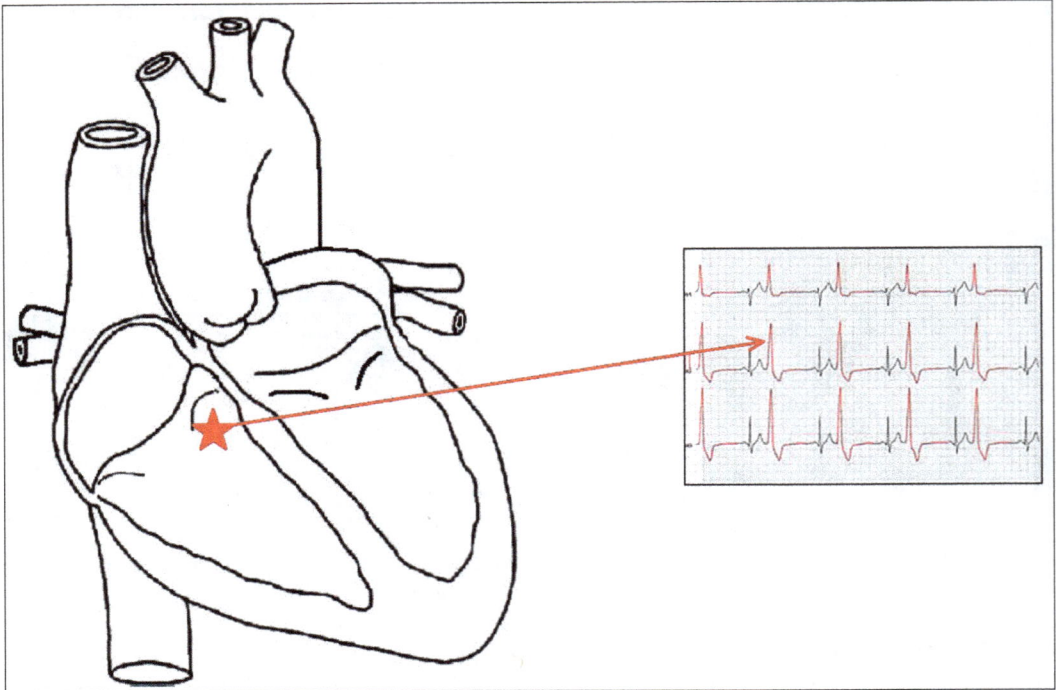

Figure 20.19 RVOT premature ventricular contractions have a specific QRS morphology, with superior axis, and precordial transition after V2. In Holter ECG, the three channels CH1, CH2 and CH3 cannot be used to differentiate between different types of PVCs as they are not standardized ECG leads.

BIBLIOGRAPHY

1. He W, Lu Z, Bao M, et al. Autonomic involvement in idiopathic premature ventricular contractions. *Clinical Research in Cardiology*. 2013; 102(5): 361–370. doi:10.1007/s00392-013-0545-6

2. Hamon D, Abehsira G, Gu K, et al. Circadian variability patterns predict and guide premature ventricular contraction ablation procedural inducibility and outcomes. *Heart Rhythm*. 2018; 15(1): 99–106. doi:10.1016/j.hrthm.2017.07.034

3. Jeyaraj D, Haldar SM, Wan X, et al. Circadian rhythms govern cardiac repolarization and arrhythmogenesis. *Nature*. 2012; 483(7387): 96–99. doi:10.1038/nature10852

4. Ruben MD, Wu G, Smith DF, et al. A database of tissue-specific rhythmically expressed human genes has potential applications in circadian medicine. *Science Translational Medicine*. 2018; 10(458) doi:10.1126/scitranslmed.aat8806

5. Yamashita T, Sekiguchi A, Iwasaki Y-K, et al. Circadian variation of cardiac K+ channel gene expression. *Circulation*. 2003; 107(14): 1917–1922. doi:10.1161/01.CIR.0000058752.79734.F0

6. Schroder EA, Burgess DE, Zhang X, et al. The cardiomyocyte molecular clock regulates the circadian expression of Kcnh2 and contributes to ventricular repolarization. *Heart Rhythm*. 2015; 12(6): 1306–1314. doi:10.1016/j.hrthm.2015.02.019

7. Black N, D'Souza A, Wang Y, et al. Circadian rhythm of cardiac electrophysiology, arrhythmogenesis, and the underlying mechanisms. *Heart Rhythm*. 2019; 16(2): 298–307. doi:10.1016/j.hrthm.2018.08.026

8. Patton KK, Hellkamp AS, Lee KL, et al. Unexpected deviation in circadian variation of ventricular arrhythmias. *Journal of the American College of Cardiology*. 2014; 63(24): 2702–2708. doi:10.1016/j.jacc.2013.11.072

9. Miyake CY, Asaki SY, Webster G, et al. Circadian variation of ventricular arrhythmias in catecholaminergic polymorphic ventricular tachycardia. *JACC: Clinical Electrophysiology*. 2017; 3(11): 1308–1317. doi:10.1016/j.jacep.2017.05.004

10. Matsuo K, Kurita T, Inagaki M, et al. The circadian pattern of the development of ventricular fibrillation in patients with Brugada syndrome. *European Heart Journal*. 1999; 20(6): 465–470. doi:10.1053/euhj.1998.1332

11. Bonnemeier H, Wiegand UK, Braasch W, Brandes A, Richardt G, Potratz J. Circadian profile of QT interval and QT interval variability in 172 healthy volunteers. *Pacing and Clinical Electrophysiology*. 2003; 26: 377–382. doi:10.1046/j.1460-9592.2003.00053.x

12. Martino T, Arab S, Straume M, Belsham DD, Tata N, Cai F, Liu P, Trivieri M, Ralph M, Sole MJ. Day/night rhythms in gene expression of the normal murine heart. *Journal of Molecular Medicine*. 2004; 82: 256–264. doi:10.1007/s00109-003-0520-1

13. Durgan DJ, Young ME. The cardiomyocyte circadian clock: Emerging roles in health and disease. *Circulation Research*. 2010; 106: 647–658. doi:10.1161/CIRCRESAHA.109.209957

14. Portaluppi F, Hermida RC. Circadian rhythms in cardiac arrhythmias and opportunities for their chronotherapy. *Advanced Drug Delivery Reviews*. 2007; 59: 940–951. doi:10.1016/j.addr.2006.10.011

15. Przybylski R, Meziab O, Gauvreau K, Dionne A, DeWitt ES, Bezzerides VJ, Abrams DJ. Premature ventricular contractions in children and young adults: Natural history and clinical implications. *Europace*. 2024 Mar. 1; 26(3): euae052. doi: 10.1093/europace/euae052. PMID: 38441283; PMCID: PMC10927167.

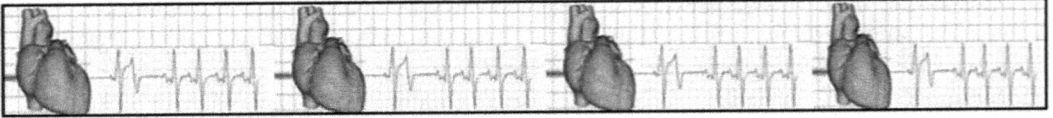

Case 21 PVCs in a Neonate

Sorin Andreica, Camelia Vidrea, Raluca Hudrea, and Delia Ghinga

CLINICAL CASE

A male baby was born at term by vaginal delivery. His Apgar score was 10 (1 min)/10 (5 min) and no irregular beats were heard on cardiac examination. However in the neonatal department the nurse noted irregular heartbeats and monitoring of the patient revealed premature ventricular contractions. Echocardiography was normal with a patent ductus arteriosus and a patent foramen ovale, which were normal for his age. Holter ECG revealed high burden premature ventricular contractions.

Concluzie

Ritm cardiac		
Total bătăi	173 455	(0% paced)
HR max / min	**210 / 79 bpm**	
Media HR	**Ø 135 bpm**	
HR Max / Min Sinus	210 / 91 bpm	
Media HR (Treaz/Adormit)	136 / 132 bpm	
Index circadian	1,03	
Tahicardie / Bradicardie	2 % / 44 %	

Pauze	
RR Max	**1 932 ms**
Pauze (>2000ms)	0

Fibrilație atrială / Flutter atrial	
Total AF	-
AF HR Max	0 bpm
Cel mai lung AF	-

Bradicardie		
Cea mai mică	Ø 79 bpm	6 sec
Cea mai mare	Ø 120 bpm	01:46:31

ST		
St ridicare max	0,50 mV	V4
ST depresurizare max	-0,38 mV	V1

Ectopie ventriculară		
V Total	32327	(19%)
V / Ora Max	2 606	pe oră
Episoade Tahicardie V	32 Σ 00:02:17	
Cea mai rapidă Tahicardie V	Ø - bpm	5 sec
V Cea mai lungă secvență	Ø 83 bpm	00:01:19
Triplete / Execută	0 Σ 0 bătăi	
Cuplete	598 Σ 1196 bătăi	
Bigeminism	2925 Σ 13176 bătăi	
Trigeminism	1041 Σ 2428 bătăi	

Ectopie supraventriculară		
S Tot	0	(< 1%)
Episoade Tahicardie SV	-	
Cea mai rapidă Tahicardie SV	-	
S Cea mai lungă secvență	-	
Triplete / Execută	-	
Cuplete	0 Σ 0 bătăi	

Figure 21.1 The summary page shows a maximum heart rate of 210 bpm and a minimum rate of 79 bpm. The PVC burden in high: 19% on 24 hours with episodes of bigeminy, trigeminy, couplets. The longest VT episode had 5 seconds duration. The longest recorder pause was 1.9 seconds.

DOI: 10.1201/9781003545040-21

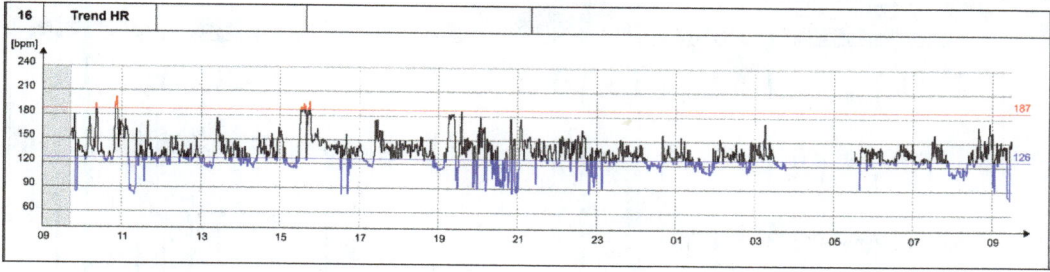

Figure 21.2 The heart rate histogram shows average rates between 90 and 180 bpm with several episodes of tachycardia.

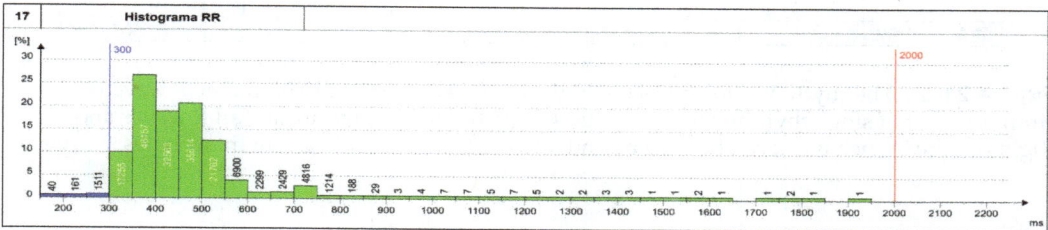

Figure 21.3 The RR histogram shows short RR intervals < 300 ms marked with blue color, and mean RR intervals 300 to 2000 ms marked with green color. There is no long interval above 2000 ms.

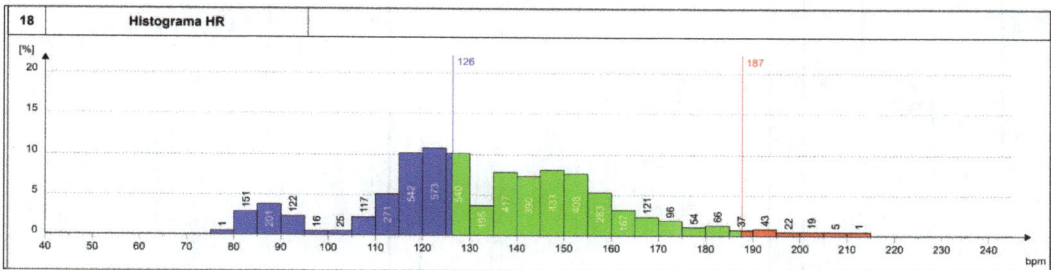

Figure 21.4 The HR histogram shows 3 types of rates: low< 128bpm with blue color, mean 128–187 bpm marked with green color and high >187 bpm marked with red color.

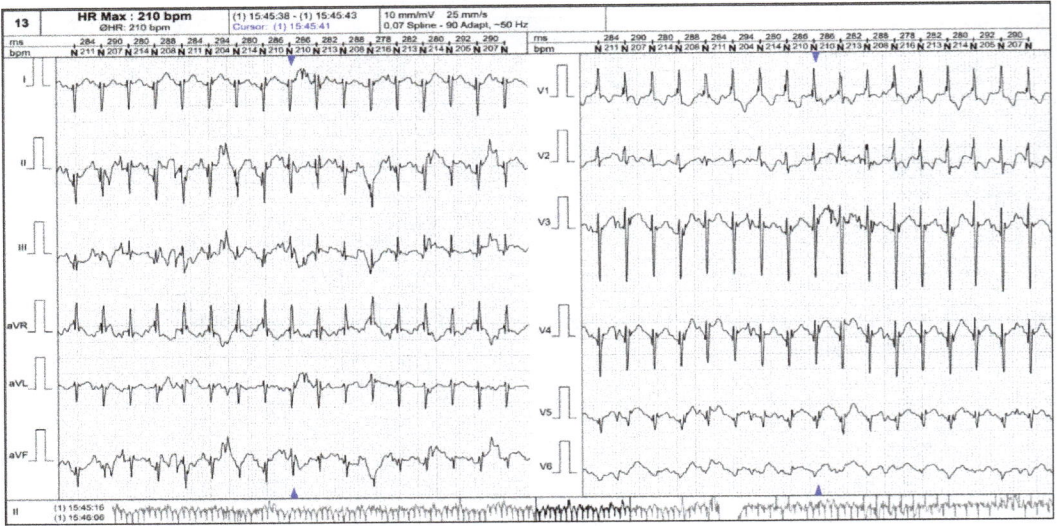

Figure 21.5   The rhythm strip shows the highest rate recorded of 210 bpm. The P wave is similar to that of sinus rhythm; therefore, this should be sinus tachycardia. Tall R waves and Right bundle branch block can be seen in lead V1 which is a normal variant in neonates.

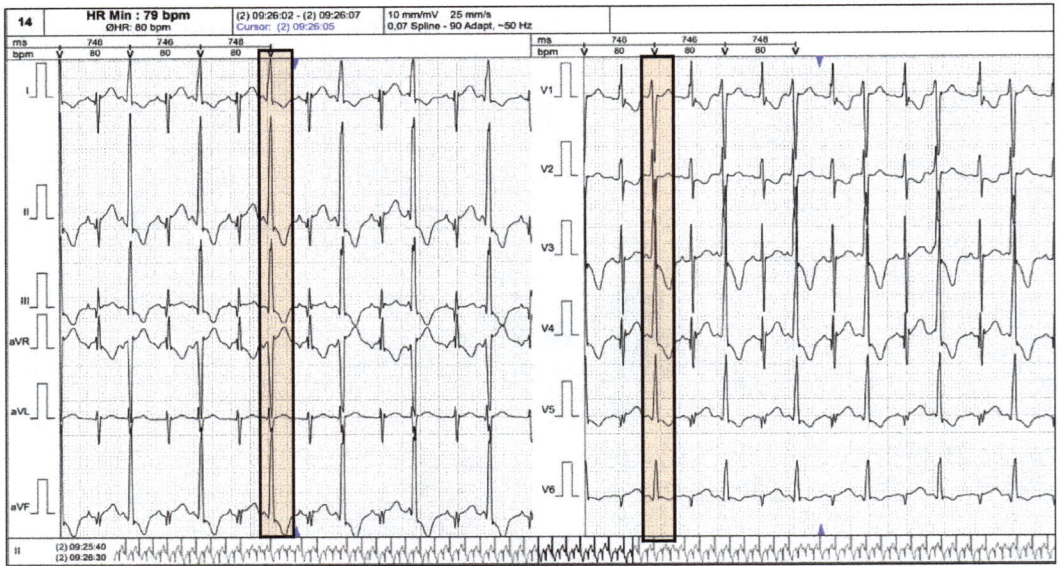

Figure 21.6   The tracing shows the lowest recorded rate of 79 bpm. The rhythm strip shows ventricular bigeminy: every second beat is a premature ventricular contraction; PVCs have a left bundle branch block morphology with inferior axis, suggesting an RVOT origin. However, the heart rate is double: 158 bpm because only the second beat is counted by the software.

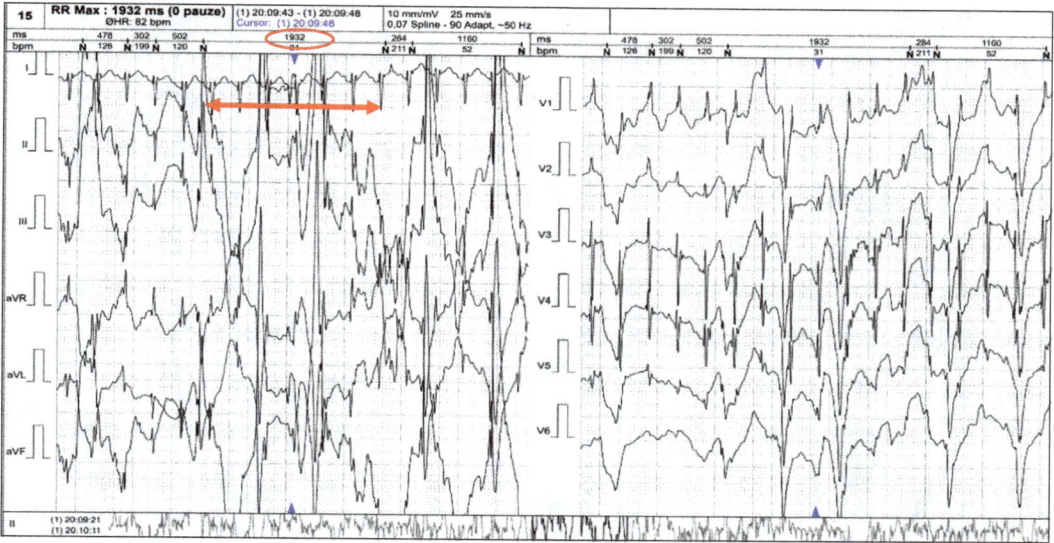

Figure 21.7 The rhythm strip shows the longest recorded pause of 1.932 seconds, which is obviously an artifact due poor electrical contact to seen in all precordial and limb leads.

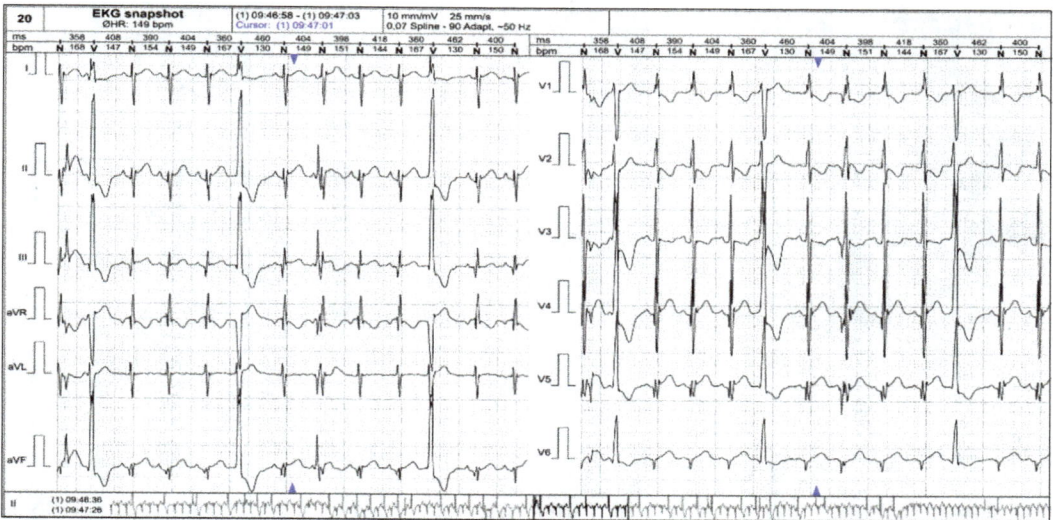

Figure 21.8 The rhythm strip shows ventricular quadrigeminy (characterized by every fourth beat being a premature ventricular contraction) and pentageminy (which has a premature beat every fifth beat).

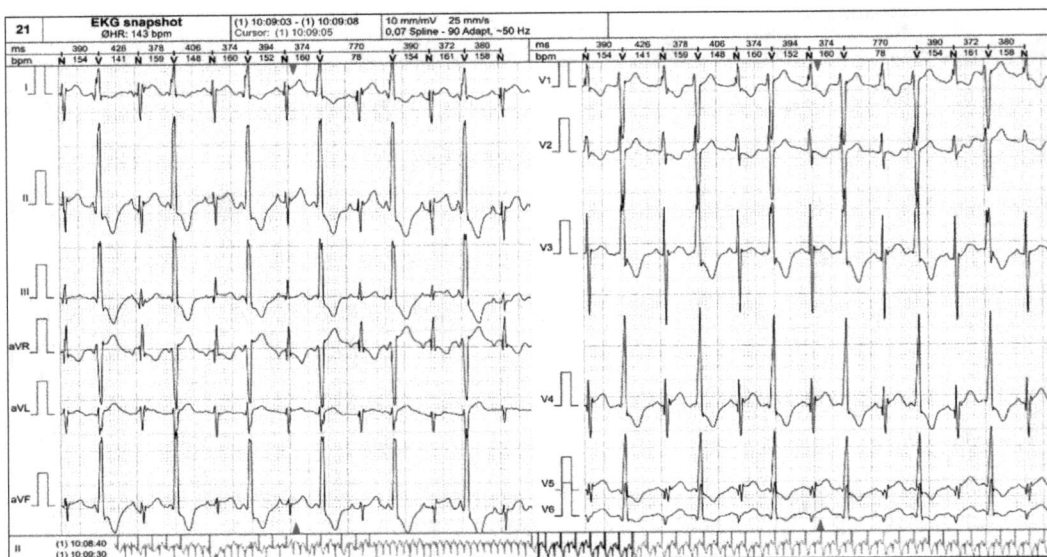

Figure 21.9 The rhythm strip shows ventricular bigeminy: every second beat is a premature ventricular contraction; PVCs have a left bundle branch block morphology with inferior axis, suggesting an RVOT origin. This is an example of late PVCs occurring after the preceding P wave.

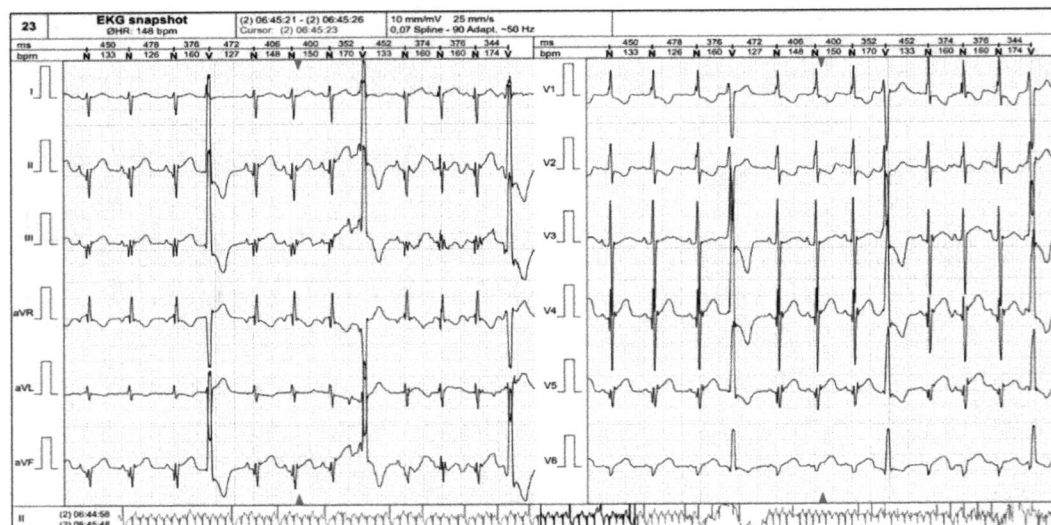

Figure 21.10 The rhythm strip shows ventricular quadrigeminy, with every fourth beat being a premature ventricular contraction.

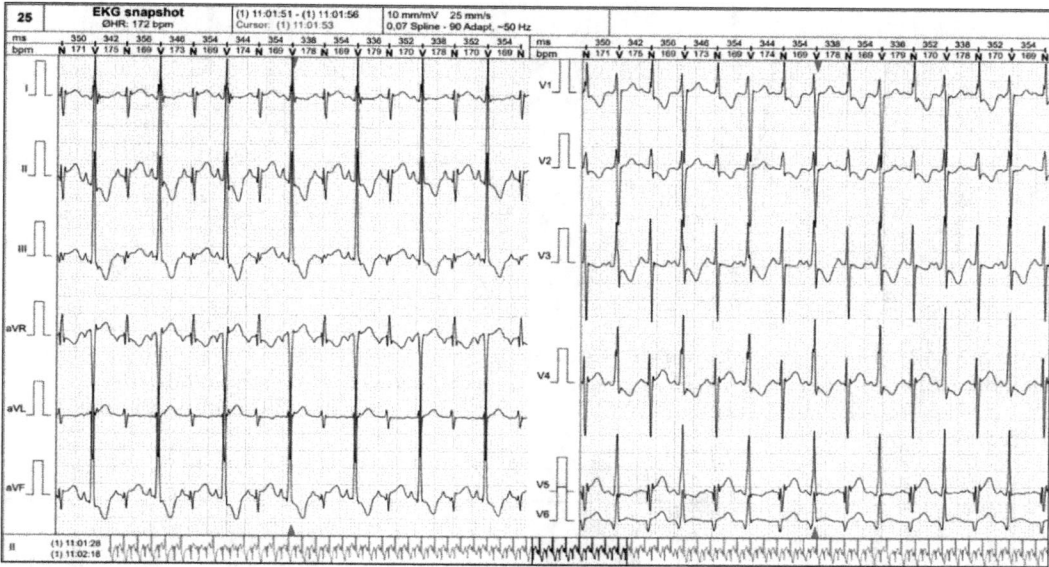

Figure 21.11 The rhythm strip shows ventricular bigeminy with PVCs occurring after the preceding P wave a pattern that should be differentiated from ventricular preexcitation.

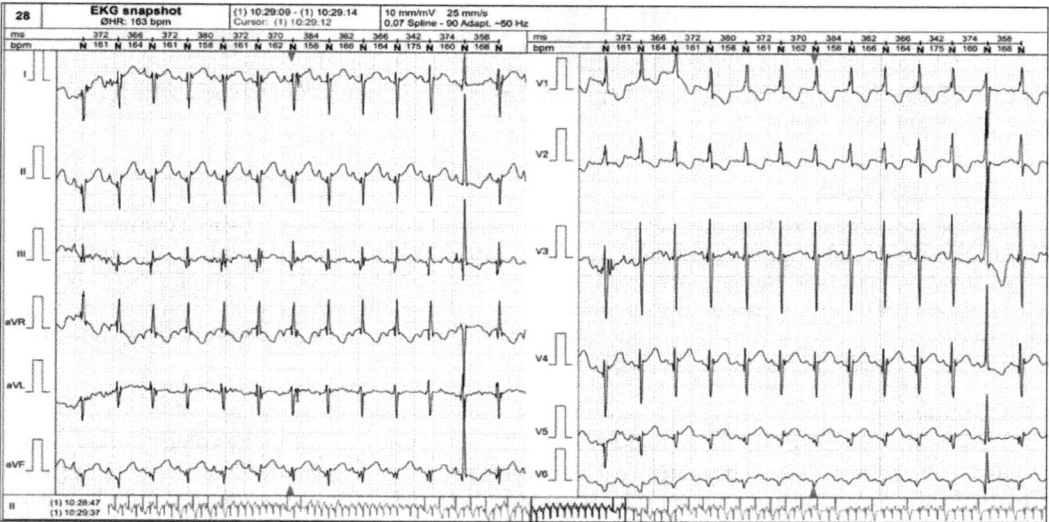

Figure 21.12 The rhythm strip shows one premature ventricular contraction.

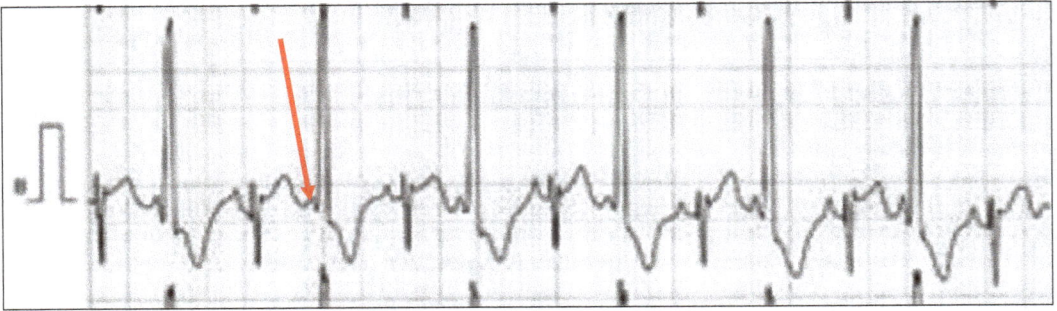

Figure 21.13 The tracing shows late PVCs occurring after the preceding P wave. This pattern should be differentiated from a WPW pattern. However previous rhythm strips showed no relationship between the P waves and PVCs. Red arrow shows that the PVC occurs after the preceding P wave.

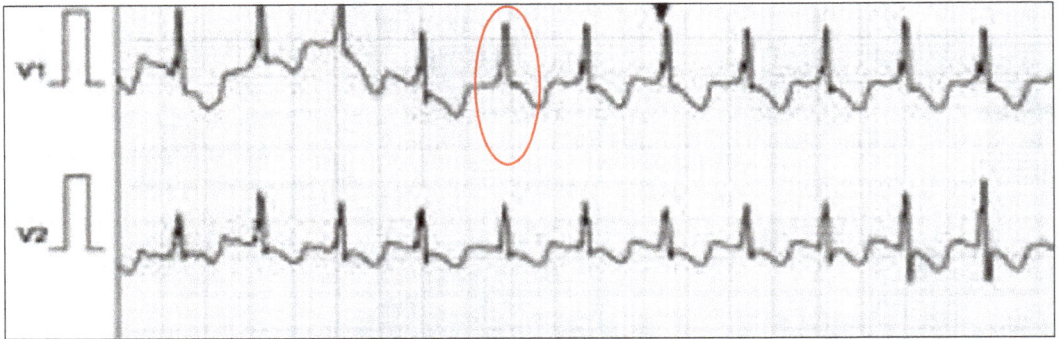

Figure 21.14 During sinus rhythm the patient has a right bundle branch block, which is a normal variant in neonates.

HOLTER SUMMARY

During the monitoring period the maximum heart rate was 210 bpm during sinus tachycardia. The minimum rate of 79 bpm is incorrect as the rhythm was ventricular bigeminy and only the second beat was counted by the software. The newborn had a high PVC burden of 19 %/24 hours with episodes of bigeminy, trigeminy, quadrigeminy and pentageminy. The PVC morphology suggest origin in the right ventricular outflow tract. The longest reported pause of 1.9 seconds is incorrect as it resulted from electrical artifacts.

DISCUSSION

PVCs are frequently reported in neonates in up to 20% of cases. The pathophysiology of neonatal PVCs is believed to be due to immature cardiac conduction tissue and autonomic nervous system growth. With advancing age, they tend to disappear. They may rarely be associated with hypokalemia, acidemia, hypoxemia, myocarditis, and the maternal consumption of caffeine and nicotine, which are excreted in breast milk. Almost always PVCs are benign in neonates. They are usually discovered "by chance" on the monitoring of the newborn. In case of high burden PVCs > 24 %/24 hours, an echocardiogram should be performed for the dimensions and the systolic function of the left ventricle.

PVCs generally have a larger QRS complex; however, in neonates, they may present as narrow, complicating the differentiation from supraventricular premature beats.

PVCs can occur in specific patterns:

- pairs or couplets when 2 sequential PVCs occur

- runs: 3 or more PVCs also known as ventricular tachycardia if rate above 120 bpm

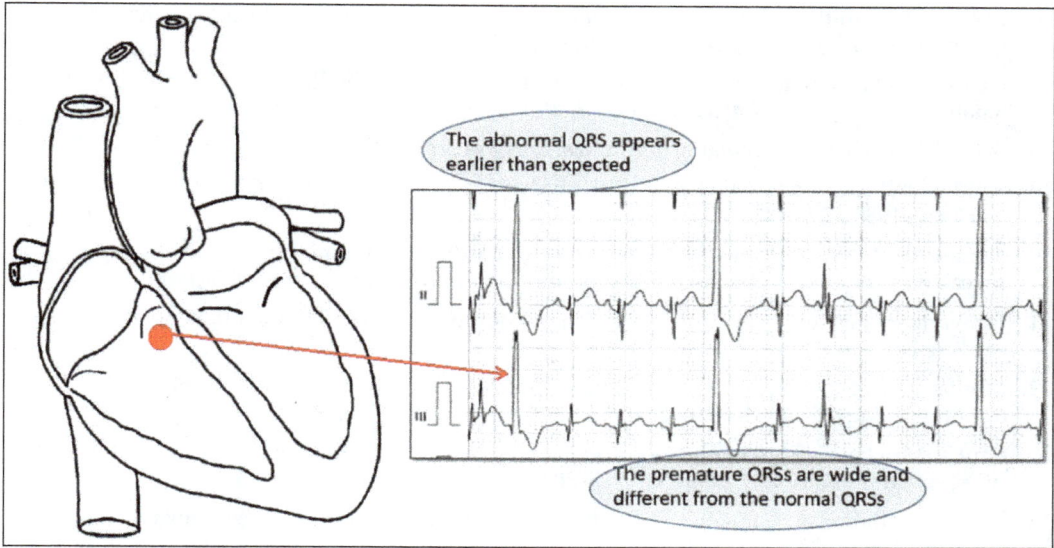

Figure 21.15 Premature ventricular contractions originate in the ventricular myocardium and give abnormal QRS complexes that occur earlier than the following sinus beat. The QRS is wide and different from the normal QRS complexes. Following the abnormal beat there is a pause, followed by a normal sinus beat. The T wave is also abnormal, opposite to the normal QRS complex.

- bigeminy: Every other beat is a PVC
- trigeminy: every third beat is a PVC
- quadrigeminy: every fourth beat is a PVC
- pentageminy: every fifth beat is a PVC.

Treatment of ventricular premature beats in neonates is not often indicated. If a drug is to be given it may be preferable to start with a beta blocker such as Propranolol rather than more effective drugs such as Amiodarone or class I antiarrhythmics: Flecainide.

De Rosa et al. evaluated 16 newborns with ventricular arrhythmias: PVCs, couplets and ventricular tachycardia with a follow-up at 1, 3, 6 and 12 months and yearly afterwards. Six of the patients had a LBBB morphology and 10 of the patients had an RBBB morphology. The PVC burden was 8000/24 hours in the PVC group, 53000/24 hours in the couplets group and 40000/24 hours in the VT group. In the PVC group, all PVCs disappeared at a mean age of 2.1 months, in the couplets group PVCs disappeared at a mean age of 6.5 months and in the VT group, PVCs disappeared at a mean age of 1.7 months.

BIBLIOGRAPHY

1. De Rosa G, Butera G, Chessa M, et al. Outcome of newborns with asymptomatic monomorphic ventricular arrhythmia. *Arch Dis Child Fetal Neonatal Ed* 2006;91:F419–F422.

2. Jaeggi E, Öhman A. Fetal and neonatal arrhythmias. *Clin Perinatol* 2016;43:99–112. doi:10.1016/j.clp.2015.11.007

3. Tsuji A, Nagashima M, Hasegawa S, et al. Long-term follow-up of idiopathic ventricular arrhythmias in otherwise normal children. *Jpn Circ J* 1995;59:654–662. doi:10.1253/jcj.59.654

4. Saudubray JM, Garcia-Cazorla À. Inborn errors of metabolism overview: pathophysiology, manifestations evaluation, and management. *Pediatr Clin North Am* 2018;65:179–208.

5. Ban JE. Neonatal arrhythmias: diagnosis, treatment, and clinical outcome. *Korean J Pediatr* 2017;60:344. doi:10.3345/kjp.2017.60.11.344

6. Benson DW, Smith WM, Dunnigan A, et al. Mechanism of regular, wide QRS tachycardia in infants and children. *Am J Cardiol* 1982 May 1;49(7):1778–1788.

7. Hamilton RM, Gow RM. Disorders of heart rate and rhythm. In: Freedom RM, Benson LN, Smallhorn JF, eds. *Neonatal heart disease*. Berlin: Springer Verlag, 1992777–1992805.

8. Batra A, Silka MJ. Ventricular arrhythmias. *Prog Pediatr Cardiol* 2000;11:39–45.

9. Southall DP, Richards J, Mitchell P, et al. Study of cardiac rhythm in healthy newborn infants. *Br Heart J* 1980;43:14–20.

10. Nagashima M, Matsushima M, Ogawa A, et al. Cardiac arrhythmias in healthy children revealed by 24-hour ambulatory ECG monitoring. *Pediatr Cardiol* 1987;8:103–108.

11. Schwartz PJ, Garson A, Jr, Paul T, et al. Guidelines for the interpretation of the neonatal electrocardiogram. *Eur Heart J* 2002;23:329–344.

12. Montague TJ, McPherson DD, MacKenzie BR, et al. Frequent ventricular ectopic activity without underlying cardiac disease: analysis of 45 subjects. *Am J Cardiol* 1983;52:980–984.

13. Paul T, Marchal C, Garson A., Jr. Ventricular couplets in the young: prognosis related to underlying substrate. *Am Heart J* 1990;119:577–582.

14. Waldo AL, Biblo LA, Carlson MD. Ventricular arrhythmias in perspective: a current view. *Am Heart J* 1992;123:1140–1147.

15. Pfammater J P, Paul T. Idiopathic ventricular tachycardia in infancy and childhood: a multicenter study on clinical profile and outcome. *J Am Coll Cardiol* 1999;33:2067–2072.

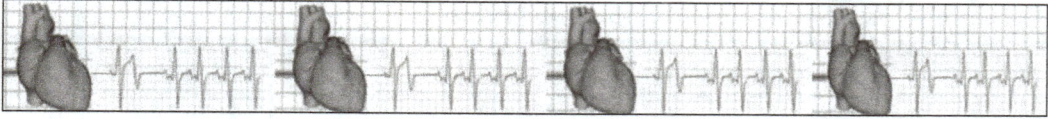

Case 22 Incessant Focal Atrial Tachycardia Originating from the Crista Terminalis

Lucian Muresan

CLINICAL CASE

A 16-year-old male adolescent with no past medical history undergoes a 24-hour Holter ECG monitoring because of a suspicion of a cardiac arrhythmia. He had presented to the Emergency Department a few days prior complaining of pre-syncope occurring at rest, light-headedness and an unusual state of fatigue, that had occurred after an intense physical effort (cycling for several hours). There was no associated chest pain, palpitations, or dyspnea. There was no history of sudden cardiac death in his family. He was on no chronic medication at home, and he denied any illicit drug use or alcohol consumption. An ECG recorded at admittance to the Emergency Department demonstrated an irregular rhythm with a variable heart rate (between 38 and 100 bpm) and the patient was transferred to the Cardiology Department. At physical examination, his blood pressure was 121/78 mmHg, his heart rhythm was irregular, his heart rate varied between 42 and 100 bpm, his SpO2 was 99–100% breathing room air, his height was 165 cm, his weight was 85 kg, BMI = 31.22 kg/m², there were no audible murmurs, lung auscultation was unremarkable, and there were no signs of left or right heart failure. A transthoracic echocardiography was performed, which found no argument in favor of a structural heart disease. Blood workup was unremarkable. A 24-hour Holter ECG was performed, and the results are presented in Figures 22.1–22.5.

Figure 22.1 The summary of the 24-hour Holter ECG showing the presence of a total of 102753 QRS complexes, of which 51496 are labeled "Premature atrial contractions" (red rectangle in the left lower corner of the image). There were also 9 pauses recorded (red rectangle in the center of the image), of which 2 were of a duration of more than 3 seconds. The average heart rate recorded was 73 bpm, the highest heart rate was 142 bpm, and the lowest heart rate was 23 bpm.

DOI: 10.1201/9781003545040-22

Heure hh:mn	Temps Anal. (mn)	Nb. total de QRS	Fréq.cardiaque (bpm) Moyenne	Min	Max	Pause	Période Longue	ESSV Isolée	Doublet	Salve	Total	ESV Isolée	Doublet	Salve	Total
(1)13:07	57	5335	93	40	127	0	144	0	33	216	1622	0	0	0	0
(1)14:07	59	4755	80	41	128	0	107	0	29	295	2200	0	0	0	0
(1)15:07	58	4885	83	43	135	0	85	0	12	324	2334	0	0	0	0
(1)16:07	59	4463	75	39	113	0	87	0	13	400	2583	0	0	0	0
(1)17:07	59	4567	76	40	127	0	17	0	19	405	2394	0	0	0	0
(1)18:07	59	4725	80	39	140	0	191	0	27	246	1627	0	0	0	0
(1)19:07	58	4902	83	38	142	0	69	0	30	298	2021	0	0	0	0
(1)20:07	57	4502	78	38	141	0	86	0	29	313	2002	0	0	0	0
(1)21:07	58	4417	75	44	113	0	10	0	28	457	2501	0	0	0	0
(1)22:07	59	4427	74	38	114	0	65	0	25	418	2366	0	0	0	0
(1)23:07	59	4306	72	37	111	0	46	0	39	416	2452	0	0	0	0
(1)00:07	59	4228	70	37	117	0	16	0	17	368	2160	0	0	0	0
(1)01:07	59	4081	68	35	104	0	11	0	12	431	2475	0	0	0	0
(1)02:07	59	3801	64	33	106	0	159	0	20	347	1997	0	0	0	0
(1)03:07	59	3801	63	39	100	0	1	0	39	390	2113	0	0	0	0
(1)04:07	59	3994	66	38	102	0	4	0	29	352	2084	0	0	0	0
(1)05:07	59	4073	68	37	110	0	40	0	15	376	2299	0	0	0	0
(1)06:07	55	3703	66	37	102	0	18	0	14	311	2139	0	0	0	0
(1)07:07	59	4095	68	26	110	4	66	0	13	301	2288	0	0	0	0
(1)08:07	59	3935	65	34	112	0	19	0	12	355	2192	0	0	0	0
(1)09:07	59	3920	65	23	106	5	26	0	10	275	1861	0	0	0	0
(1)10:07	59	4139	69	35	113	0	131	0	16	313	2232	0	0	0	0
(1)11:07	59	4433	74	35	127	0	57	0	28	273	1905	0	0	0	0
(1)12:07	44	3266	73	37	123	0	13	0	17	270	1649	0	0	0	0
Total	23:23	102753	72	23	142	9	1468	0	526	8150	51496	0	0	0	0

Figure 22.2 Hourly distribution of all premature atrial contractions recorded, ranging from 1622/hour to 2583/hour, for a total of 51496 over 23 hours and 23 minutes ("ESSV" column, red rectangle). There were also 9 pauses longer than 2.5 seconds recorded, with 1468 pauses of less than 2.5 seconds ("Pause" column). This finding might raise suspicion of tachycardia–bradycardia syndrome.

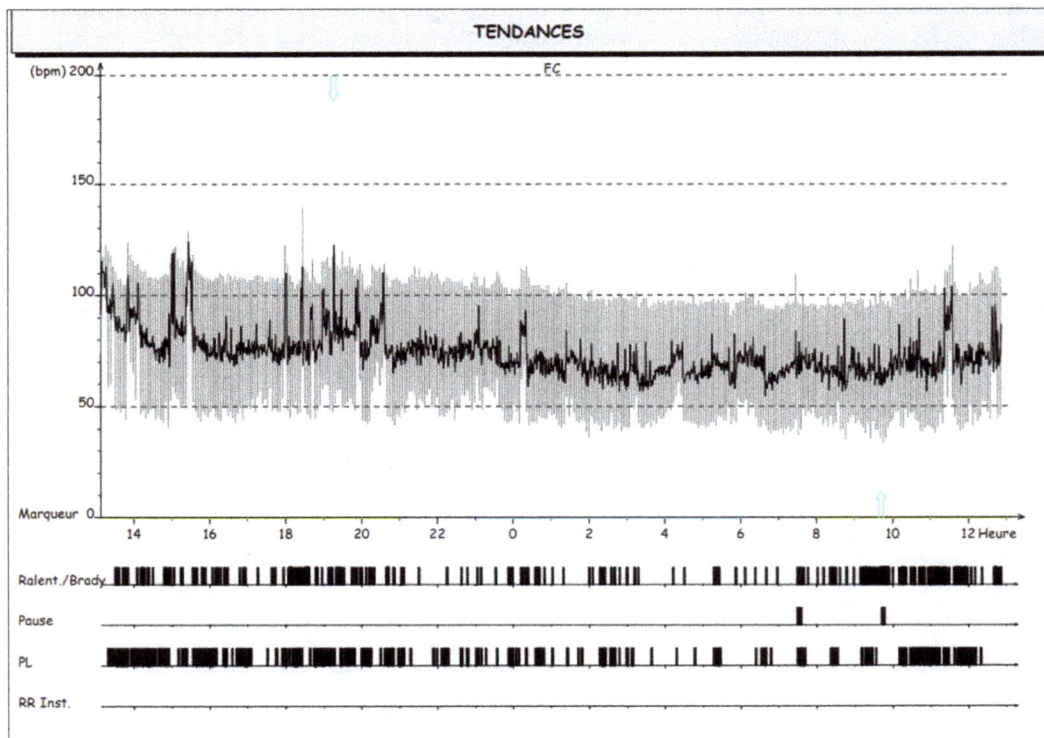

Figure 22.3 Heart rate variation over the 24-hour recording period, demonstrating the absence of significant overall differences, with a slightly lower heart rate recorded at night.

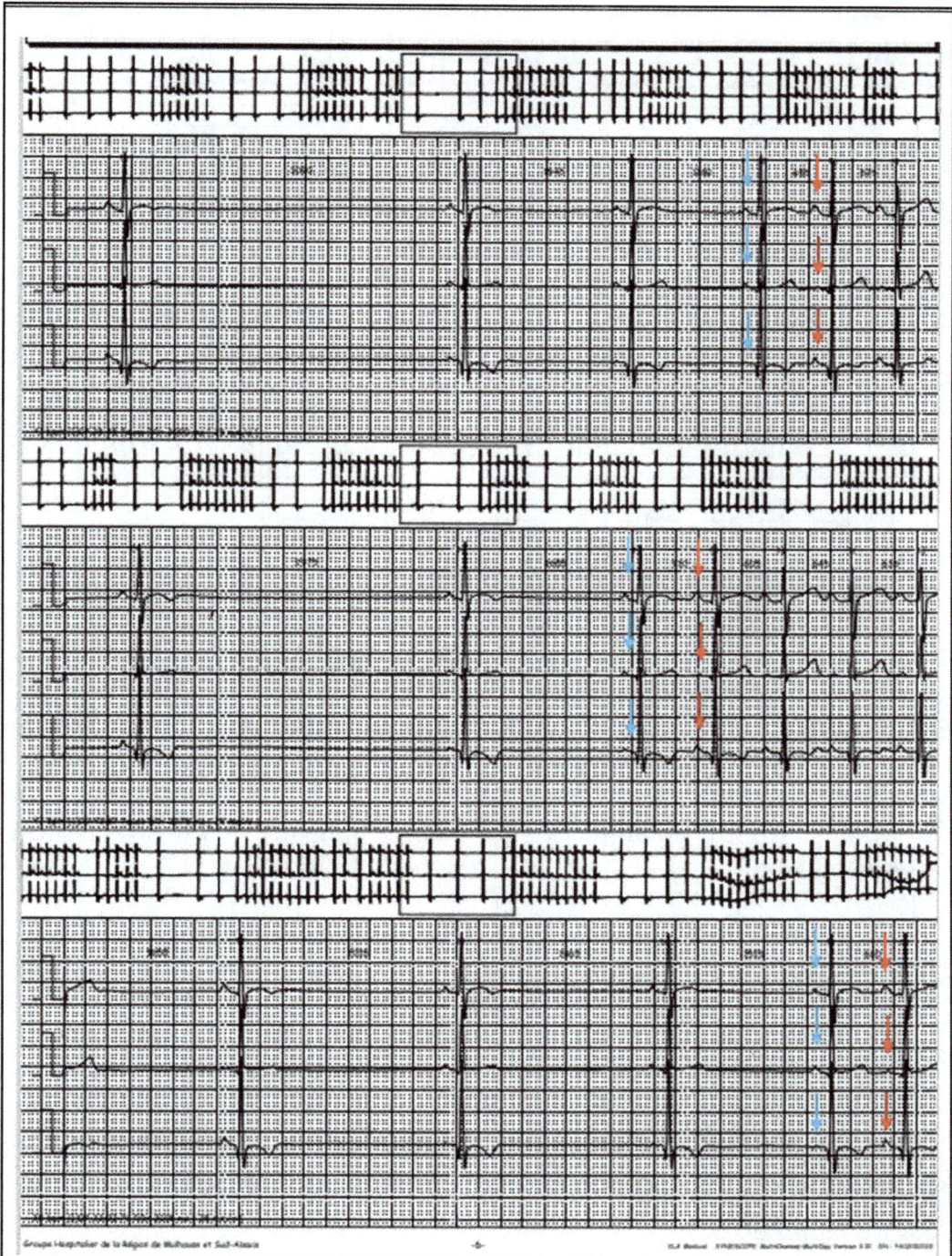

Figure 22.4 Three excerpts from the 24-hour Holter ECG recording, showing the alternance between high and low heart rates. Of note, the P wave morphology during low heart rates (blue arrows) is slightly different from the P wave morphology during high heart rates (red arrows), suggesting two different origins of atrial depolarizations.

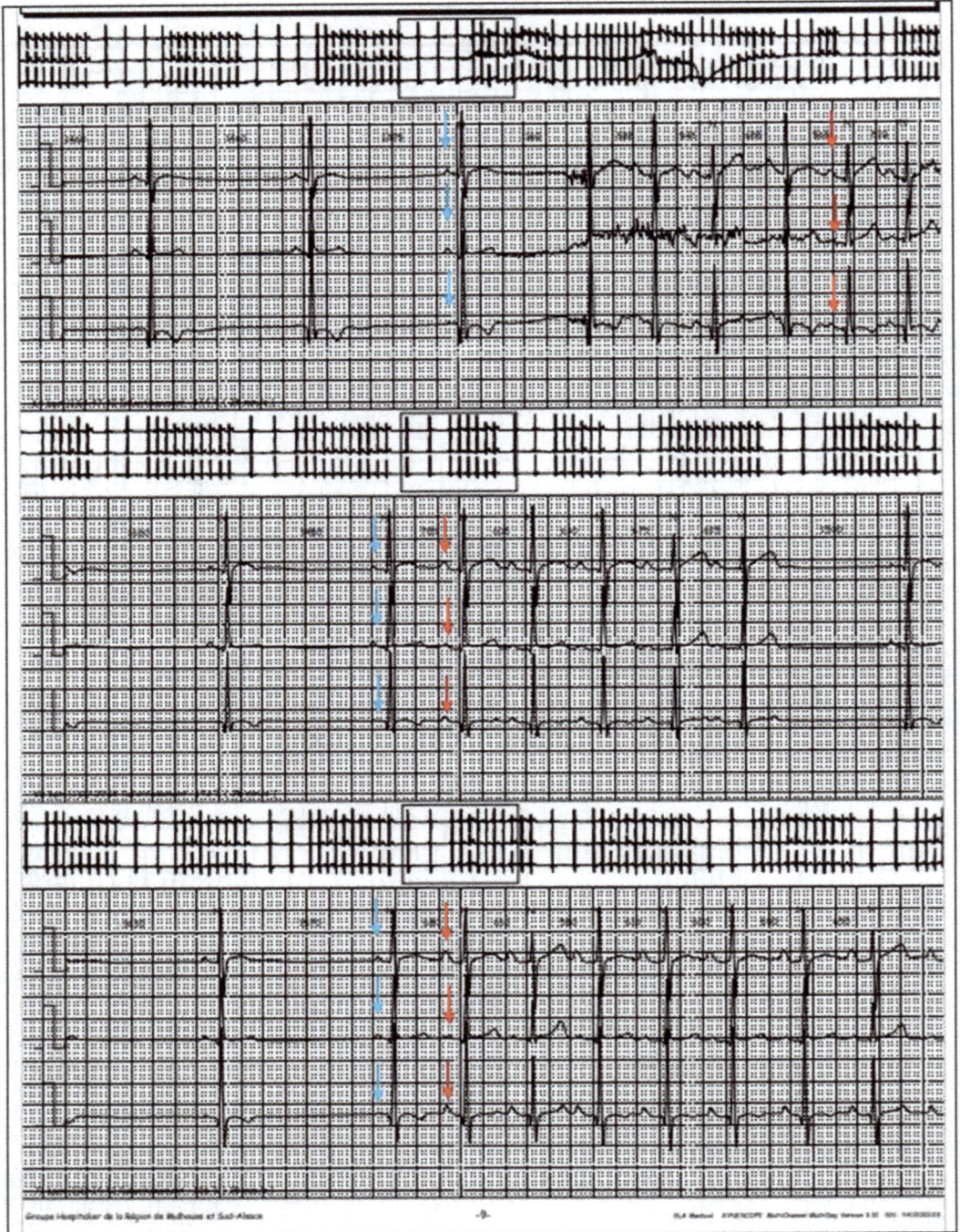

Figure 22.5 Three excerpts from the 24-hour Holter ECG recording, showing as in Figure 22.4, the alternance between high and low heart rates. Of note, the P wave morphology during low heart rates (blue arrows) is slightly different from the P wave morphology during high heart rates (red arrows), suggesting two different origins of atrial depolarizations.

HOLTER SUMMARY

The 24-hour Holter ECG shows the presence of alternating periods of high heart rates and of low heart rates. The average heart rate recorded was 73 bpm, with a highest heart rate of 142 bpm and a lowest rate of 23 bpm. As can be seen in Figures 22.4 and 22.5, there are 2 different P wave morphologies, compatible with 2 different origins of atrial depolarizations: the one present during the low heart rates has likely a sinus node origin; the other is compatible with an ectopic origin provoking incessant runs of atrial tachycardia. This is therefore a fine example of an incessant (very likely focal) atrial tachycardia.

DISCUSSION

The present case illustrates an example of an incessant focal atrial tachycardia in a 16-year-old adolescent with no underlying structural heart disease. The patient underwent an electrophysiological study using a three-dimensional electro-anatomical mapping system, which confirmed the diagnosis and which identified the origin of the tachycardia at the level of the postero-lateral right atrium in its superior part, at the level of the crista terminalis. The patient underwent a successful catheter ablation procedure.

The 24-hour Holter ECG played an important part in establishing the correct diagnosis of incessant atrial tachycardia, showing repeated alternance between short periods of regular low-heart rate episodes (corresponding to sinus rhythm) and incessant runs of higher heart rate episodes, corresponding to incessant runs of focal atrial tachycardia. This might be missed on a 12-lead standard ECG recording, given its short recording time. Another important advantage of the 24-hour Holter ECG monitoring is its potential to demonstrate the absence of significant variations between daytime and nighttime heart rates, a finding supporting the diagnosis of incessant atrial tachycardia (in normal individuals, because of an increased vagal tone during nighttime, there is a significant decrease in heart rate compared to the daytime period).

Even though only 3 leads were recorded by the Holter ECG (compared to a standard 12-lead ECG), they were enough to demonstrate that the morphology of the P wave was clearly different between episodes of low vs high heart rates. This fact is in favor of 2 different origins of atrial depolarizations: one at the level of the sinus node, recorded during low heart rates, and the other being an ectopic origin, recorded during higher heart rates, corresponding to a focal atrial tachycardia.

It is important to correctly establish the diagnosis of incessant focal atrial tachycardia and differentiate it from sinus (respiratory) arrhythmia, since the former requires the administration of antiarrhythmic drugs of catheter ablation, while the latter is a normal finding in adolescents and requires no treatment.

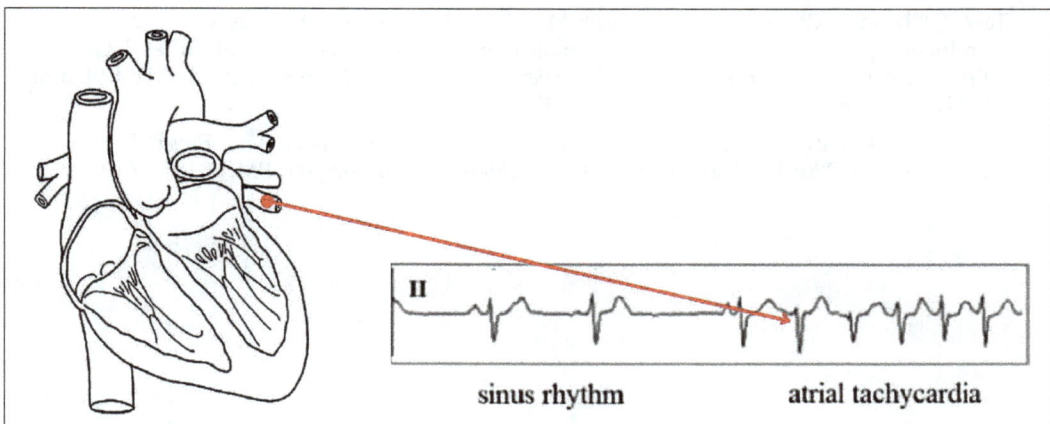

Figure 22.6   Focal atrial tachycardia originating from the left inferior pulmonary vein. The most common origins of focal atrial tachycardias are: the pulmonary veins, the crista terminalis, the ostium of the coronary sinus, the right and the left atrial appendage and the mitral and the tricuspid annulus.

Atrial tachycardia represents around 10% of supraventricular tachycardias, the other 90% being represented by AVNRT and AVRT. The mechanism of atrial tachycardia can be reentry, increased trigger activity, or increased automaticity. They can be reentrant (macro-reentrant or micro-reentrant), or they can be focal. They can originate both in the right atrium and in the left atrium. The most common origins of focal atrial tachycardias are: the pulmonary veins, the crista terminalis, the ostium of the coronary sinus, the right and the left atrial appendage and the mitral and the tricuspid annulus. The best treatment option is catheter ablation.

BIBLIOGRAPHY

1. Schmitt C, Pustowoit A, Schneider M. Focal atrial tachycardia. *Catheter Ablation of Cardiac Arrhythmias*. 2006: 165–181.

2. Balla C, Foresti S, Ali H, Sorgente A, Egidy Assenza G, De Ambroggi G, et al. Long-term follow-up after radiofrequency ablation of ectopic atrial tachycardia in young patients. *Journal of Arrhythmia*. 2019; 35(2): 290–295.

3. Huo Y, Braunschweig F, Gaspar T, Richter S, Schonbauer R, Sommer P, et al. Diagnosis of atrial tachycardias originating from the lower right atrium: Importance of P-wave morphology in the precordial leads V3-V6. *Europace: European Pacing, Arrhythmias, and Cardiac Electrophysiology: Journal of the Working Groups on Cardiac Pacing, Arrhythmias, and Cardiac Cellular Electrophysiology of the European Society of Cardiology*. 2013; 15(4): 570–577.

4. Morris GM, Segan L, Wong G, Wynn G, Watts T, Heck P, et al. Atrial tachycardia arising from the crista terminalis, detailed electrophysiological features and long-term ablation outcomes. *JACC Clinical Electrophysiology*. 2019; 5(4): 448–458.

5. Li-jun J, Xue-yin L, Cong-xin H, Bo Y, Sha-ning Y, Gang W, Qiang X, Huang-jun L. Electrophysiologic characteristics of the Crista terminalis and implications on atrial tachycardia in rabbits. *Cell Biochem Biophys*. 2012 Mar; 62(2): 267–271. doi: 10.1007/s12013-011-9290-5. PMID: 21938558.

6. Liskov S, Milstein JA, Barth AS, Cedars A, Mettler BA, Gottlieb Sen D, Aronis KN. Epicardial Mapping and Ablation of Focal Atrial Tachycardia from the Crista Terminalis During Cardiac Surgery. *JACC Clin Electrophysiol*. 2025 May; 11(5): 1074–1079. doi: 10.1016/j.jacep.2024.12.021. Epub 2025 Feb 19. PMID: 39985524.

7. Jia YH, Wang FZ, Gao DS, Chu JM, Pu JL, Ren XQ, Hua W, Zhang S. Right phrenic injury after radiofrequency catheter ablation of atrial tachycardia at crista terminalis. *Chin Med J (Engl)*. 2011 May; 124(10): 1588–1589. PMID: 21740824.

8. Liwanag M, Willoughby C. Atrial Tachycardia. 2023 Jun 26. In: StatPearls [Internet]. Treasure Island (FL): StatPearls Publishing; 2025 Jan–. PMID: 31194392.

9. Tai CT, Chen SA, Chen YJ, Yu WC, Hsieh MH, Tsai CF, Chen CC, Ding YA, Chang MS. Conduction properties of the crista terminalis in patients with typical atrial flutter: Basis for a line of block in the reentrant circuit. *J Cardiovasc Electrophysiol*. 1998 Aug; 9(8): 811–819. doi: 10.1111/j.1540-8167.1998.tb00120.x. PMID: 9727659.

10. Patel A, Markowitz SM. Atrial tachycardia: Mechanisms and management. *Expert Rev Cardiovasc Ther*. 2008 Jul; 6(6): 811–822. doi: 10.1586/14779072.6.6.811. PMID: 18570619.

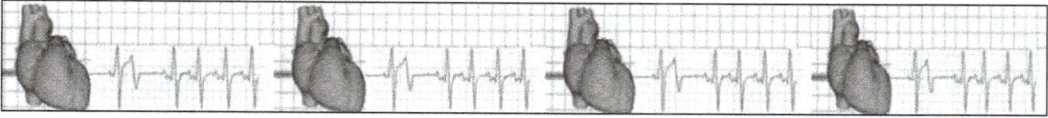

Case 23 Sinus Node Disease in a Newborn With V141M Mutation

Alice Maltret

CLINICAL CASE

A 3-week-old female neonate, with a prenatal diagnosis of fetal bradycardia, was found to be bradycardic, prompting a recommendation for a Holter ECG. Genetic study identified a V141M variation in the KCNQ1 gene which is associated with fetal bradycardia, sinus node dysfunction, and atrial fibrillation. It may also be linked to Short QT syndrome. Following multiple Holter monitorings, she received a dual chamber pacemaker implantation at the age of 3 due to symptomatic bradycardia, accompanied by growth failure and exercise intolerance.

RESULTATS (Tous)

FREQUENCE CARDIAQUE : (Nombre total de QRS : 104334)   (Temps Heure : 23:38)

Moyenne : 74 bpm	FC Max : 147 bpm à (1)20:01:47	RR Max : 1005 ms à (1)17:02:39
Jour (08:00 - 21:00) : 76 bpm	FC Min : 60 bpm à (1)04:10:01	RR Min : 405 ms à (1)20:01:47
Nuit (23:00 - 06:00) : 72 bpm		

BRADYCARDIE : 0   **PAUSES : 0**   **PERIODES LONGUES : 0**

EVENEMENTS VENTRICULAIRES :
EXTRASYSTOLES :   **BI & TRIGEMIN. : 0 & 0**   **TACHYCARDIE : 0**

Isolées : 0	0.0 %
Doublets : 0	0.0 %
Salves : 0	0.0 %
Total : 0	

EVENEMENTS SUPRAVENTRICULAIRES :
EXTRASYSTOLES :   **BI & TRIGEMIN. : 0 & 0**   **TACHYCARDIE : 0**   **RR INSTABLE : 0**

Isolées : 13	0.0 %
Doublets : 0	0.0 %
Salves : 0	0.0 %
Total : 13	

Figure 23.1   The summary page shows a maximum heart rate of 147 and a minimum rate of 60 bpm. The mean heart rate was 74 bpm which is too low for a newborn.

DOI: 10.1201/9781003545040-23

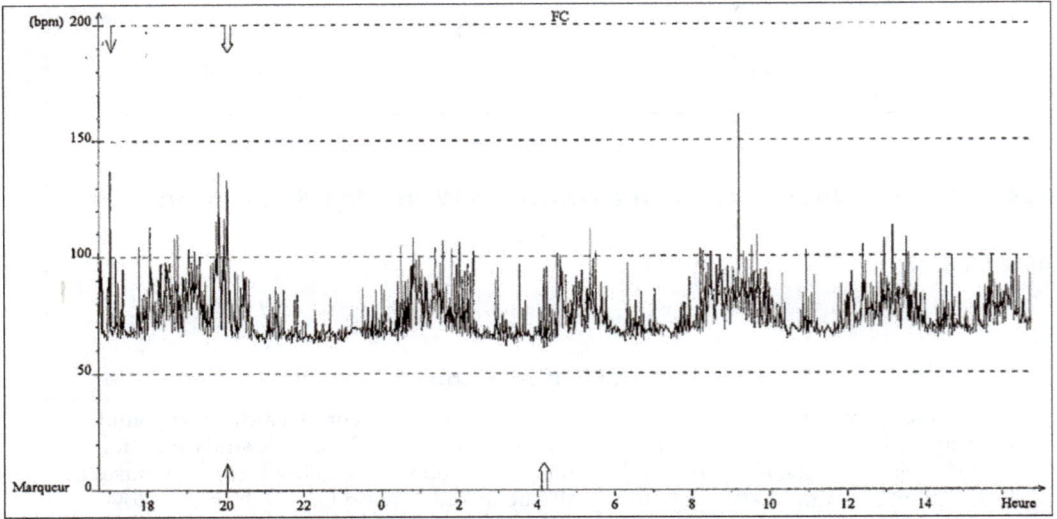

Figure 23.2   The heart rate graph shows a mean rate of 75 bpm.

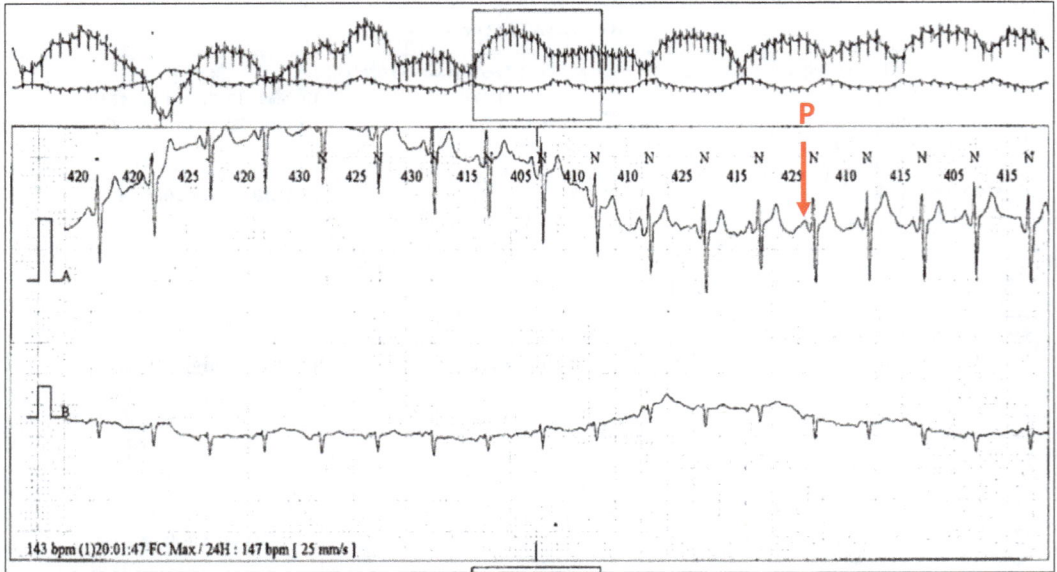

Figure 23.3   The tracing shows the maximum heart rate recorded, which is sinus rhythm 147 bpm. P wave is present before every QRS complex.

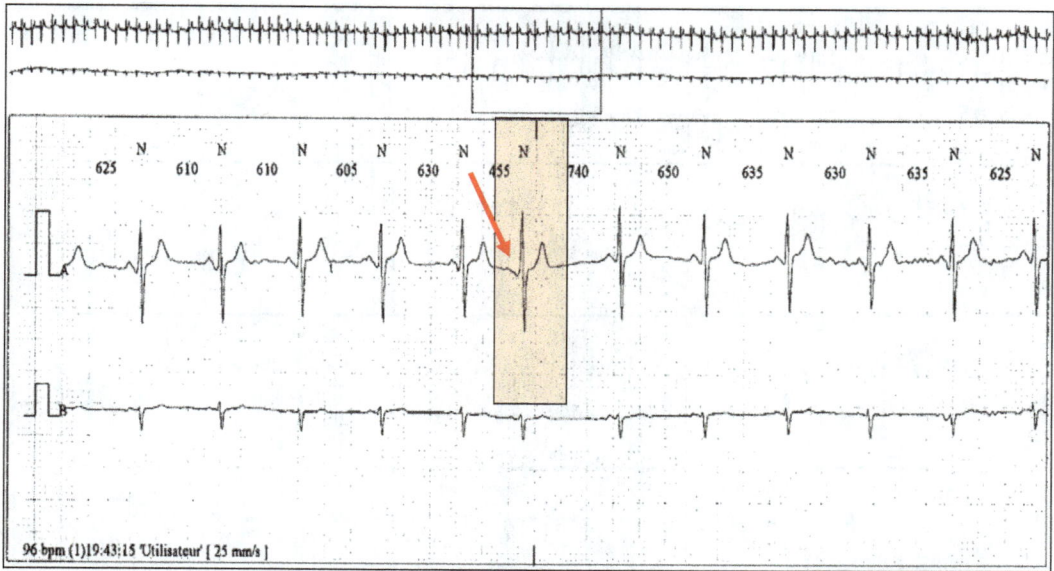

Figure 23.4   The tracing shows sinus rhythm 96 bpm with an atrial premature contraction which has a P wave with a different morphology compared to sinus P wave.

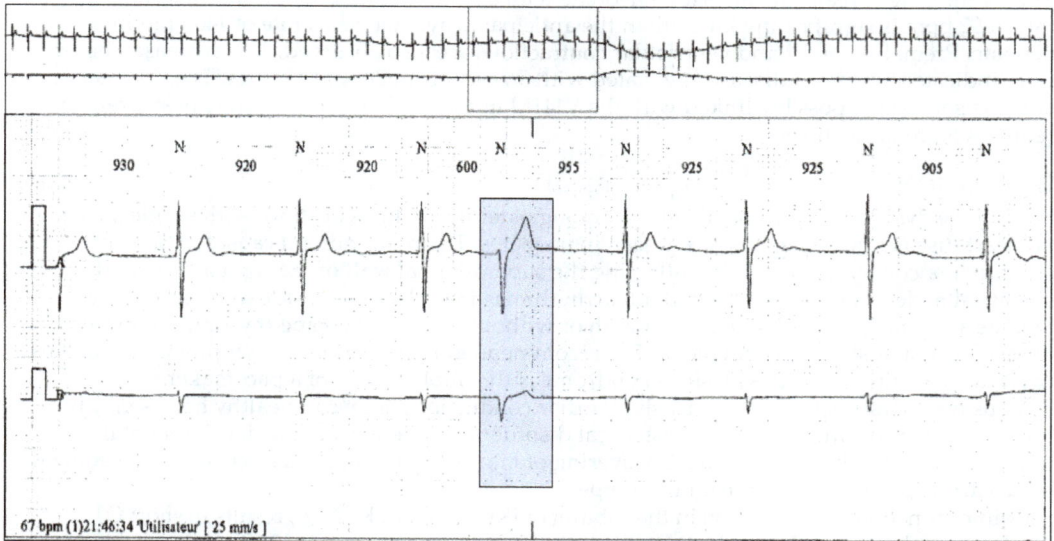

Figure 23.5   The tracing shows junctional rhythm 67bpm with absent P wave. A PVC is evident in the center of the tracing.

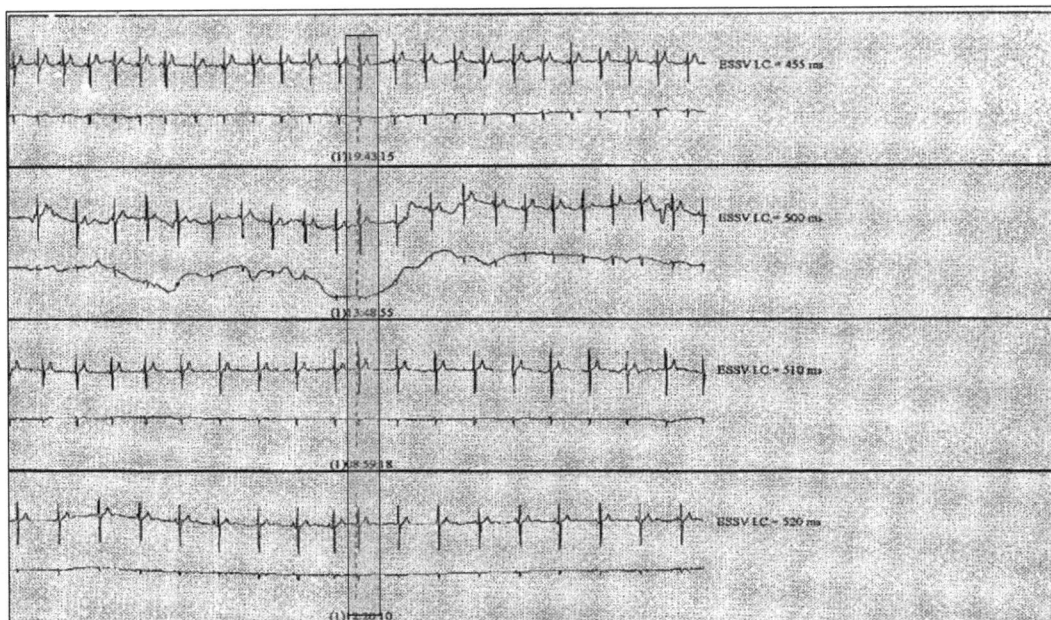

Figure 23.6 The tracing shows premature atrial contractions and the RR interval preceding the PAC: 455, 500, 510 and 520 ms.

HOLTER SUMMARY

The monitoring reveals low rates for a neonate with episodes of junctional rhythm. The average rate of 92 bpm is significantly lower than the anticipated average heart rate of 140 bpm in a neonate. Premature atrial and ventricular contractions are also observed. The decreased heart rates indicate sinus node disease associated with an escape junctional rhythm. The QT interval appears shortened, possibly linked with the V141M mutation; however, accurate measurement requires more derivations.

DISCUSSION

Sinus node dysfunction is more common among older individuals or those with surgical congenital heart disease; however, it is rarely seen in neonates. The predominant causes of SND in children are congenital anomalies affecting the supero-lateral wall of the right atrium and sinoatrial node artery impairment. Bradyarrhythmias in patients with sick sinus syndrome include sinus bradycardia, sinus arrest with or without junctional escape rhythm, ectopic atrial bradycardia, and sinoatrial exit block. The recommended intervention for symptomatic bradyarrhythmias in children with sick sinus syndrome is the implantation of a pacemaker.

Sinus node dysfunction or progressive cardiac conduction disease in healthy hearts may be hereditary, manifesting as primary electrical disorders. A recent dramatic development in molecular genetics has allowed the uncovering of many genetic causes associated with neonatal bradycardia, particularly of the familial type.

Gain-of-function-type mutation in the subunit of IKs channels, KCNQ1, results in short QT syndrome and severe arrhythmias. Nonetheless, the mechanism by which mutant IKs channels induce SQTS remains ambiguous. The V141M mutation in KCNQ1 results in a gain-of-function of the IKs and is associated with SQT2 characterized by a short QT interval, fetal bradycardia, sinus bradycardia, atrioventricular block after birth, and atrial fibrillation. The V141M mutation causes higher current density, accelerated activation, and delayed deactivation, resulting in the accumulation of IKs. The mutation results in KCNQ1 channels being persistently open which has several actions:

1. The V141M KCNQ1 mutation affects the sinoatrial nodal pacemaker rate due to its pronounced impact on IKs over the membrane potential. The sinus node cells ceased spontaneous activity and in the absence of pacemaker activity, atrial electrical activity would begin in the atrioventricular node, elucidating the bradycardia and junctional rhythm observed in those cases.

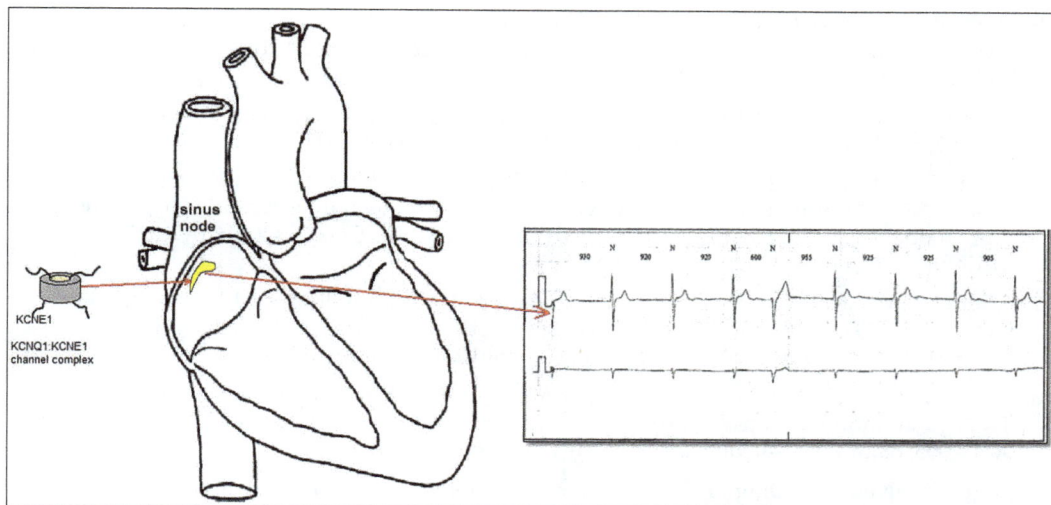

Figure 23.7 V141M mutation of KCNQ1 results in a gain-of-function of the IKs with decreased pacemaker activity of the sino-atrial node and the occurrence of junctional rhythm from the AV node.

2. The V141M mutation reduces atrial action potentials, reduces the atrial effective refractory period and induces atrial fibrillation in the affected child.

In the study of G. Garcia Ordonez et al. on 56 patients with Short QT syndrome, 13 had a V141M KCNQ1 mutation. Most of the patients were female (77%). Patients that were positive for the mutation had sinus node disease in 36% of cases, compared to none from the negative mutation group. Almost all of the patients with V141M had atrial fibrillation associated with sinus node disease and AV block, but none of them had ventricular arrhythmias. In addition, all V141M patients had a history of fetal bradycardia, compared with none from the mutation negative group. Therefore, the authors suggest classifying individuals with Short QT syndrome into V141M positive and V141M negative groups based on phenotypic distinctions.

BIBLIOGRAPHY

1. Garcia Ordonez G, Reyes-Quintero AE, Garcia A, Nava S, Levinstein MJ, Villarreal-Molina MT, Iturralde P. KCNQ1 V141M and short QT syndrome: Are we dealing with a different entity? *Eur Heart J.* 2020; 41(Supplement_2): ehaa946.0453.

2. Montague TJ, Taylor PG, Stockton R, Roy DL, Smith ER. The spectrum of cardiac rate and rhythm in normal newborns. *Pediatr Cardiol.* 1982; 2(1): 33–38.

3. Kramer MR, Shilo S, Hershko C. Atrioventricular and sinoatrial block in thyrotoxic crisis. *Br Heart J.* 1985; 54(6): 600–602.

4. Scagliotti D, Deal BJ. Arrhythmias in the tiny, premature infant. *Clin Perinatol.* 1986; 13(2): 339–350.

5. Beder SD, Gillette PC, Garson Jr. A, Porter CB, McNamara DG. Symptomatic sick sinus syndrome in children and adolescents as the only manifestation of cardiac abnormality or associated with unoperated congenital heart disease. *Am J Cardiol.* 1983; 51(7): 1133–1136.

6. Taylor PV, Scott JS, Gerlis LM, Esscher E, Scott O. Maternal antibodies against fetal cardiac antigens in congenital complete heart block. *New Engl J Med.* 1986; 315(11): 667–672.

7. Lahidheb D, Fehri W, Smiri Z, Gharbi M, Barakett N, Haouala H, Guediche M. Dysfonction sinusale à "coeur sain"chez l'enfant. A propos d'un cas [Sinus node dysfunction in a "healthy heart" in an infant. A case report]. *Tunis Med.* 2002 Dec; 80(12): 793–796. French. PMID: 12664508.

8. De Roy L. Maladie de l'oreillette [Sick sinus syndrome]. *Arch Mal Coeur Vaiss.* 2005 Dec; 98 Spec No 5: 42–47. French. PMID: 16433242.

9. Baruteau AE, Perry JC, Sanatani S, Horie M, Dubin AM. Evaluation and management of bra-dycardia in neonates and children. *Eur J Pediatr*. 2016 Feb; 175(2): 151–161. doi:10.1007/s00431-015-2689-z. Epub 2016 Jan 16. PMID: 26780751.

10. Sidhu S, Marine JE. Evaluating and managing bradycardia. *Trends Cardiovasc Med*. 2020 Jul; 30(5): 265–272. doi:10.1016/j.tcm.2019.07.001. Epub 2019 Jul 9. PMID: 31311698.

11. Lee HC, Rudy Y, Liang H, Chen CC, Luo CH, Sheu SH, Cui J. Pro-arrhythmogenic effects of the V141M KCNQ1 mutation in short QT syndrome and its potential therapeutic targets: Insights from modeling. *J Med Biol Eng*. 2017 Oct; 37(5): 780–789. doi:10.1007/s40846-017-0257-x. Epub 2017 Jul 5. PMID: 29213224; PMCID: PMC5714284.

12. Maltret A, Wiener-Vacher S, Denis C, Extramiana F, Morisseau-Durand MP, Fressart V, et al. Type 2 short QT syndrome and vestibular dysfunction: Mirror of the Jervell and Lange-Nielsen syndrome? *Int J Cardiol*. 2014; 171(2): 291–293. doi:10.1016/j.ijcard.2013.11.078

13. Hong K, Piper DR, Diaz-Valdecantos A, Brugada J, Oliva A, Burashnikov E, et al. De novo KCNQ1 mutation responsible for atrial fibrillation and short QT syndrome in utero. *Cardiovasc Res*. 2005; 68(3): 433–440. doi:10.1016/j.cardiores.2005.06.023

14. Righi D, Silvetti MS, Drago F. Sinus bradycardia, junctional rhythm, and low-rate atrial fibril-lation in Short QT syndrome during 20 years of follow-up: three faces of the same genetic problem. *Cardiol Young*. 2016 Mar.; 26(3): 589–592. doi: 10.1017/S1047951115001432. Epub 2015 Aug 17. PMID: 26279191.

15. Benson DW, Wang DW, Dyment M, Knilans TK, Fish FA, Strieper MJ, Rhodes TH, George AL Jr. Congenital sick sinus syndrome caused by recessive mutations in the cardiac sodium channel gene (SCN5A). *J Clin Invest*. 2003 Oct.; 112(7): 1019–1028. doi: 10.1172/JCI18062. PMID: 14523039; PMCID: PMC198523.

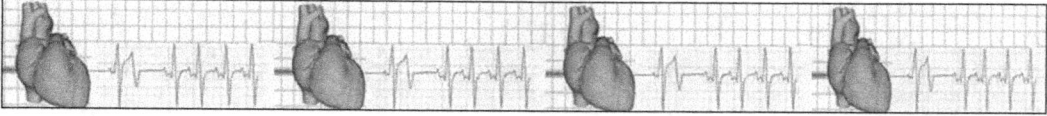

Case 24 Arrhythmia in a Patient with Pulmonary Nodule

Lavinia Oniga, Nicoleta Motoc, and Emanuel Palade

CLINICAL CASE

While hospitalized in the Pneumology Department, a male patient with a lung nodule exhibited arrhythmia during auscultation. He had 8 kg weight loss during the last 6 weeks and no cardiac symptoms. The arrhythmia was identified as premature ventricular contractions by a 12-lead ECG. The echocardiogram was unremarkable. A Holter ECG indicated the presence of atrial and ventricular premature contractions and an episode of atrial fibrillation of 2 minutes 36 seconds. An anticoagulant treatment with Eliquis 2 × 5 mg/day was started. No relationship was found between the lung nodule and the cardiac arrhythmia.

The examination lasted for 20:32:40.
Is started on 04-07-24 11:49.

In the recorded ECG detected:
- 95573 beats
- The average Heart Rate was 79
- Maximum Heart Rate was 160
- Minimum Heart Rate was 43

Moreover SupraVentricular beats were detected:
- 3407 Single Premature SupraVentricular beats,
- 20 segments of PSVT,
- 855 segments of SupraVentricular tachycardia,
- 1 segments of SupraVentricular bradycardia,
- 1 segments of SupraVentricular irregular rhythm,
- 15 Cardiopauses,
- 7 AFib,
- 0 Wenckebach Block.

Moreover 5770 Ventricular beats were detected
- 4446 Single Premature Ventricular beats,
- 0 segments of Ventricular tachycardia,
- 0 segments of IVR,
- 11 segments of Salvo events,
- 130 segments of bigeminy,
- 50 segments of trigeminy,
- 309 Ventricular couplets.

Figure 24.1 The summary page shows the presence of both PVCs and PACs. The PACs were 3407 with atrial salvos and episodes of atrial fibrillation.

DOI: 10.1201/9781003545040-24

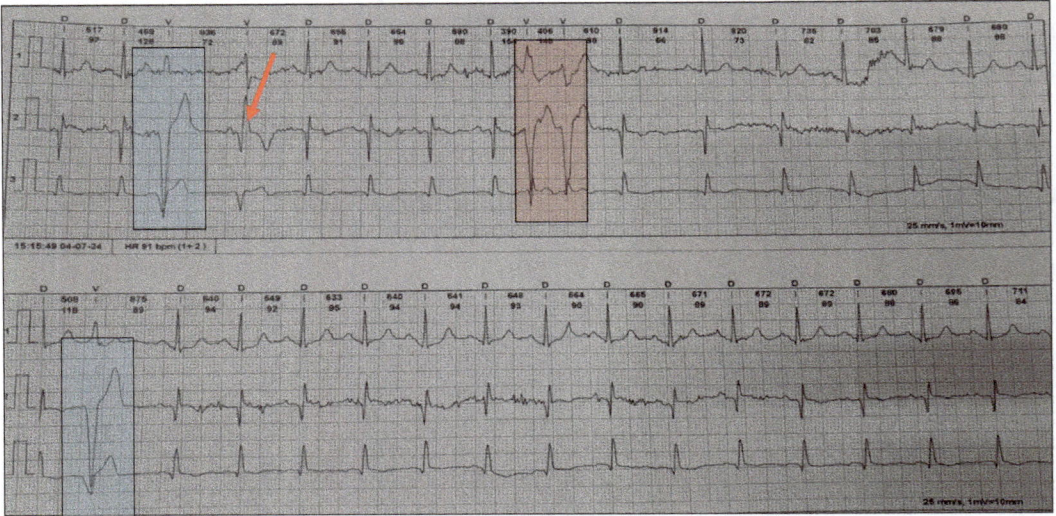

Figure 24.2 The tracing shows sinus rhythm and PVCs marked with blue square, and a ventricular couplet (red square). The fourth beat of the tracing, marked with an arrow is a fusion beat, occurring after a P wave.

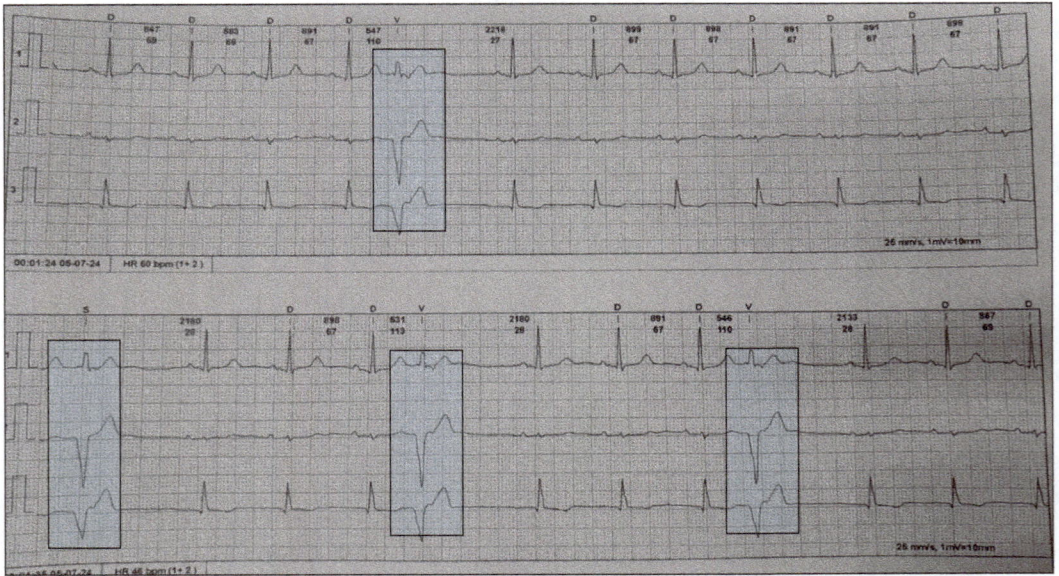

Figure 24.3 The tracing shows sinus rhythm with monomorphic PVCs marked with a blue square.

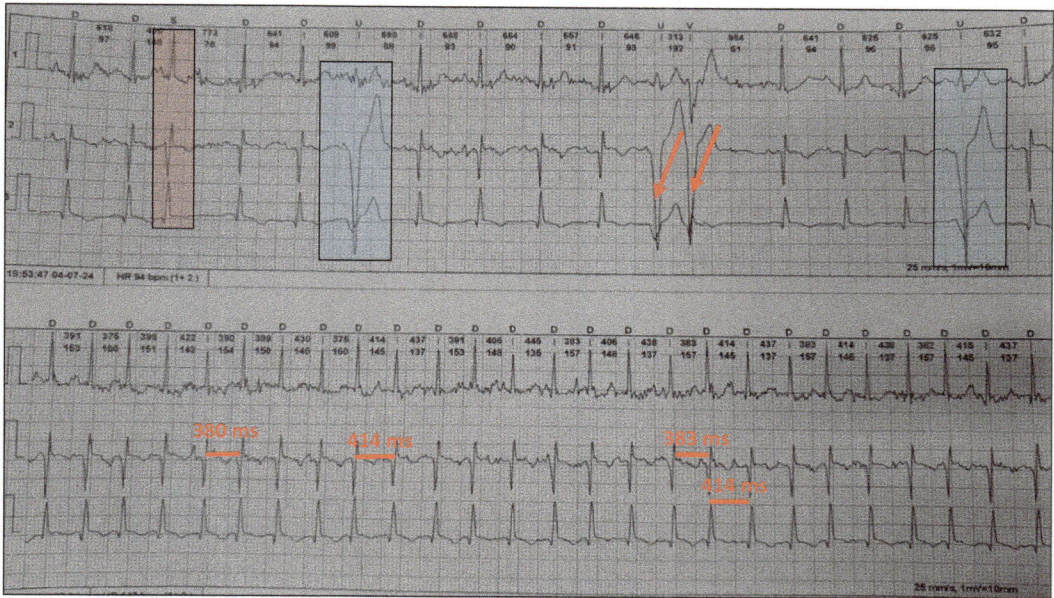

Figure 24.4 The upper part of the tracing shows one premature atrial contractions (red square), monomorphic PVCs (blue square) and a couplet made of 2 different PVCs (arrows). The lower part shows atrial fibrillation with irregular RR intervals (383 to 445 ms).

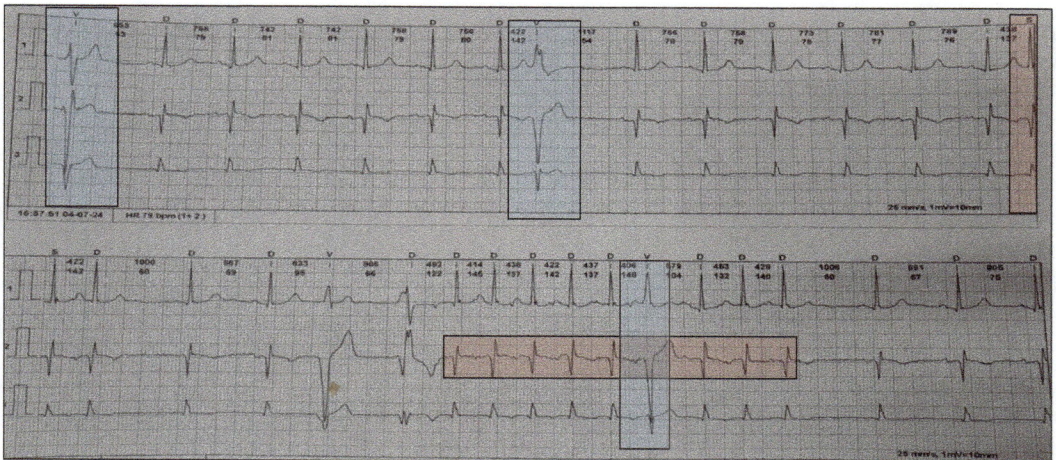

Figure 24.5 The upper part of the tracing shows one PAC and 2 PVCs with distinct morphologies. The lower part of the tracing shows an atrial salvo of 8 consecutive beats and a PVC that does not stop the atrial arrhythmia.

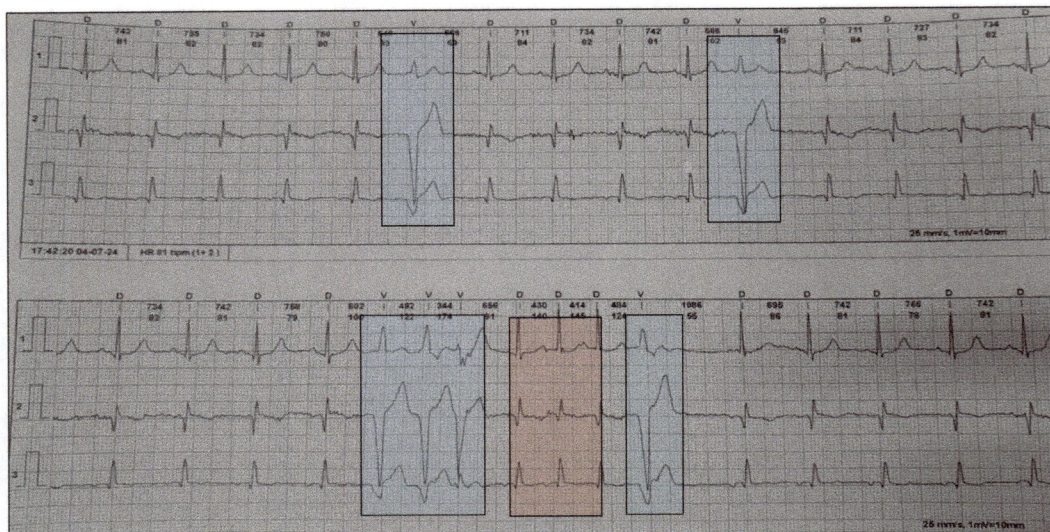

Figure 24.6 The tracing shows single premature ventricular contractions and a triplet marked with blue color.

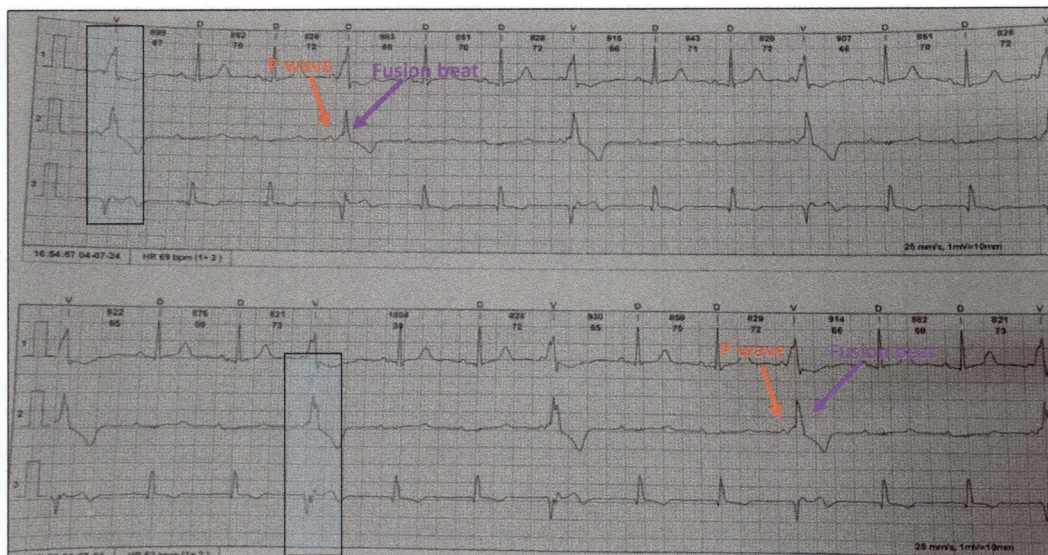

Figure 24.7 The tracing shows ventricular trigeminy: 2 normal beats followed by a premature ventricular contraction. The blue square marks a rhythm that should be differentiated from low idioventricular rhythm. The red arrow indicates the presence of normal QRS complexes, although of low amplitude, mimicking an isoelectric line between the large QRS complexes.

HOLTER SUMMARY

The monitoring reveals 3% of premature atrial contractions and 5% of premature ventricular contractions, accompanied by an episode of atrial fibrillation. At certain points, the atrial fibrillation rhythm appeared organized and regular, resembling a left atrial flutter. Given the atrial fibrillation episode duration of 2 minutes and 36 seconds and a CHADSVASc score of 3, the patient was initiated on anticoagulants, namely Eliquis at a dosage of 2 x 5 mg daily.

DISCUSSION

The primary lung cancer in children is uncommon. Adenocarcinoma is the predominant form of lung cancer in adolescents. Delays typically occur between the presentation and the certain diagnosis of pediatric lung cancer. Numerous studies indicate that nonspecific presenting symptoms, such as long-term cough, are often managed with multiple antibiotic treatments prior to identification, and only a small percentage of children are truly asymptomatic at presentation. Additional symptoms and clinical signs include chest discomfort, wheezing, and hemoptysis. Radiological anomalies like a lung nodule that is persistent upon multiple X-ray examinations, or incidental discoveries during screening X ray imaging could possibly end in a diagnosis of cancer. Weight loss is a consequence of a systemic pro-inflammatory state in children with lung cancer.

Cardiac arrhythmia has been recognized as a possible adverse effect of radiation exposure during the treatment of lung cancer. Atrial tachyarrhythmias, including premature atrial contractions, focal atrial tachycardia, and atrial fibrillation, represent the most prevalent rhythm abnormalities encountered in general cardio-oncology clinics. Supraventricular and ventricular arrhythmias, atrioventricular blocks, and sinus node dysfunction are very uncommon adverse effects of anticancer treatment. Nonetheless, certain antineoplastic agents are recognized for their direct or indirect ability to induce arrhythmias.

The etiology of arrhythmias remains largely ambiguous; numerous instances have indicated a direct impact of the tumor on the heart. A tumor exerting pressure on the right or left atrium may result in atrial fibrillation or atrial tachycardia. Identical arrhythmias arise when there is invasion at the pulmonary veins, specifically at the junction of the atrial muscular sleeves and the venous endothelium. Pericardial inflammation caused by a lung tumor may result in symptomatic pericarditis and atrial arrhythmias originating from the myocardium beneath the inflamed pericardium. Nevertheless, increasing data indicates the interplay of many mechanisms contributing to the cardiotoxic effects of anticancer drugs. These likely include alterations in the membrane activity of Na, K and Ca ion channels, abnormal calcium homeostasis inside cardiomyocytes leading to modifications in their electrophysiological characteristics (as for anthracyclines: daunorubicin, doxorubicin, taxanes: docetaxel, antimetabolites: methotrexate, 5 fluorouracyl, alkylating agents: cyclophosphamide, ifosfamide, melphalan), and their impact on the functioning

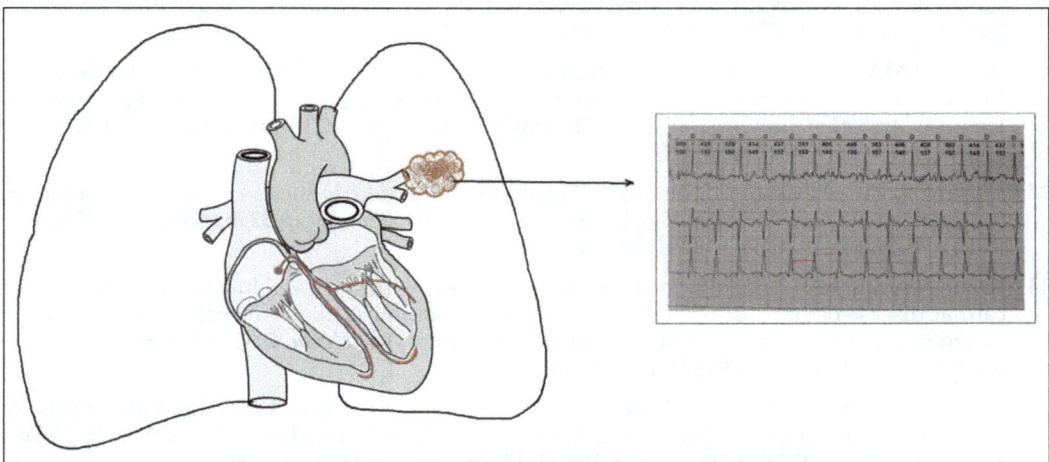

Figure 24.8 Lung tumors can cause atrial fibrillation either through a direct influence on the pulmonary veins and left atrium or as a consequence of an inflamed atrial pericardium or due to the side effects of radiotherapy/chemotherapy.

of ion channels and cellular signaling pathways (tyrosine kinase inhibitors: imatinib, dasatinib, sunitinib). In patients receiving immunotherapy (Rituximab, Trastuzumab), arrhythmias primarily arise due to myocarditis induced by these agents; still, the occurrence of such episodes is rare. Arrhythmias may manifest in cancer survivors experiencing many years of post-oncological treatment completion.

BIBLIOGRAPHY

1. Beardsley JM. Primary carcinoma of the lung in a child. *Can Med Assoc J*. 1933; 29: 257–259.

2. Hirsch FR, Scagliotti GV, Mulshine JL, et al. Lung cancer: Current therapies and new targeted treatments. *Lancet*. 2017; 389: 299–311.

3. Rojas Y, Shi YX, Zhang W, et al. Primary malignant pulmonary tumors in children: A review of the national cancer data base. *J Pediatr Surg*. 2015; 50: 1004–1008.

4. Neville HL, Hogan AR, Zhuge Y, et al. Incidence and outcomes of malignant pediatric lung neoplasms. *J Surg Res*. 2009; 156: 224–230.

5. Yu DC, Grabowski MJ, Kozakewich HP, et al. Primary lung tumors in children and adolescents: A 90-year experience. *J Pediatr Surg*. 2010; 45: 1090–1095.

6. Lee C, Maan A, Singh JP, Fradley MG. Arrhythmias and device therapies in patients with cancer therapy-induced cardiomyopathy. *Heart Rhythm*. 2021; 18: 1223–1229. doi:10.1016/j.hrthm.2021.02.017

7. Fradley MG, Beckie TM, Brown SA, Cheng RK, Dent SF, Nohria A, Patton KK, Singh JP, Olshansky B. Recognition, prevention, and management of arrhythmias and autonomic disorders in cardio-oncology: A scientific statement from the American Heart Association. *Circulation*. 2021; 144: e41–e55. doi:10.1161/CIR.0000000000000986

8. Buza V, Rajagopalan B, Curtis AB. Cancer treatment–induced arrhythmias. *Circ Arrhythm Electrophysiol*. 2017; 10: e005443. doi:10.1161/CIRCEP.117.005443

9. Huang Y, Guo FZ, Dai S, Hu HY, Fu SY, Liu JW, Luo F. Clinical insights into cisplatin-induced arrhythmia in a patient with locally advanced non-small cell lung cancer: A case report. *Eur Rev Med Pharmacol Sci*. 2022; 26: 6–10. doi:10.26355/eurrev_202201_27741

10. Guo GG, Luo X, Zhu K, Li LL, Ou YF. Fatal ventricular arrhythmias after osimertinib treatment for lung adenocarcinoma: A case report. *J Geriatr Cardiol*. 2023; 20: 242–246. doi:10.26599/1671-5411.2023.03.009

11. Gawlik M, Zimodro JM, Gąsecka A, Filipiak KJ, Szmit S. Cardiac arrhythmias in oncological patients-epidemiology, risk factors, and management within the context of the new ESC 2022 guidelines. *Curr Oncol Rep*. 2023 Oct; 25(10): 1107–1115. doi:10.1007/s11912-023-01445-x. Epub 2023 Aug 17. PMID: 37589940; PMCID: PMC10556148.

12. Agarwal MA, Sridharan A, Pimentel RC, Markowitz SM, Rosenfeld LE, Fradley MG, Yang EH. Ventricular arrhythmia in cancer patients: Mechanisms, treatment strategies and future avenues. *Arrhythm Electrophysiol Rev*. 2023 May 29; 12: e16. doi:10.15420/aer.2023.04. PMID: 37457438; PMCID: PMC10345968.

13. Hawryszko M, Sławiński G, Tomasik B, Lewicka E. Cardiac arrhythmias in patients treated for lung cancer: A review. *Cancers (Basel)*. 2023 Dec 6; 15(24): 5723. doi:10.3390/cancers15245723. PMID: 38136269; PMCID: PMC10741954.

14. Raabe NK, Storstein L. Cardiac arrhythmias in patients with small cell lung cancer and cardiac disease before, during and after doxorubicin administration. An evaluation of acute cardiotoxicity by continuous 24-hour Holter monitoring. *Acta Oncol*. 1991; 30(7): 843–846. doi:10.3109/02841869109091832. PMID: 1662523.

15. Gong J, Wang X, Liu Z, Yao S, Xiao Z, Zhang M, Zhang Z. Risk factors and survival analysis of arrhythmia following lung cancer surgery: A retrospective study. *J Thorac Dis*. 2021 Feb; 13(2): 847–860. doi:10.21037/jtd-20-2740. PMID: 33717558; PMCID: PMC7947489.

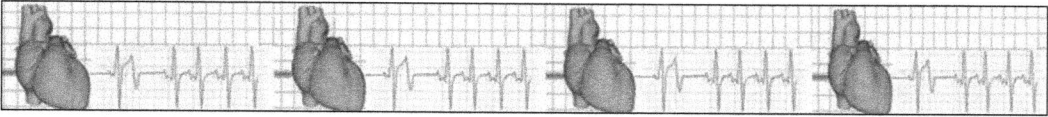

Case 25 WPW Syndrome with Orthodromic Tachycardia in a Newborn

Sorin Andreica, Camelia Vidrea, Raluca Hudrea, and Delia Ghinga

CLINICAL CASE

A male neonate presented multiple episodes of tachycardia at a rate of 230 bpm after birth. Digoxin and Propranolol treatment was ineffective in preventing the arrhythmia. Following intravenous administration of Flecainide, episodes of arrhythmia were handled and he was discharged with a prescription for oral Flecainide to be taken twice daily.

Concluzie

Ritm cardiac		
Total bătăi	168 068	(0% paced)
HR max / min	**247 / 89 bpm**	
Media HR	**Ø 126 bpm**	
HR Max / Min Sinus	171 / 89 bpm	
Media HR (Treaz/Adormit)	123 / 131 bpm	
Index circadian	0,94	
Tahicardie / Bradicardie	5 % / 75 %	

Pauze	
RR Max	**980 ms**
Pauze (>2000ms)	**0**

Fibrilaţie atrială / Flutter atrial	
Total AF	-
AF HR Max	0 bpm
Cel mai lung AF	-

Bradicardie		
Cea mai mică	Ø 106 bpm	17 sec
Cea mai mare	Ø 117 bpm	01:01:36

ST		
St ridicare max	0,49 mV	II
ST depresurizare max	-0,71 mV	V3

Ectopie ventriculară		
V Total	0	(< 1%)
V / Ora Max	0	pe oră
Episoade Tahicardie V		-
Cea mai rapidă Tahicardie V		-
V Cea mai lungă secvenţă		-
Triplete / Execută		0 Σ 0 bătăi
Cuplete		0 Σ 0 bătăi
Bigeminism		0 Σ 0 bătăi
Trigeminism		0 Σ 0 bătăi

Ectopie supraventriculară		
S Tot	14269	(8%)
Episoade Tahicardie SV		14 Σ 01:02:27
Cea mai rapidă Tahicardie SV	Ø 230 bpm	00:33:01
S Cea mai lungă secvenţă	Ø 230 bpm	00:33:01
Triplete / Execută		1 Σ 4 bătăi
Cuplete		1 Σ 2 bătăi

Figure 25.1 The summary page shows a maximum heart rate of 247 bpm and 14 episodes of supraventricular tachycardia.

DOI: 10.1201/9781003545040-25

2		Bradicardii				Primele 5 episoade cu media HR > 124 bpm
Începe de la	Ritm	HR Media	HR Min	HR Max	Durata
(2) 01:48:11	Bradicardie	106	89	116	00:00:17
(1) 11:46:07	Bradicardie	110	101	123	00:02:22
(1) 11:23:09	Bradicardie	110	101	123	00:22:44
(1) 14:33:27	Bradicardie	111	104	123	00:02:30
(1) 16:50:05	Bradicardie	111	97	123	00:03:34

3		Tahicardii				Primele 5 episoade cu media HR > 169 bpm
Începe de la	Ritm	HR Media	HR Min	HR Max	Durata
(2) 01:15:10	Tahicardie	230	217	247	00:33:01
(1) 16:07:19	Tahicardie	229	212	241	00:12:21
(2) 01:08:24	Tahicardie	229	229	229	00:00:09
(2) 01:04:23	Tahicardie	227	224	232	00:01:13
(2) 01:05:36	Tahicardie	227	226	228	00:00:14

4		Secventa V				secvența cea mai lungă 5
Începe de la	Ritm	HR Media	HR Min	HR Max	Durata

5		Secventa S				Primele 5 cele mai lungi secvențe
Începe de la	Ritm	HR Media	HR Min	HR Max	Durata
(2) 01:15:10	7595 x S	230	217	247	00:33:01
(1) 16:07:19	2831 x S	229	212	241	00:12:21
(2) 01:11:28	825 x S	225	206	236	00:03:40
(2) 01:05:51	571 x S	224	218	228	00:02:33
(2) 01:08:35	485 x S	226	215	233	00:02:08

6		Episoadele V Tach				Toate episoadele cu media HR > 169 bpm
Începe de la	Ritm	HR Media	HR Min	HR Max	Durata

Figure 25.2 The summary table shows episodes of bradycardia, tachycardia, and supraventricular arrhythmia. The longest supraventricular tachycardia had a duration of 33 minutes and a rate of 247 bpm.

7		Ectopii						Run-uri V sunt compuse din mai puțin de 5 bătăi. Run-uri S sunt compuse din mai puțin de 20 bătăi.													
Interval		TOTAL	act.	HR[bpm]			Bătăi V							Bătăi S						Pauza	Buton
De la	Dur.	Bătai	[%]	Min	Media	Max	Σ Individui	Bi	Tri	Cvadr	Cupl	Tripl	Ruleaz	Σ Individui	Bi	Tri	Cvadr	Cupl	Tripl Ruleaz		
(1) 08:36	00:23	2882	4,00	95	125	143	0	0	0	0	0	0	0	0	0	0	0	0	0 0	0	0
(1) 09:00	01:00	7124	3,00	107	119	136	0	0	0	0	0	0	0	0	0	0	0	0	0 0	0	0
(1) 10:00	01:00	6889	3,00	103	115	135	0	0	0	0	0	0	0	0	0	0	0	0	0 0	0	0
(1) 11:00	01:00	7012	7,00	98	117	158	0	0	0	0	0	0	0	0	0	0	0	0	0 0	0	0
(1) 12:00	01:00	7739	6,00	103	129	157	0	0	0	0	0	0	0	0	0	0	0	0	0 0	0	0
(1) 13:00	01:00	7080	3,00	101	118	144	0	0	0	0	0	0	0	0	0	0	0	0	0 0	0	0
(1) 14:00	01:00	7524	13,00	98	126	149	0	0	0	0	0	0	0	0	0	0	0	0	0 0	0	0
(1) 15:00	01:00	7545	8,00	101	126	164	0	0	0	0	0	0	0	0	0	0	0	0	0 0	0	0
(1) 16:00	01:00	8638	5,00	97	144	241	0	0	0	0	0	0	0	2831	0	0	0	0	0 0	0	0
(1) 17:00	01:00	7289	5,00	103	123	164	0	0	0	0	0	0	0	0	0	0	0	0	0 0	0	0
(1) 18:00	01:00	7057	3,00	93	118	135	0	0	0	0	0	0	0	0	0	0	0	0	0 0	0	0
(1) 19:00	01:00	7002	3,00	106	117	135	0	0	0	0	0	0	0	0	0	0	0	0	0 0	0	0
(1) 20:00	01:00	6976	3,00	101	116	139	0	0	0	0	0	0	0	0	0	0	0	0	0 0	0	0
(1) 21:00	01:00	7764	3,00	102	129	171	0	0	0	0	0	0	0	0	0	0	0	0	0 0	0	0
(1) 22:00	01:00	7292	3,00	105	122	139	0	0	0	0	0	0	0	0	0	0	0	0	0 0	0	0
(1) 23:00	01:00	7209	3,00	102	120	137	0	0	0	0	0	0	0	0	0	0	0	0	0 0	0	0
(2) 00:00	01:00	8418	3,00	102	140	229	0	0	0	0	0	0	0	1440	3	1	1	0	1 0	0	0
(2) 01:00	01:00	12043	10,00	89	204	247	0	0	0	0	0	0	0	9998	0	2	4	0	0 1	0	0
(2) 02:00	01:00	7351	5,00	108	123	145	0	0	0	0	0	0	0	0	0	0	0	0	0 0	0	0
(2) 03:00	01:00	7124	3,00	97	119	149	0	0	0	0	0	0	0	0	0	0	0	0	0 0	0	0
(2) 04:00	01:00	6943	3,00	99	116	133	0	0	0	0	0	0	0	0	0	0	0	0	0 0	0	0
(2) 05:00	01:00	7009	3,00	98	117	137	0	0	0	0	0	0	0	0	0	0	0	0	0 0	0	0
(2) 06:00	00:52	6158	4,00	97	118	151	0	0	0	0	0	0	0	0	0	0	0	0	0 0	0	0
Σ adormit	08:52	69547	4,00	89	131	247	0	0	0	0	0	0	0	11438	3	3	5	0	1 1	0	0
Σ treaz	13:23	98521	5,00	93	123	241	0	0	0	0	0	0	0	2831	0	0	0	0	0 0	0	0
TOTAL	22:16	168068	5,00	89	126	247	0	0	0	0	0	0	0	14269	3	3	5	0	1 1	0	0

Figure 25.3 The summary table shows several episodes of supraventricular tachycardia at 16:00, 00:00, and 01:00.

9		Ritmuri bazale								Limita bradicardiei = 124 [bpm]; Limita tahicardiei = 169 [bpm]				
Interval		TOTAL	Bradicardie			Normal			Tahicardie			Neanalizat	
De la	Dur.	Batai	Durata	%	HR	Durata	%	HR	Durata	%	HR	Durata	%
(1) 08:36	00:23	2882	00:13:53	60	119	00:09:14	40	133	00:00:00	0	-	00:00:00	0
(1) 09:00	01:00	7124	00:58:50	98	119	00:01:10	2	132	00:00:00	0	-	00:00:00	0
(1) 10:00	01:00	6889	00:59:10	99	115	00:00:50	1	132	00:00:00	0	-	00:00:00	0
(1) 11:00	01:00	7012	00:49:23	82	112	00:10:37	18	141	00:00:00	0	-	00:00:00	0
(1) 12:00	01:00	7739	00:25:01	42	119	00:34:59	58	136	00:00:00	0	-	00:00:00	0
(1) 13:00	01:00	7080	00:48:32	81	115	00:11:28	19	133	00:00:00	0	-	00:00:00	0
(1) 14:00	01:00	7524	00:31:06	52	115	00:28:50	48	137	00:00:00	0	-	00:00:04	< 1
(1) 15:00	01:00	7545	00:34:00	57	118	00:26:00	43	136	00:00:00	0	-	00:00:00	0
(1) 16:00	01:00	8638	00:35:29	59	117	00:12:08	20	136	00:12:21	21	229	00:00:00	0
(1) 17:00	01:00	7289	00:45:06	75	116	00:14:19	24	143	00:00:00	0	-	00:00:34	< 1
(1) 18:00	01:00	7057	00:59:10	99	118	00:00:50	1	135	00:00:00	0	-	00:00:00	0
(1) 19:00	01:00	7002	00:59:40	> 99	117	00:00:20	< 1	133	00:00:00	0	-	00:00:00	0
(1) 20:00	01:00	6976	00:58:04	97	116	00:01:56	3	131	00:00:00	0	-	00:00:00	0
(1) 21:00	01:00	7764	00:27:20	46	117	00:32:04	53	140	00:00:36	1	169	00:00:00	0
(1) 22:00	01:00	7292	00:54:38	91	121	00:05:22	9	130	00:00:00	0	-	00:00:00	0
(1) 23:00	01:00	7209	00:57:08	95	120	00:02:52	5	131	00:00:00	0	-	00:00:00	0
(2) 00:00	01:00	8418	00:24:59	42	118	00:28:33	48	141	00:06:24	11	224	00:00:03	< 1
(2) 01:00	01:00	12043	00:01:49	3	120	00:14:22	24	135	00:43:40	73	229	00:00:06	< 1
(2) 02:00	01:00	7351	00:50:52	85	121	00:09:08	15	134	00:00:00	0	-	00:00:00	0
(2) 03:00	01:00	7124	00:44:13	74	115	00:15:47	26	130	00:00:00	0	-	00:00:00	0
(2) 04:00	01:00	6943	00:59:34	> 99	116	00:00:26	< 1	132	00:00:00	0	-	00:00:00	0
(2) 05:00	01:00	7009	00:55:22	92	116	00:04:38	8	129	00:00:00	0	-	00:00:00	0
(2) 06:00	00:52	6158	00:42:03	79	115	00:09:57	19	134	00:00:00	0	-	00:00:56	2
Σ adormit	08:52	69547	06:30:38	73	118	01:31:05	17	135	00:50:05	9	229	00:01:07	< 1
Σ treaz	13:23	98521	10:04:44	75	116	03:04:45	23	137	00:12:57	2	226	00:00:38	< 1
TOTAL	22:16	168068	16:35:23	75	117	04:35:51	21	137	01:03:03	5	228	00:01:45	< 1

Figure 25.4 The summary table shows episodes of tachycardia at 16:00, 21:00, 00:00, 01:00, the longest having 43 minutes.

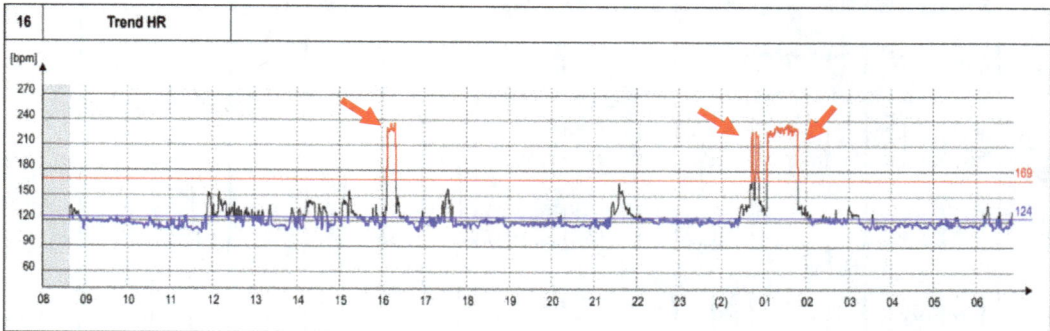

Figure 25.5 The heart rate trend shows episodes of paroxysmal supraventricular tachycardia. The onset and termination of the tachycardia are sudden.

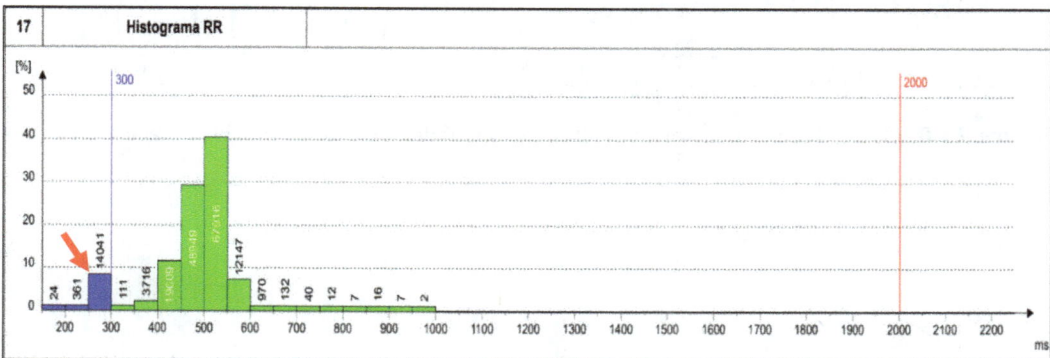

Figure 25.6 The RR histogram shows short intervals < 300 ms associated with tachycardia episodes.

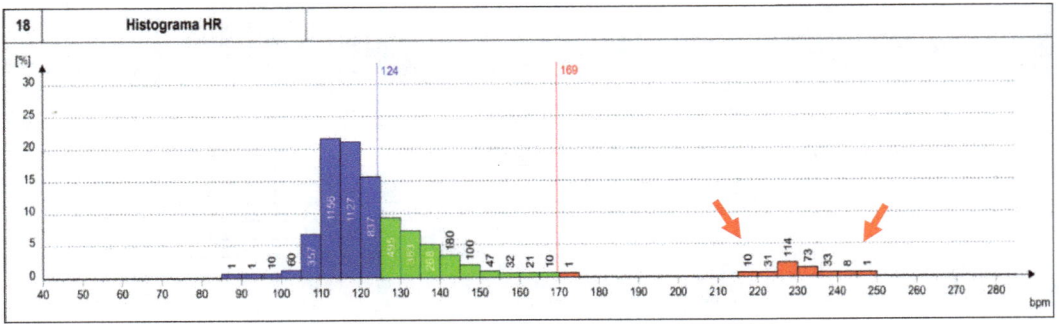

Figure 25.7 The heart rate histogram shows increased rates > 200 bpm due to tachycardia episodes.

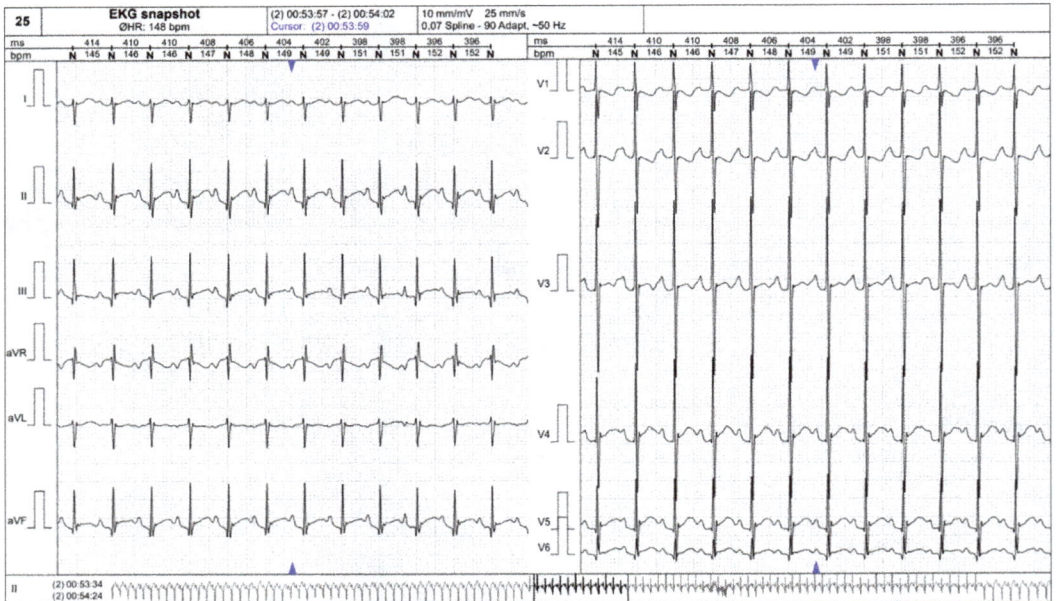

Figure 25.8 The PR interval is normal, with absence of delta waves in this ECG trace.

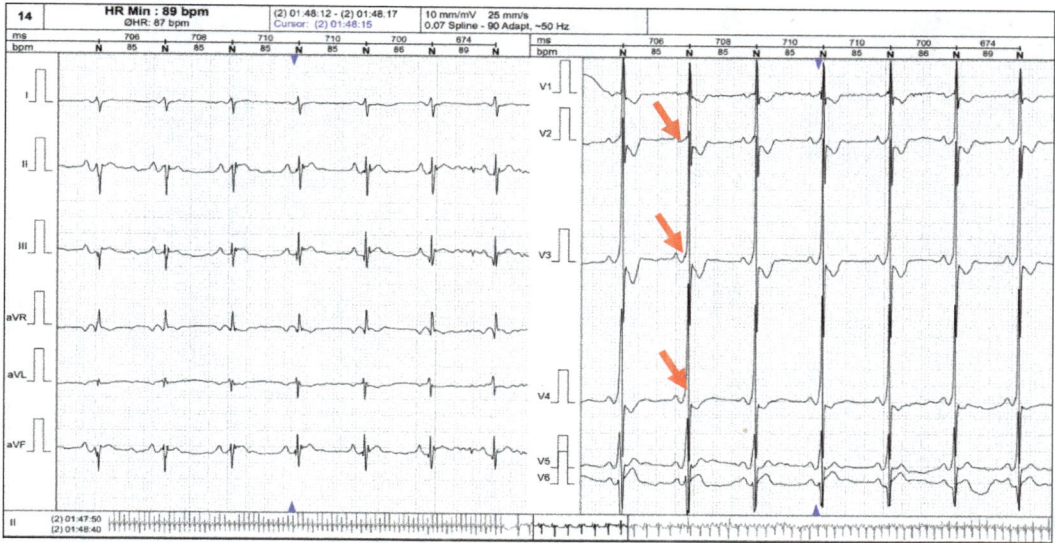

Figure 25.9 The PR interval is shorter than in the previous image, with delta waves clearly seen in the precordial derivations.

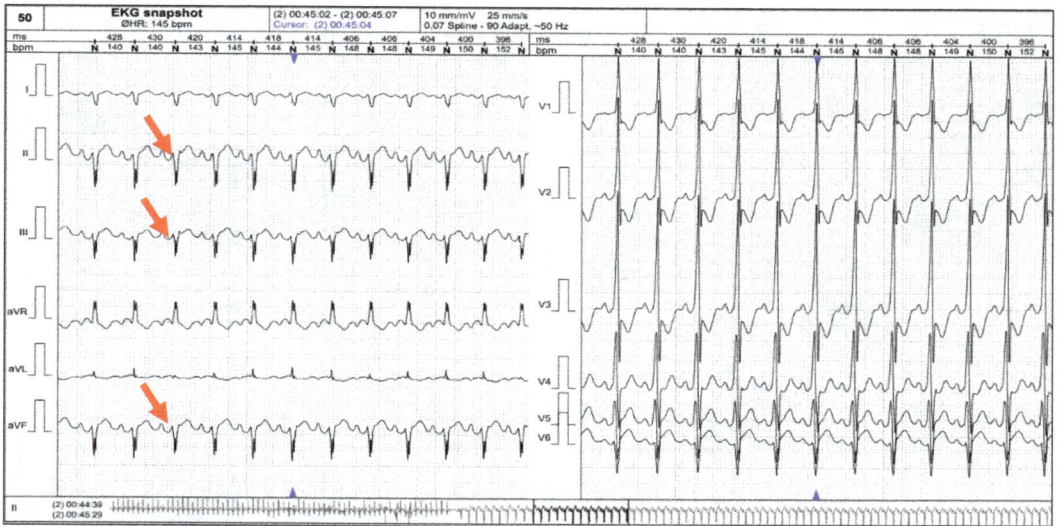

Figure 25.10 The PR interval is short, and a delta wave is visible in all leads. Nonetheless, this does not constitute maximal pre-excitation, as the inferior leads exhibit a minor R wave preceding the S wave. The antegrade conduction from the sinus node to the ventricles occurs both via the AV node and the accessory pathway.

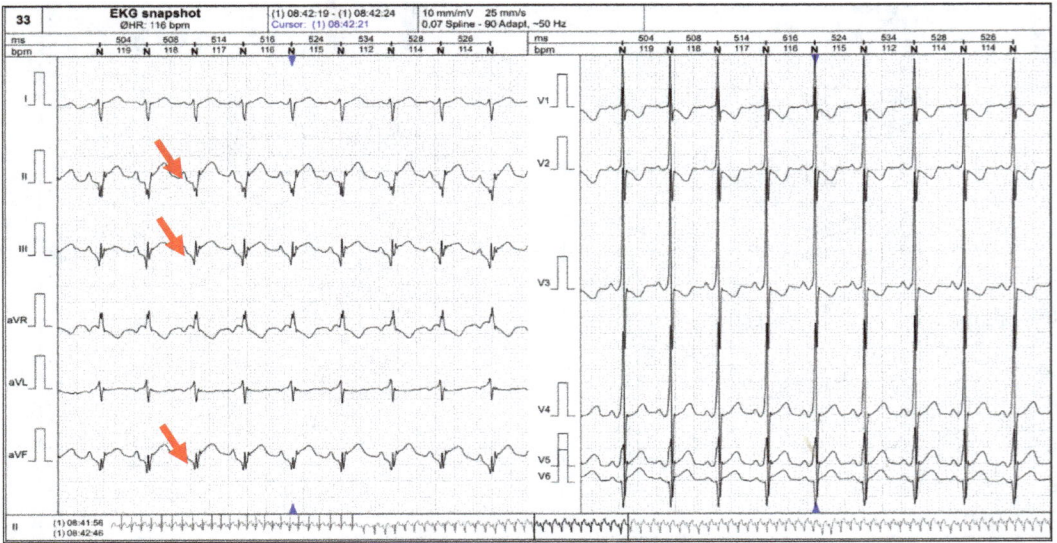

Figure 25.11 The PR interval is short and delta waves are seen in all leads. This appears to be maximal pre-excitation. The negative delta wave in inferior leads and positive in lead V1 suggests a left posterior accessory pathway.

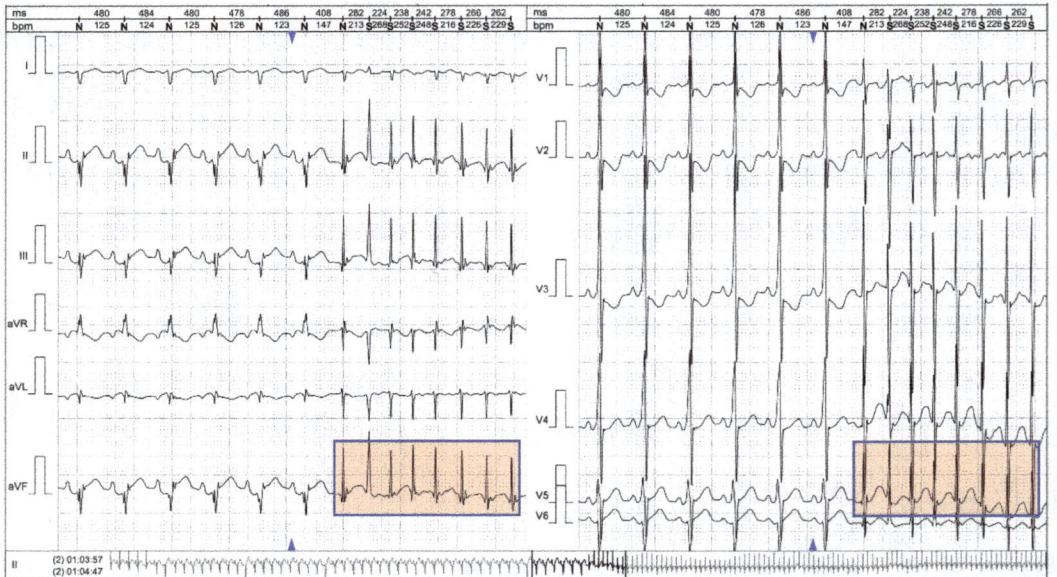

Figure 25.12 Onset of paroxysmal supraventricular tachycardia. There is sinus rhythm on the first half of the image and PSVT on the second half (red square).

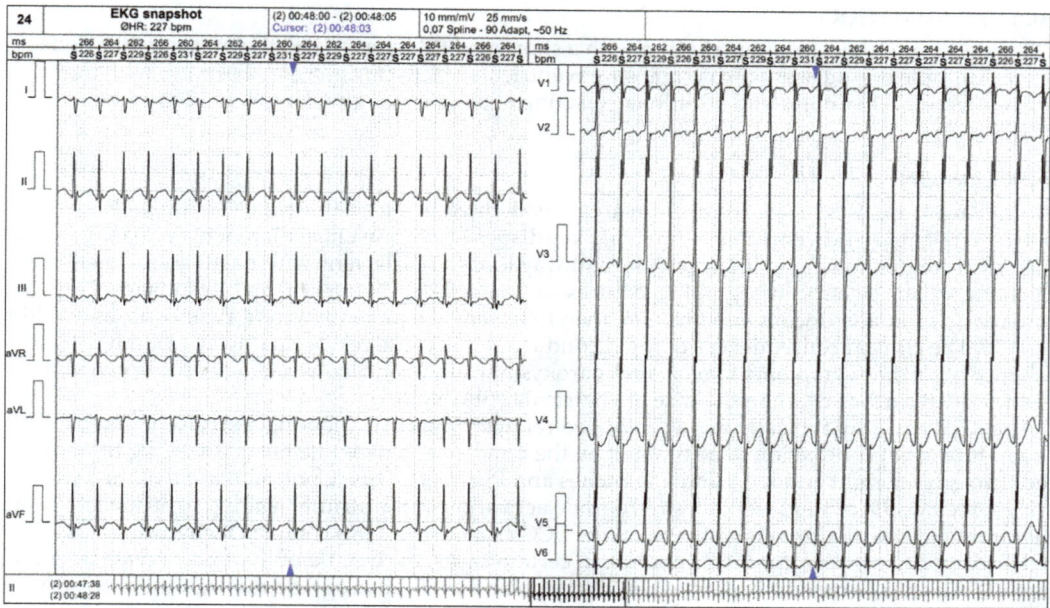

Figure 25.13   Supraventricular tachycardia with a narrow QRS and a rate of 227 bpm. It is an ORT (orthodromic reentrant tachycardia using an accessory pathway).

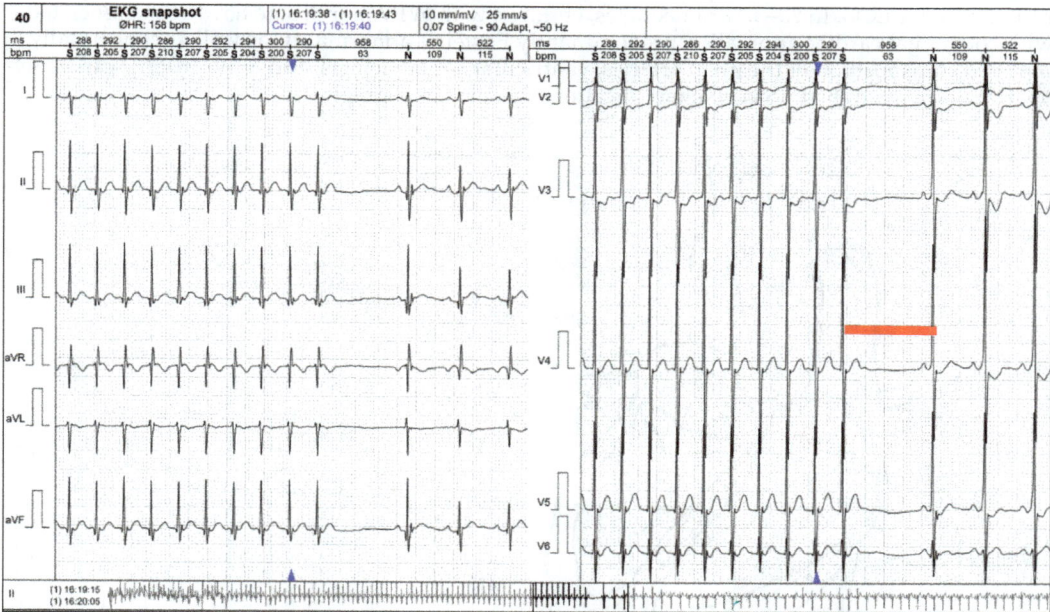

Figure 25.14   Tachycardia ends with a pause (which is equivalent to sinus rhythm recovery time = SNRT), after which sinus rhythm resumes.

HOLTER SUMMARY

The monitoring indicates sinus rhythm with a shortened PR interval and the presence of a delta wave. Multiple episodes of paroxysmal supraventricular tachycardia were observed, with the longest lasting 33 minutes and additional sustained episodes ranging from 2 to 12 minutes in duration.

DISCUSSION

Wolff–Parkinson–White syndrome is an anomaly defined by an additional electrical pathway between the atria and ventricles, which may predispose to supraventricular tachycardias. Electrical conduction along the accessory pathway leads to early ventricular activation, resulting in characteristic electrocardiographic features such as a short PR interval and delta wave. The disease was initially documented in 1915, then followed by a paper by Wolff, Parkinson, and White in 1930. The clinical consequences of rapid conduction via the accessory pathway can range from absence of cardiac symptoms to recurrent paroxysmal supraventricular tachycardia, syncope, and even sudden cardiac death in the case of ventricular fibrillation.

The Kent pathway typically has a prolonged refractory period, allowing a precisely timed premature atrial contraction to be blocked by the bundle of Kent, while normally being transmitted through the right and left bundle branches and Purkinje fibers. Upon activation of the ventricles, the bundle of Kent facilitates retrograde activation of the atrium, leading to atrioventricular reentrant tachycardia, which is shown on the ECG as a narrow QRS complex tachycardia (ORT=orthodromic reentrant tachycardia). In certain cases, the bundle of Kent may create re-entry circuits via anterograde activation, when the impulse travels anterograde through the accessory pathway followed by retrograde conduction through the bundle of His and the AV node. This condition, although rare, leads to broad QRS complex PSVT that resembles ventricular tachycardia called antidromic reentrant tachycardia (ART).

Determining the accurate prevalence of a WPW pattern in neonates is difficult, with prior research from Japan, Belgium, Canada, and the United States indicating prevalence ranging from 0.03% to 0.5%.

The pre-excitation pattern may be subtle, intermittent, or concealed, limiting its detection on a 24-hour Holter ECG. In 20–37% of neonates, children with WPW syndrome have been associated with congenital cardiac anomalies, predominantly Ebstein's abnormality, as well as congenitally repaired transposition of the great arteries, ventricular septal defects, and hypertrophic cardiomyopathy. Our patient had no visible modifications in echocardiography.

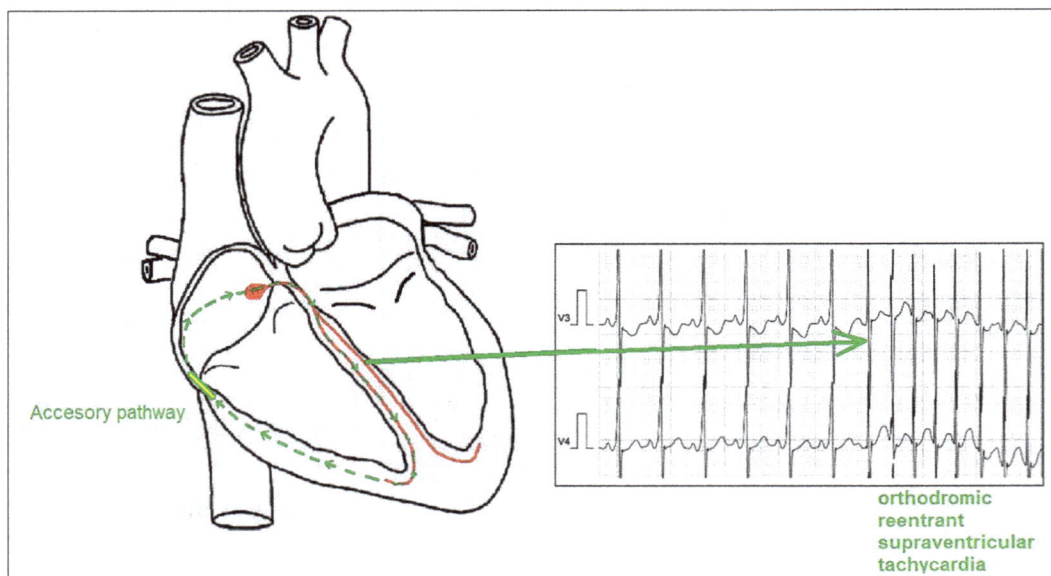

Figure 25.15 The mechanism of accessory-pathway mediated orthodromic reentrant tachycardia.

Multiple investigations examining pediatric patients with WPW syndrome indicated that spontaneous resolution of ventricular pre-excitation occurred in up to 36% of the cohorts, implying a disappearance of anterograde conduction. Additional studies indicate that SVT became non-inducible in a comparable proportion of WPW patients, implying a loss of retrograde conduction as well. Patients who lost the pre-excitation pattern exhibited a prolonged anterograde effective refractory period and reduced rate of conduction through the accessory pathway compared to those with a persistent pre-excitation pattern.

The optimal treatment of children with WPW syndrome remains controversial, with some physicians choosing a conservative approach and others promoting early catheter ablation. Nevertheless, as ablation techniques have advanced, radiofrequency catheter ablation is increasingly performed in children, particularly if they experience episodes of paroxysmal supraventricular tachycardia.

The precise identification of accessory pathway locations by ECG features is a crucial first step prior to radiofrequency catheter ablation, aiding in the effective planning of mapping and ablation techniques. Numerous algorithms with good sensitivity and specificity have been created for pediatric patients. Upon applying proven algorithms to our newborn, we identified a left posterior accessory pathway pattern. However, none of the algorithms were explicitly designed for newborns, and in the majority of these algorithms, the initial step relies on the amplitudes of the R- and S-waves in lead V1. Nevertheless, neonates typically display pronounced R-waves in lead V1. Moreover, we lack invasive electrophysiological testing in our neonates to verify the localization.

BIBLIOGRAPHY

1. Pærregaard MM, Hartmann J, Sillesen AS, Pihl C, Dannesbo S, Kock TO, Pietersen A, Raja AA, Iversen KK, Bundgaard H, Christensen AH. The Wolff–Parkinson–White pattern in neonates: results from a large population-based cohort study. *Europace*. 2023 Jul. 4; 25(7): euad165. doi:10.1093/europace/euad165. PMID: 37465966; PMCID: PMC10354624.

2. Chambers S, Jnah A, Newberry D. The pathophysiology, diagnosis, and management of Wolff–Parkinson–White syndrome in the neonate. *Adv Neonatal Care*. 2021 Jun 1; 21(3): 178–188. doi:10.1097/ANC.0000000000000785. PMID: 32826411.

3. Jadczak EA, Jnah AJ. Wolff–Parkinson–White syndrome in the preterm neonate. *Neonatal Netw*. 2024 Aug. 1; 43(4): 212–223. doi:10.1891/NN-2023-0076. PMID: 39164096.

4. Hoeffler CD, Krenek ME, Brand MC. Wolff–Parkinson–White syndrome in a term infant presenting with cardiopulmonary arrest. *Adv Neonatal Care*. 2016 Feb.; 16(1): 44–51. doi:10.1097/ANC.0000000000000246. PMID: 26742096.

5. Hermosura T, Bradshaw WT. Wolff–Parkinson–White syndrome in infants. *Neonatal Netw*. 2010 Jul.–Aug.; 29(4): 215–223. doi:10.1891/0730-0832.29.4.215. PMID: 20630836.

6. Valderrama AL. Wolff–Parkinson–White syndrome: Essentials for the primary care nurse practitioner. *J Am Acad Nurse Pract*. 2004 Sep.; 16(9): 378–383. doi:10.1111/j.1745-7599.2004.tb00387.x. PMID: 15495691.

7. Perry JC, Garson Jr A. Supraventricular tachycardia due to Wolff–Parkinson–White syndrome in children: Early disappearance and late recurrence. *J Am Coll Cardiol*. 1990 Nov.; 16(5): 1215–1220. doi:10.1016/0735-1097(90)90555-4. PMID: 2229769.

8. Calkins H, Sousa J, el-Atassi R, Rosenheck S, de Buitleir M, Kou WH, Kadish AH, Langberg JJ, Morady F. Diagnosis and cure of the Wolff-Parkinson-White syndrome or paroxysmal supraventricular tachycardias during a single electrophysiologic test. *N Engl J Med*. 1991 Jun. 6; 324(23): 1612–1618. doi:10.1056/NEJM199106063242302. PMID: 2030717.

9. Inoue K, Igarashi H, Fukushige J, Ohno T, Joh K, Hara T. Long-term prospective study on the natural history of Wolff–Parkinson–White syndrome detected during a heart screening program at school. *Acta Paediatr*. 2000 May; 89(5): 542–545. doi:10.1080/080352500750027817. PMID: 10852188.

10. Jemtrén A, Saygi S, Åkerström F, Asaad F, Bourke T, Braunschweig F, Carnlöf C, Drca N, Insulander P, Kennebäck G, Nordin AP, Sadigh B, Rickenlund A, Saluveer O, Schwieler J, Svennberg E, Tapanainen J, Turkmen Y, Bastani H, Jensen-Urstad M. Risk assessment in

patients with symptomatic and asymptomatic pre-excitation. *Europace*. 2024 Feb. 1; 26(2): euae036. doi:10.1093/europace/euae036. PMID: 38363996; PMCID: PMC10873488.

11. Lowenstein SR, Halperin BD, Reiter MJ. Paroxysmal supraventricular tachycardias. *J Emerg Med*. 1996 Jan.–Feb.; 14(1): 39–51. doi:10.1016/0736-4679(95)02061-6. PMID: 8655936.

12. Ornato JP. Management of paroxysmal supraventricular tachycardia. *Circulation*. 1986 Dec.; 74(6 Pt 2): IV108-10. PMID: 3536156.

13. Kadish A, Passman R. Mechanisms and management of paroxysmal supraventricular tachycardia. *Cardiol Rev*. 1999 Sep.–Oct.; 7(5): 254–264. doi:10.1097/00045415-199909000-00009. PMID: 11208235.

14. Verdú Solans J, Soler Costa M, Molero Arcos A, Ojeda Cuchillero I. Taquicardia paroxística supraventricular (TPSV): dos presentaciones. Dos aproximaciones [Paroxysmal supraventricular tachycardia (PSVT): Two presentations. Two approaches]. *Semergen*. 2017 Apr.; 43(3): 240–242. Spanish. doi:10.1016/j.semerg.2016.04.006. Epub 2016 Jun 27. PMID: 27365225.

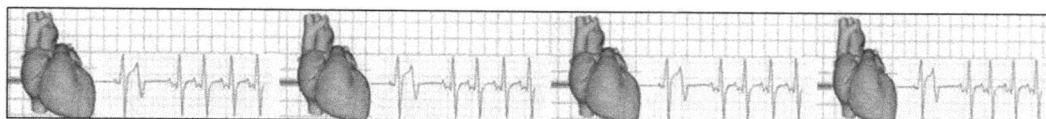

Case 26 Focal Atrial Tachycardia

Andrei Mihordea, Adrian Stef, and Cismaru Gabriel

CLINICAL CASE

A 13-year-old obese male patient with anxiety experienced multiple episodes of tachycardia (220 bpm), beginning two years prior to his presentation. During the preceding year, he had experienced 7 episodes of tachycardia. His electrocardiogram was normal, and echocardiogram revealed a normal heart. His complete blood count and biochemistry were carried out; these were also normal. A Holter ECG was performed, confirming the arrhythmia, and the patient started treatment with Propranolol and Flecainide. Due to recurrent arrhythmias under medication, an electrophysiological study was performed. Under General Anesthesia using the three-dimensional mapping method Carto 3, a diagnosis of parahisian focal atrial tachycardia was established, and catheter ablation was carried out. At the seven-month follow-up, the patient experienced no additional episodes of arrhythmia.

Concluzie

Ritm cardiac		
Total bătăi	74 233	(0% paced)
HR max / min	**209 / 51 bpm**	
Media HR	**Ø 88 bpm**	
HR Max / Min Sinus	166 / 51 bpm	
Media HR (Treaz/Adormit)	89 / 80 bpm	
Index circadian	1.11	
Tahicardie / Bradicardie	36 % / - %	

Pauze	
RR Max	**1 326 ms**
Pauze (>2000ms)	**0**

Fibrilație atrială / Flutter atrial	
Total AF	-
AF HR Max	0 bpm
Cel mai lung AF	-

Bradicardie	
Cea mai mică	-
Cea mai mare	-

ST		
St ridicare max	0.31 mV	I
ST depresurizare max	-0.28 mV	aVR

Ectopie ventriculară		
V Total	26	(< 1%)
V / Ora Max	13	pe oră
Episoade Tahicardie V		2 Σ 3 sec
Cea mai rapidă Tahicardie V	Ø 175 bpm	2 sec
V Cea mai lungă secvență	Ø 175 bpm	2 sec
Triplete / Execută		1 Σ 4 bătăi
Cuplete		2 Σ 4 bătăi
Bigeminism		1 Σ 2 bătăi
Trigeminism		1 Σ 2 bătăi

Ectopie supraventriculară		
S Tot	244	(< 1%)
Episoade Tahicardie SV		7 Σ 51 sec
Cea mai rapidă Tahicardie SV	Ø 208 bpm	7 sec
S Cea mai lungă secvență	Ø 199 bpm	9 sec
Triplete / Execută		7 Σ 51 bătăi
Cuplete		4 Σ 8 bătăi

Figure 26.1 The summary page shows a maximum heart rate of 209 bpm and a minimum rate of 51 bpm. PVC and PAC burden are low < 1%/24 hours. There were 7 episodes of supraventricular arrhythmia with a duration of up to 9 seconds and a rate of up to 208 bpm.

DOI: 10.1201/9781003545040-26

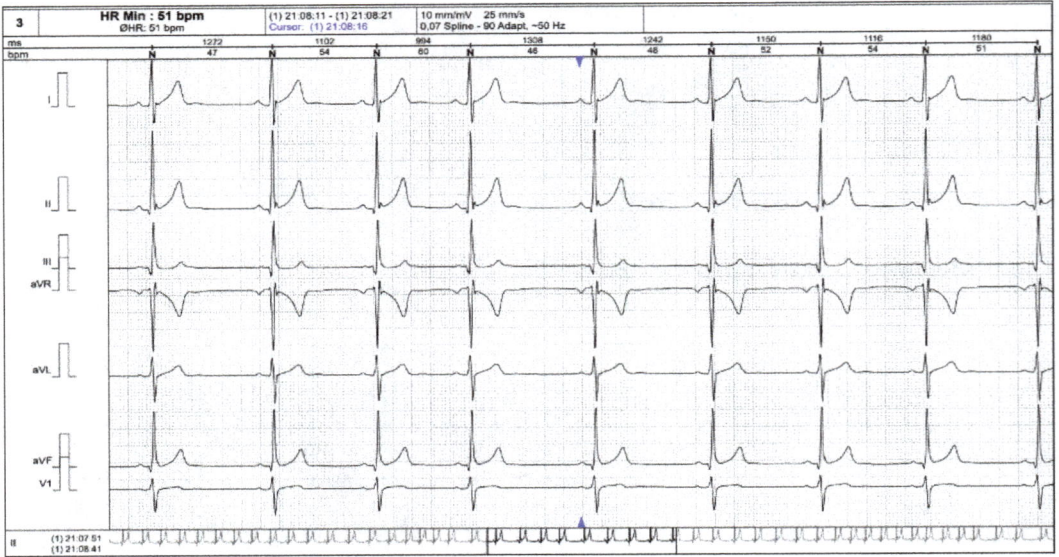

Figure 26.2   The tracing shows normal sinus rhythm with a rate of 51 bpm.

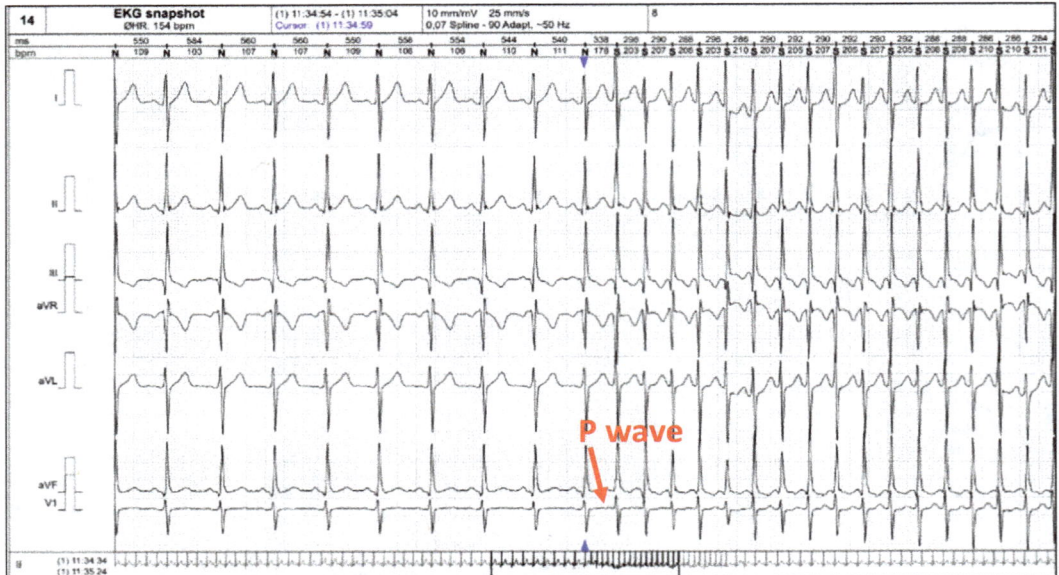

Figure 26.3   The tracing shows an episode of paroxysmal supraventricular tachycardia, with narrow QRS complexes, initiated by a premature atrial contraction (arrow).

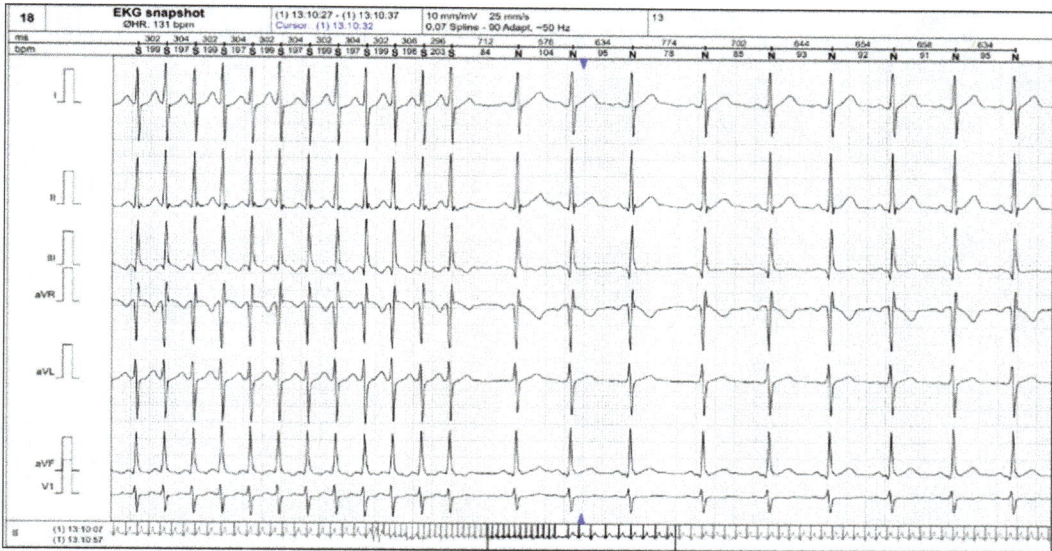

Figure 26.4   Arrhythmia stops and is followed by normal sinus rhythm.

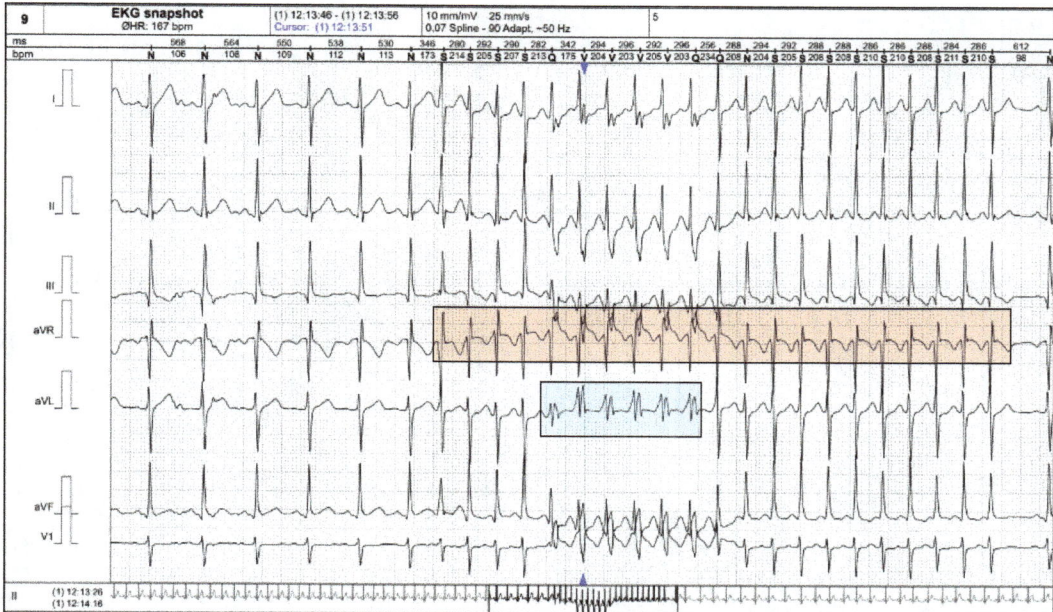

Figure 26.5   The tracing shows an episode of paroxysmal supraventricular tachycardia, with narrow QRS complexes, initiated by a premature atrial contraction. During the episode, 6 beats are conducted with larger QRS due to RBBB aberrancy.

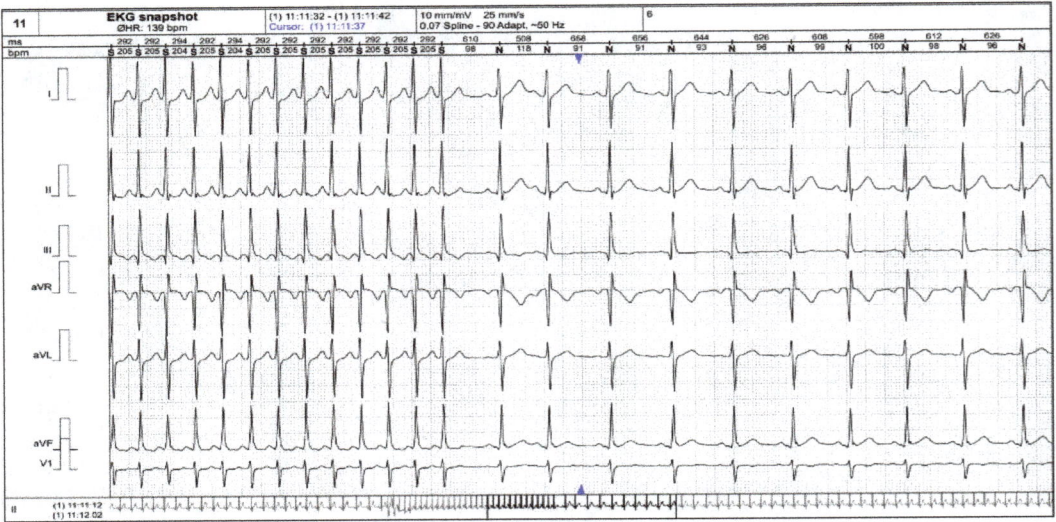

Figure 26.6 The arrhythmia stops with a ventricular activation (QRS complex). An arrhythmia that stops with an atrial activation (P wave) would exclude an atrial tachycardia.

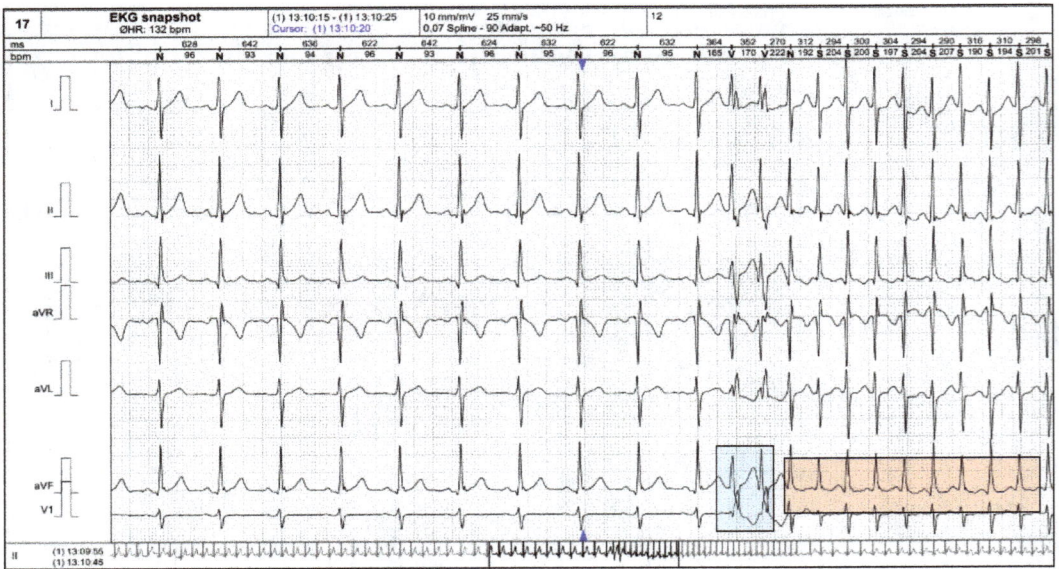

Figure 26.7 The tracing shows an episode of atrial tachycardia, initiated by 2 PACs conducted with an aberrant RBBB ventricular complex.

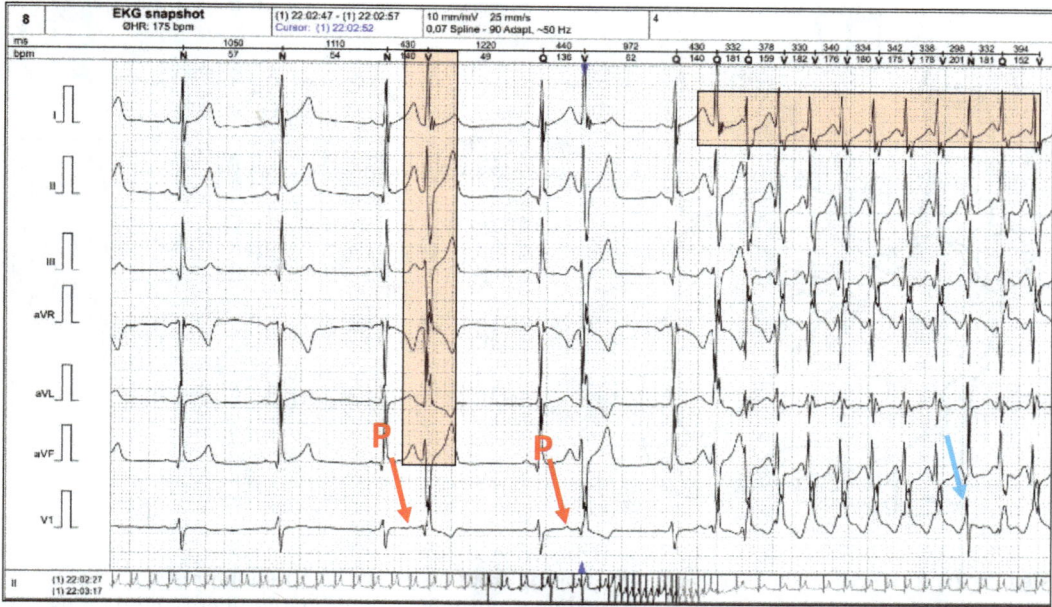

Figure 26.8 The tracing shows 2 PACs conducted with RBBB aberrancy and an episode of atrial tachycardia with intermittent RBBB.

HOLTER SUMMARY

The monitoring indicates episodes of supraventricular tachycardia, with a rate reaching 209 bpm and lasting up to 9 seconds. The tachycardia has narrow QRS complexes; nonetheless, a right bundle branch block is intermittently observed, attributed to aberrant ventricular conduction. Two premature atrial contractions were detected, exhibiting a longer PR interval compared to the sinus rhythm, in addition to RBBB aberrancy.

DISCUSSION

Focal atrial tachycardia is a rare cause of tachycardia in pediatric patients, originating from an atrial focus with increased automaticity. The term focal atrial tachycardia is often used interchangeably with atrial tachycardia, which is a broader designation for any type of supraventricular tachycardia originating in the atria other than the sinus node. It is dictated by a singular ectopic focus. The mechanism includes: automaticity, triggered activity, or reentry. It may be either paroxysmal or persistent arrhythmia. Persistent atrial tachycardia may progress to tachycardia-induced cardiomyopathy. Although they constitute a minor portion of SVT types, they represent the predominant amount of tachycardia-induced cardiomyopathy observed in newborns and young children.

ECG characteristics of focal atrial tachycardia are:

- Atrial rate above 100 bpm;
- Abnormal P wave morphology and axis;
- Unifocal, identical P waves;
- Isoelectric baseline (as opposed to atrial flutter);
- Normal QRS morphology, except in cases of rate-related aberrant conduction.

Pharmacological intervention has been the main approach for FAT, particularly in newborns, infants and small children who are more prone to spontaneous remission. Numerous antiarrhythmic agents have been used; however, FAT frequently exhibits resistance to pharmacological treatment. β-blockers and class Ic antiarrhythmics (Flecainide, Propafenone) are effective for managing atrial tachycardia, in contrast to other drugs such as Digoxin, Amiodarone, or Sotalol,

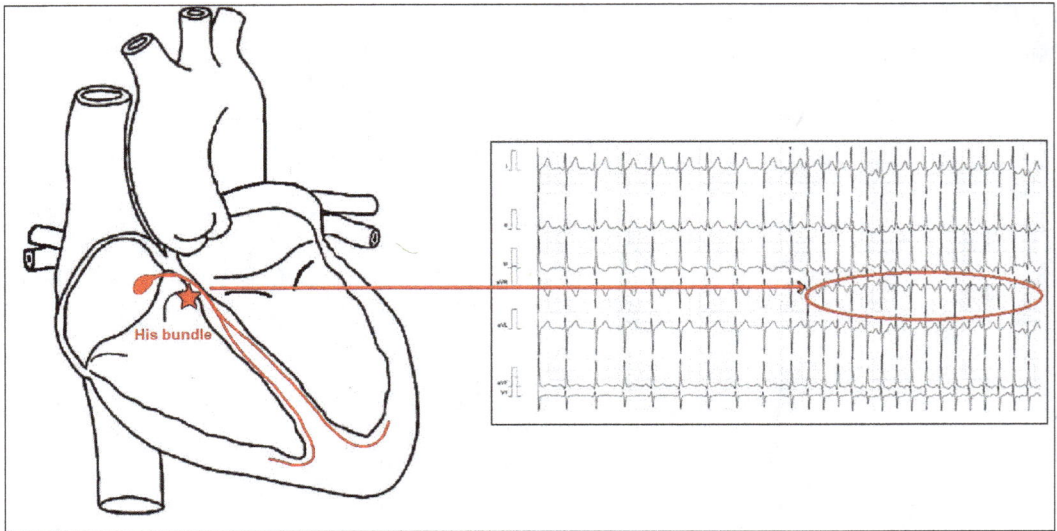

Figure 26.9 Focal atrial tachycardia originating from the parahisian region presents a risk of atrioventricular block during catheter ablation. Consequently, alternative energy modalities may be employed, such as cryotherapy or ablation from adjacent areas, like the left septum or noncoronary aortic cusps.

which have proven less efficacious. Radiofrequency ablation has been successfully employed for definitive treatment of the arrhythmia. The integration of three-dimensional electroanatomic mapping systems for catheter ablation has facilitated increased rates of both acute and long-term results.

Symptomatic atrial tachycardias occasionally originate from the parahisian area. The mapping and ablation of these arrhythmias present particular challenges, as successful ablation sites may be situated near the His bundle, carrying a minor yet substantial risk of damaging the AV conduction system and necessitating pacemaker insertion. Consequently, alternative methods were implemented, such as ablation from the left side of the atrial septum or the non-coronary cusp. Several algorithms utilizing P-wave morphology in the 12-lead ECG have been created to determine the origin of tachycardia location on the interatrial septum; however, the intricate anatomical relationship between the interatrial septum and the aortic root renders P-wave morphology an unreliable predictor of the successful ablation site. Consequently, comprehensive mapping of both atria may be necessary in many cases. We mapped the interatrial septum and found the earliest atrial activation near the His bundle. We conducted the ablation in this patient from the right atrium, with 10, 15 and 20 watt, noting a prolongation of the AH conduction time during the procedure, with complete resolution of the arrhythmia and without any permanent complication. At the seven-month follow-up, there was no recurrence of the arrhythmia. The primary problem in ablating parahisian atrial tachycardias is to prevent complete AV block, a risk that is amplified in pediatric patients due to their small body surface area and small Koch triangle. An alternative method involves using cryoablation in the right atrium near the His bundle, permitting titration of cryoenergy to prevent irreversible damage to the AV node and the implantation of a pacemaker.

BIBLIOGRAPHY

1. Mehta AV, Sanchez GR, Sacks EJ, Casta A, Dunn JM, Donner RM. Ectopic automatic atrial tachycardia in children: Clinical characteristics, management and follow-up. *J Am Coll Cardiol*. 1988; 11: 379–385.

2. Naheed ZJ, Strasburger JF, Benson DW, Deal BJ. Natural history and management strategies of automatic atrial tachycardia in children. *Am J Cardiol*. 1995; 75: 405–407.

3. von Bernuth G, Engelhardt W, Kramer HH, Singer H, Schneider P, Ulmer H, Brodherr-Heberlein S, Kienast W, Lang D, Lindinger A. Atrial automatic tachycardia in infancy and childhood. *Eur Heart J*. 1992; 13: 1410–1415.

4. Cummings RM, Mahle WT, Strieper MJ, Campbell RM, Costello L, Balfour V, Burchfield A, Frias PA. Outcomes following electroanatomic mapping and ablation for the treatment of ectopic atrial tachycardia in the pediatric population. *Pediatr Cardiol*. 2008; 29: 393–397.

5. Dhala AA, Case CL, Gillette PC. Evolving treatment strategies for managing atrial ectopic tachycardia in children. *Am J Cardiol*. 1994; 74: 283–286.

6. Grigg WS, Pearlman JD, Nagalli S. Ashman phenomenon. 2024 Sep 11. In: *StatPearls* [Internet]. Treasure Island (FL): StatPearls Publishing; 2025 Jan–. PMID: 32965982.

7. Walsh EP, Saul JP, Hulse JE, Rhodes LA, Hordof AJ, Mayer JE, Lock JE. Transcatheter ablation of ectopic atrial tachycardia in young patients using radiofrequency current. *Circulation*. 1992; 86: 1138–1146.

8. Colloridi V, Perri C, Ventriglia F, Critelli G. Oral sotalol in pediatric atrial ectopic tachycardia. *Am Heart J*. 1992; 123: 254–256.

9. Salerno JC, Kertesz NJ, Friedman RA, Fenrich AL. Clinical course of atrial ectopic tachycardia is age-dependent: Results and treatment in children < 3 or > or = 3 years of age. *J Am Coll Cardiol*. 2004; 43: 438–444.

10. Bauersfeld U, Gow RM, Hamilton RM, Izukawa T. Treatment of atrial ectopic tachycardia in infants < 6 months old. *Am Heart J*. 1995; 129: 1145–1148.

11. Chiladakis JA, Vassilikos VP, Maounis TN, Cokkinos DV, Manolis AS. Successful radiofrequency catheter ablation of automatic atrial tachycardia with regression of the cardiomyopathy picture. *Pacing Clin Electrophysiol*. 1997; 20(4 Pt 1): 953–959.

12. Koike K, Hesslein PS, Finlay CD, Williams WG, Izukawa T, Freedom RM. Atrial automatic tachycardia in children. *Am J Cardiol*. 1988; 61: 1127–1130.

13. Keane JF, Plauth WH, Nadas AS. Chronic ectopic tachycardia of infancy and childhood. *Am Heart J*. 1972; 84: 748–757.

14. Gillette PC, Garson A. Electrophysiologic and pharmacologic characteristics of automatic ectopic atrial tachycardia. *Circulation*. 1977; 56(4 Pt 1): 571–575.

15. Aras D, Cay S, Topaloglu S, Cagirci G, Ozeke O. Parahisian atrial tachycardia: cryoablation from the aortic cusp. *Indian Pacing Electrophysiol J*. 2014 Jan. 1; 14(1):49–52. doi: 10.1016/s0972-6292(16)30716-1. PMID: 24493917; PMCID: PMC3878588.

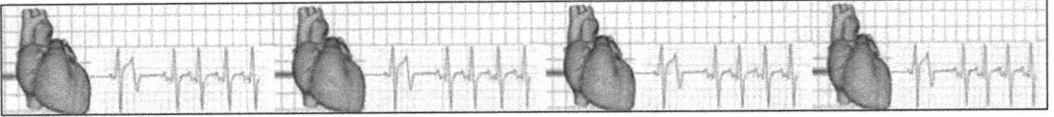

Case 27 Artifacts Mimicking Ventricular Tachycardia

Cecilia Lazea, Crina Sufana, Gabriela Kelemen, and Alexandra Popa

CLINICAL CASE

An 8-year-old female patient experienced one episode of vasovagal syncope related to micturition. Neurological examination, electrocardiogram and echocardiogram were normal. A Holter ECG monitoring found tracings suspected of ventricular tachycardia and an arrhythmological examination was requested. The patient was asymptomatic during Holter monitoring.

Concluzie

Ritm cardiac		
Total bătăi	106 666	(0% paced)
HR max / min	**220 / 53 bpm**	
Media HR	**Ø 91 bpm**	
HR Max / Min Sinus	220 / 53 bpm	
Media HR (Treaz/Adormit)	96 / 79 bpm	
Index circadian	1,22	
Tahicardie / Bradicardie	16 % / < 1 %	

Pauze	
RR Max	**1 992 ms**
Pauze (>2000ms)	**0**

Fibrilaţie atrială / Flutter atrial	
Total AF	-
AF HR Max	0 bpm
Cel mai lung AF	-

Bradicardie		
Cea mai mică	Ø 56 bpm	18 sec
Cea mai mare	Ø 56 bpm	26 sec

ST		
St ridicare max	2,46 mV	V3
ST depresurizare max	-0,65 mV	aVR

Ectopie ventriculară		
V Total	0	(< 1%)
V / Ora Max	0	pe oră
Episoade Tahicardie V		-
Cea mai rapidă Tahicardie V		-
V Cea mai lungă secvenţă		-
Triplete / Execută		0 Σ 0 bătăi
Cuplete		0 Σ 0 bătăi
Bigeminism		0 Σ 0 bătăi
Trigeminism		0 Σ 0 bătăi

Ectopie supraventriculară		
S Tot	0	(< 1%)
Episoade Tahicardie SV		-
Cea mai rapidă Tahicardie SV		-
S Cea mai lungă secvenţă		-
Triplete / Execută		0 Σ 0 bătăi
Cuplete		0 Σ 0 bătăi

Figure 27.1 The summary page displays a minimum heart rate of 53 bpm and a maximum heart rate of 220 bpm. Nevertheless, the patient had no symptoms, and this elevated rate requires meticulous verification.

DOI: 10.1201/9781003545040-27

2	**Bradicardii**					Primele 5 episoade cu media HR > 58 bpm
Începe de la	Ritm	HR Media	HR Min	HR Max		Durata
(2) 03:15:33	Bradicardie	56	54	56		00:00:18
(2) 03:16:05	Bradicardie	56	54	57		00:00:20
(2) 03:25:57	Bradicardie	56	53	57		00:00:26
(2) 03:17:27	Bradicardie	56	56	57		00:00:14
(2) 03:24:41	Bradicardie	57	57	57		00:00:12
3	**Tahicardii**					Primele 5 episoade cu media HR > 110 bpm
Începe de la	Ritm	HR Media	HR Min	HR Max		Durata
(2) 09:33:19	Tahicardie	163	114	197		00:05:18
(2) 09:28:51	Tahicardie	154	111	183		00:02:00
(2) 09:06:41	Tahicardie	151	110	220		00:04:44
(2) 09:49:03	Tahicardie	151	110	183		00:01:44
(2) 09:57:29	Tahicardie	143	95	183		00:14:24
4	**Secventa V**					secvența cea mai lungă 5
Începe de la	Ritm	HR Media	HR Min	HR Max		Durata
5	**Secventa S**					Primele 5 cele mai lungi secvențe
Începe de la	Ritm	HR Media	HR Min	HR Max		Durata
6	**Episoadele V Tach**					Toate episoadele cu media HR > 110 bpm
Începe de la	Ritm	HR Media	HR Min	HR Max		Durata

Figure 27.2 The summary table shows the highest rate of 220 bpm recorded at 9:06 and had a duration of 4:44 minutes.

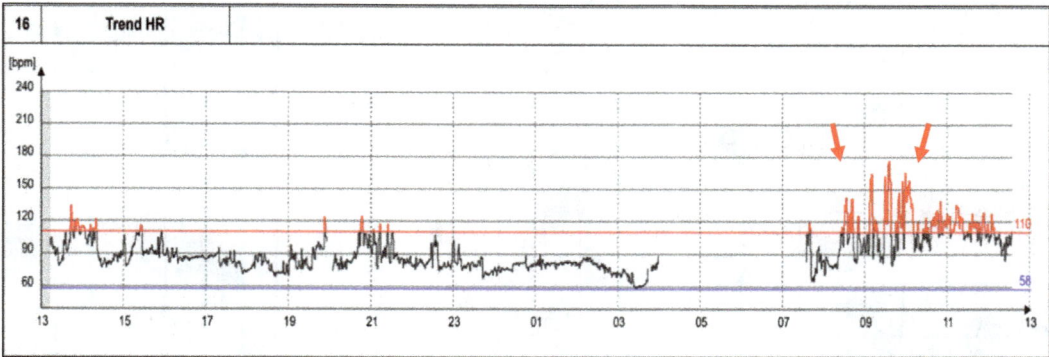

Figure 27.3 The heart rate trend shows elevated heart rates between 8:40 and 10:20 (red arrow).

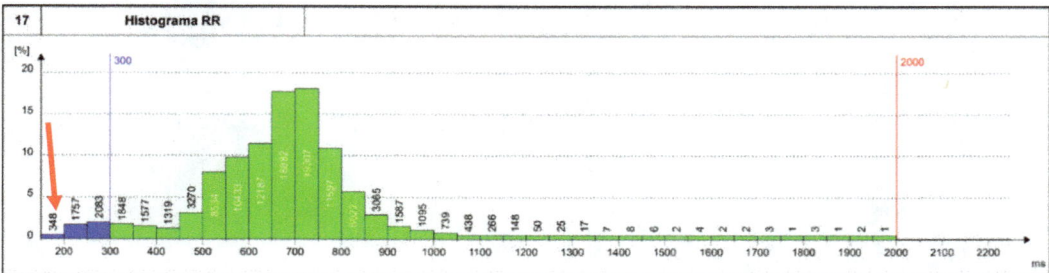

Figure 27.4 The RR histogram shows short RR intervals of < 200 ms, corresponding to heart rates of > 300 bpm.

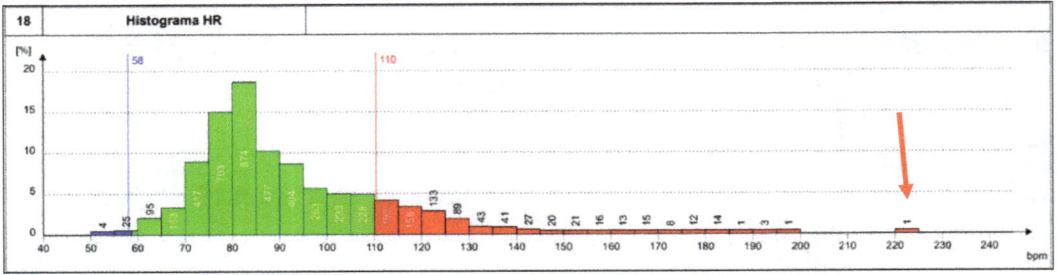

Figure 27.5 The HR histogram shows increased rates, above 180 bpm to 220 bpm.

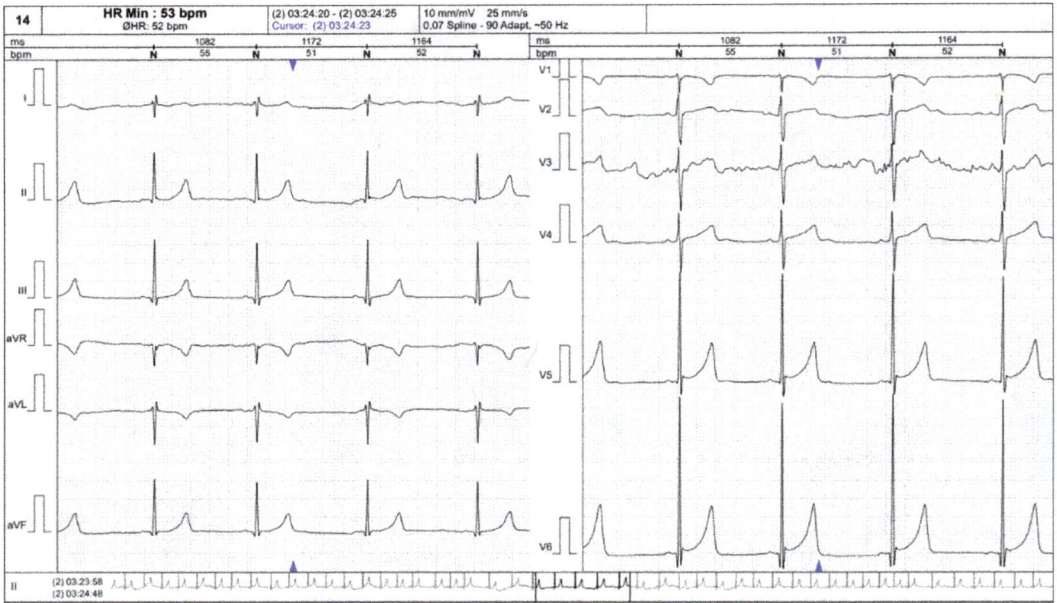

Figure 27.6 The tracing shows the minimum rate recorded during Holter monitoring.

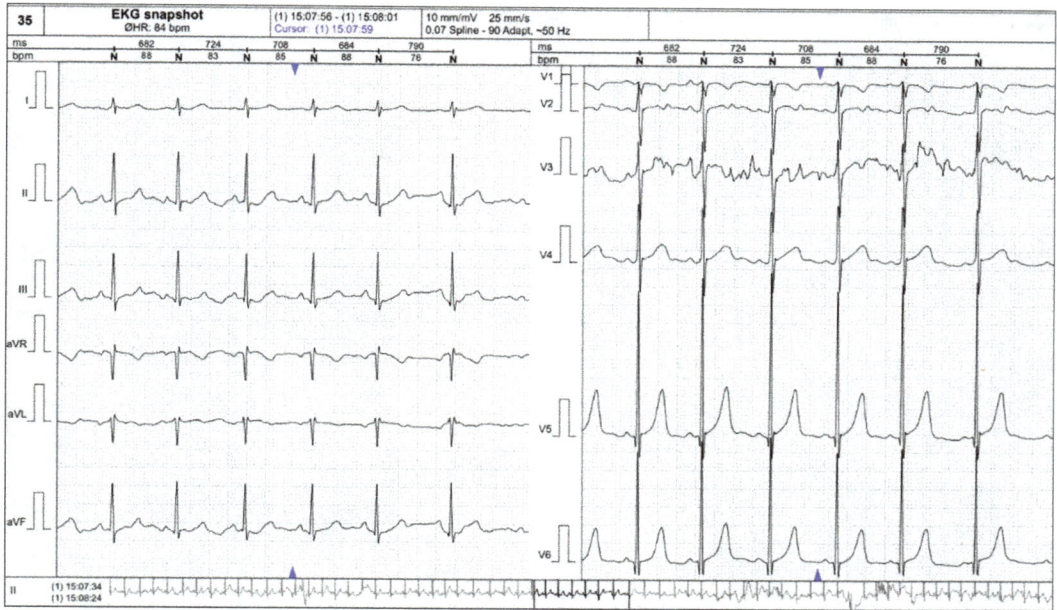

Figure 27.7 The tracing shows sinus rhythm with a rate of 84 bpm.

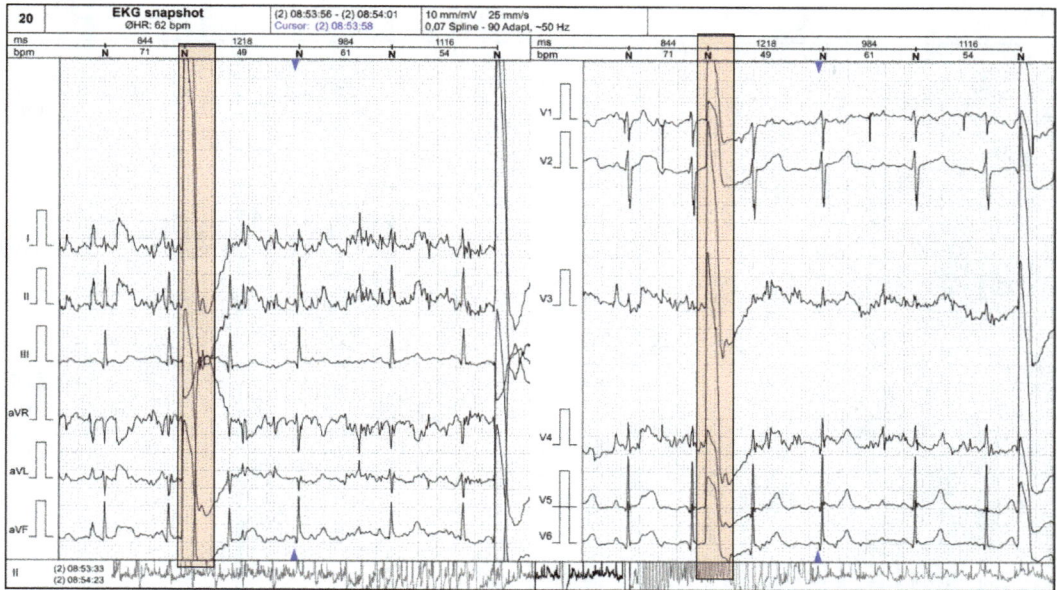

Figure 27.8 The tracing shows artifacts of the T wave, most probably due to loose electrode–skin connection.

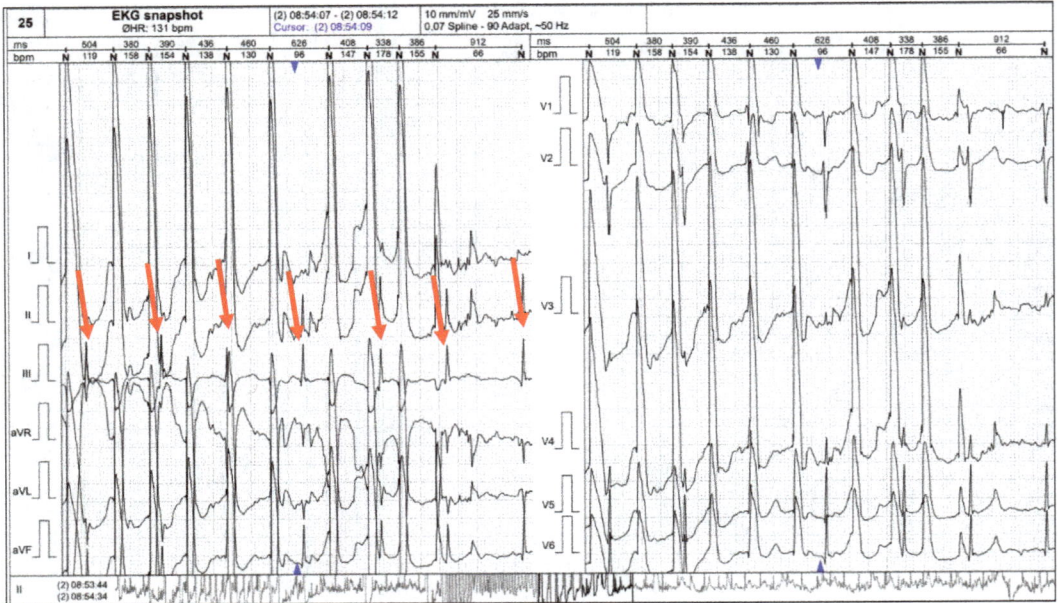

Figure 27.9 The tracing shows electrical artifacts mimicking a ventricular tachycardia. Nevertheless, the underlying sinus beat is easily identifiable (red arrows).

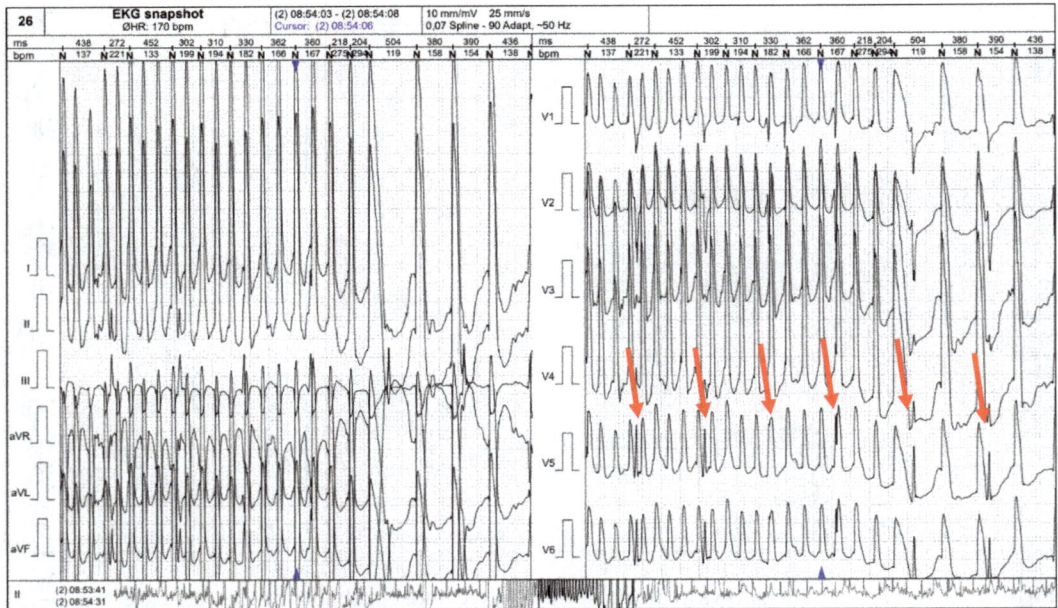

Figure 27.10 The strip shows electrical artifacts mimicking a ventricular tachycardia. Nevertheless, the underlying sinus beat is easily identifiable (red arrows).

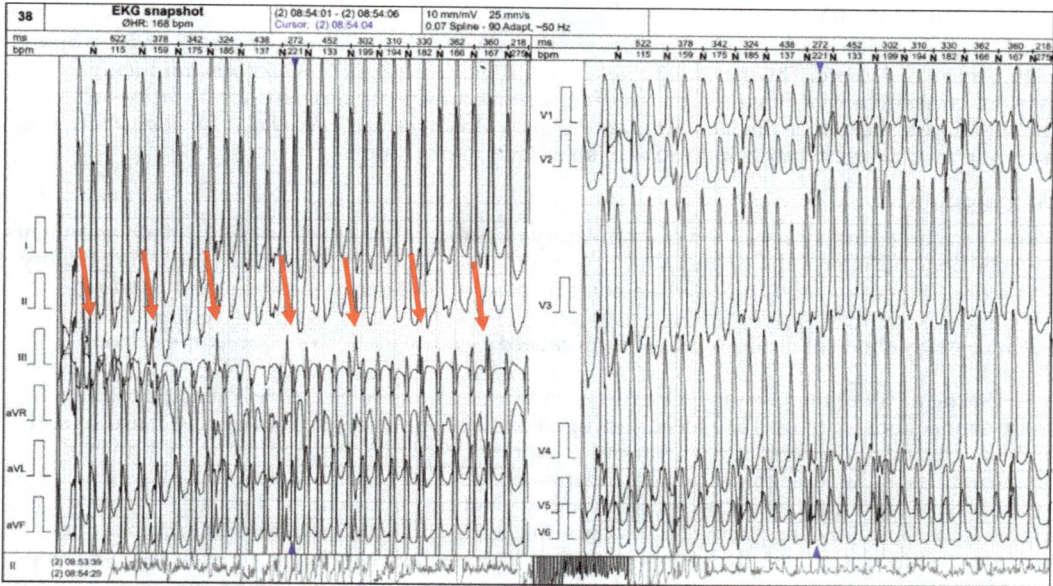

Figure 27.11   The strip shows electrical artifacts mimicking a ventricular tachycardia. Nevertheless, the underlying sinus beat is easily identifiable (red arrows).

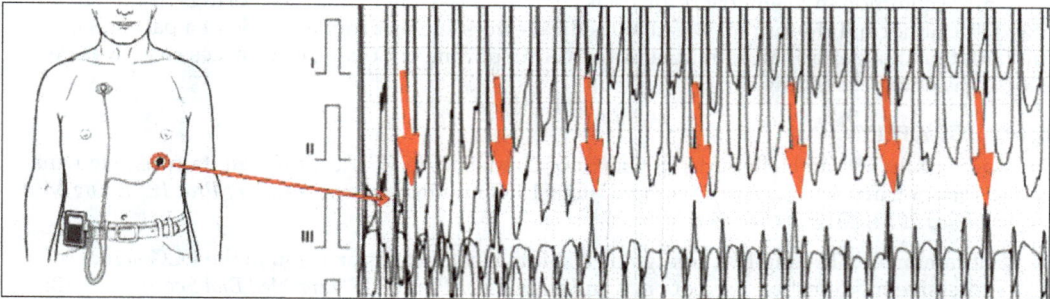

Figure 27.12   An inadequate electro-skin connection may result in electrical abnormalities that could be erroneously interpreted as ventricular tachycardia.

HOLTER SUMMARY

The 24-hour monitoring period indicates sinus rhythm with heart rates between 53 and 130 bpm, with a mean of 91 bpm. The increased rates up to 220 bpm are electrical artifacts, mimicking ventricular tachycardia. However, the accurate terminology is pseudo-ventricular tachycardia, as the signals are aberrant artifacts. In this young girl with suspected vaso-vagal syncope, there was no brady- or tachyarrhythmia indicative of an arrhythmic syncope.

DISCUSSION

Since Norman J. Holter's invention of ambulatory ECG recording in 1947, significant advancements in recording and interpretation software have taken place, leading to enhanced recording fidelity and more advanced analytical tools like Poincaré graphs, ST segment analysis, and heart rate variability. Nonetheless, recording artifacts continue to occur despite ongoing technological advancements aimed at minimizing artifacts caused by body motion or poor skin-electrode contact.

Artifacts in Holter monitoring may arise from inadequate skin–electrode contact, loose electrode connections, damaged ECG leads, myopotentials from the pectoral or deltoid muscles, and ambient electrical interference from various equipment. Artifacts may imitate arrhythmias or abnormalities in the ST segment or QRS duration.

The largest number of artifacts can be promptly identified if the doctor dedicates time to examine the simultaneous tracings across multiple leads and identify the normal rhythm under artifacts. Artifacts, particularly when just a single lead tracing is available for analysis (as in loop recorders or hand-held devices with one lead), may pose diagnostic challenges, and these artifacts are the most susceptible to generating management errors (such as the inappropriate administration of medications or implantation of devices).

Artifacts may mimic fast arrhythmias (atrial flutter, atrial fibrillation, paroxysmal supraventricular tachycardia, ventricular tachycardia, ventricular fibrillation) or bradyarrhythmias (electrical pauses, sinus node disease, atrio-ventricular block). Artifacts may infrequently be misidentified as premature atrial or ventricular contractions.

In the study of El-Sherif et al., 20 out of 500 Holter ECG recordings had artifacts, misinterpreted as atrial tachycardia, ventricular tachycardia, sinus arrest or atrioventricular block. The artifacts were more common in telemetry recordings compared to Holter ECG monitorings. If not recognized, the abnormal rhythm may lead to medical errors such as: implantation of a pacemaker; implantation of a defibrillator; treatment with Amiodarone or Sotalol; or unnecessary invasive electrophysiological testing.

BIBLIOGRAPHY

1. Kim S, Kim H, Van Helleputte N, Van Hoof C, Yazicioglu RF. Real time digitally assisted analog motion artifact reduction in ambulatory ECG monitoring system. *Conf Proc IEEE Eng Med Biol Soc 2012*; 2012: 2096–2099.

2. Subramaniam SR, Ling BW, Georgakis A. Motion artifact suppression in the ECG signal by successive modification in frequency and time. *Conf Proc IEEE, Eng Med Biol Soc 2013*; 2013: 425–428.

3. Keller KB, Lemberg L. Electrocardiographic artifacts. *Am J Crit Care* 2007; 16: 90–92.

4. Márquez MF, Colín L, Guevara M, Iturralde P, Hermosillo AG. Common electrocardiographic artifacts mimicking arrhythmias in ambulatory monitoring. *Am Heart J* 2002; 144: 187–197.

5. Knight BP, Pelosi F, Michaud GF, et al. Physician interpretation of electrocardiographic artifact that mimics ventricular tachycardia. *Am J Med* 2001; 110: 335–338.

6. Knight BP, Pelosi F, Michaud GF, et al. Clinical consequences of electrocardiographic artifact mimicking ventricular tachycardia. *N Engl J Med* 1999; 341: 1270–1274.

7. Dyke DBS, Rich PB, Morady F. Wide complex tachycardia in a critically ill patient: What is the rhythm? *J Cardiovasc Electrophysiol* 1997; 8: 1327–1328.

8. Hurst JW, Harvey WP. Iatrogenic heart disease and related problems In: Schlant RC, Alexander RW. (eds): *Hurst's the Heart*. 8th Edition New York: McGraw-Hill; 1994. p. 2111.

9. Falk RH, Knowlton AA. Atypical ventricular tachycardia or motion artifact? *Am J Cardiol* 1987; 59: 924.

10. Gardin JM, Belic N, Singer D. Pseudodysrhythmia in ambulatory ECG monitoring. *Arch Intern Med* 1979; 139: 809–812.

11. El-Sherif N, Turitto G. Ambulatory electrocardiographic monitoring between artifacts and misinterpretation, management errors of commission and errors of omission. *Ann Noninvasive Electrocardiol.* 2015 May; 20(3): 282–289. doi:10.1111/anec.12222. Epub 2014 Nov 4. PMID: 25367291; PMCID: PMC6931821.

12. Knight BP, Pelosi F, Michaud GF, Strickberger SA, Morady F. Clinical consequences of electrocardiographic artifact mimicking ventricular tachycardia. *N Engl J Med.* 1999 Oct. 21; 341(17):1270–1274. doi: 10.1056/NEJM199910213411704. PMID: 10528037.

13. Littmann L. Electrocardiographic artifact. *J Electrocardiol.* 2021 Jan.–Feb.; 64:23–29. doi: 10.1016/j.jelectrocard.2020.11.006. Epub 2020 Nov 30. PMID: 33278776.

14. Tarkin JM, Hadjiloizou N, Kaddoura S, Collinson J. Variable presentation of ventricular tachycardia-like electrocardiographic artifacts. *J Electrocardiol.* 2010 Nov.–Dec.; 43(6):691–693. doi: 10.1016/j.jelectrocard.2009.10.006. Epub 2009 Nov 25. PMID: 19932897.

15. Goldberger ZD, Rho RW, Page RL. Approach to the diagnosis and initial management of the stable adult patient with a wide complex tachycardia. *Am J Cardiol.* 2008 May 15; 101(10):1456–1466. doi: 10.1016/j.amjcard.2008.01.024. Epub 2008 Mar. 21. Erratum in: *Am J Cardiol.* 2008 Aug 1; 102(3):374. PMID: 18471458.

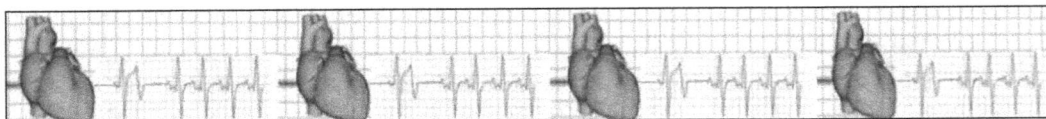

Case 28 Premature Atrial Contractions with RBBB Aberrancy, LBBB Aberrancy, and Salvos

Simona Cainap and Adrian Stef

CLINICAL CASE

She was referred to a cardiologist who confirmed the arrhythmia using a 12-lead ECG, which revealed premature atrial contractions. The echocardiogram was normal, and a Holter ECG was conducted. Following 24 hours of monitoring, no medication was considered necessary as the patient remained asymptomatic and the arrhythmia burden was classified as low to moderate. She was scheduled for an additional Holter ECG and echocardiogram at 6 months and 12 months follow-up

Concluzie

Ritm cardiac		
Total bătăi	98 620	(0% paced)
HR max / min	**141 / 50 bpm**	
Media HR	**Ø 75 bpm**	
HR Max / Min Sinus	141 / 50 bpm	
Media HR (Treaz/Adormit)	80 / 68 bpm	
Index circadian	1,18	
Tahicardie / Bradicardie	9 % / - %	

Pauze	
RR Max	**1 806 ms**
Pauze (>2000ms)	**0**

Fibrilație atrială / Flutter atrial	
Total AF	-
AF HR Max	0 bpm
Cel mai lung AF	-

Bradicardie	
Cea mai mică	-
Cea mai mare	-

ST		
St ridicare max	1,90 mV	V6
ST depresurizare max	-1,46 mV	V6

Ectopie ventriculară		
V Total	7861	(8%)
V / Ora Max	567	pe oră
Episoade Tahicardie V		-
Cea mai rapidă Tahicardie V		-
V Cea mai lungă secvență	Ø 114 bpm	1 sec
Triplete / Execută	4	Σ 14 bătăi
Cuplete	43	Σ 86 bătăi
Bigeminism	24	Σ 52 bătăi
Trigeminism	1006	Σ 3300 bătăi

Ectopie supraventriculară		
S Tot	3703	(4%)
Episoade Tahicardie SV		-
Cea mai rapidă Tahicardie SV		-
S Cea mai lungă secvență	Ø 137 bpm	3 sec
Triplete / Execută	176	Σ 639 bătăi
Cuplete	482	Σ 964 bătăi

Figure 28.1 The summary page shows a maximum heart rate of 141 bpm and a minimum rate of 50 bpm. PVC burden is moderate 7861/24 hours (8%). PAC burden is low to moderate 3703/24 hours (4%) with salvo of 3 sec. with a rate of 137 bpm.

DOI: 10.1201/9781003545040-28

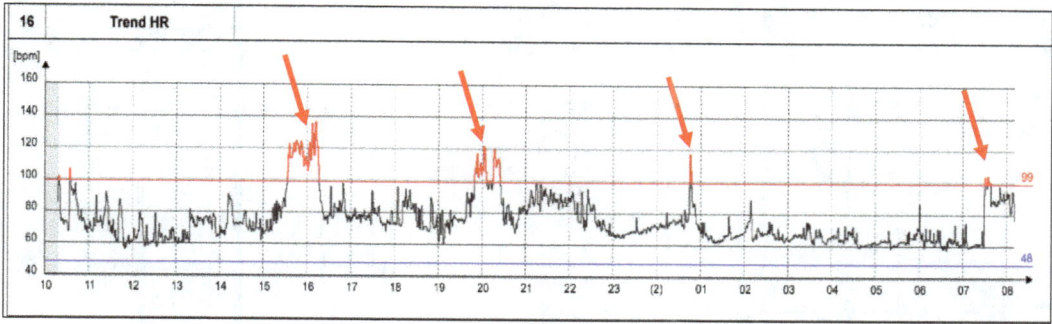

Figure 28.2   The heart rate trend shows episodes of nonsustained atrial tachycardia.

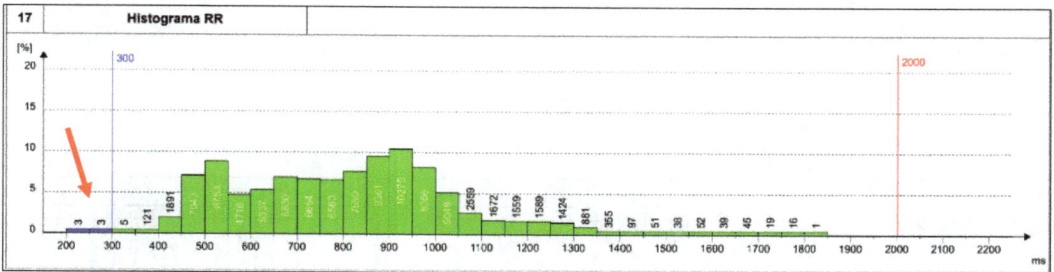

Figure 28.3   The RR histogram shows short RR intervals corresponding to episodes of nonsustained atrial tachycardia.

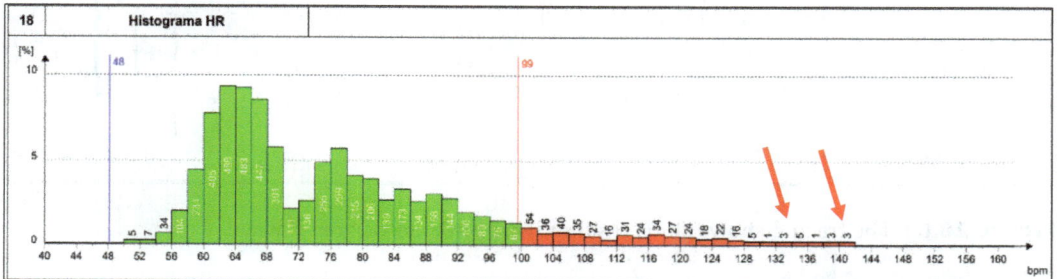

Figure 28.4   The HR histogram shows increased rates related to episodes of nonsustained atrial tachycardia.

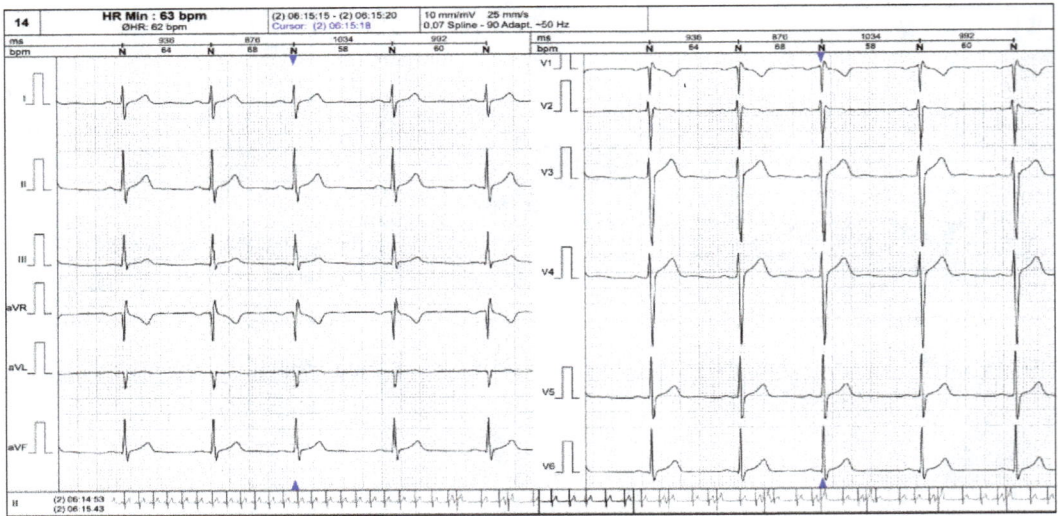

Figure 28.5 The tracing shows sinus rhythm 63 bpm.

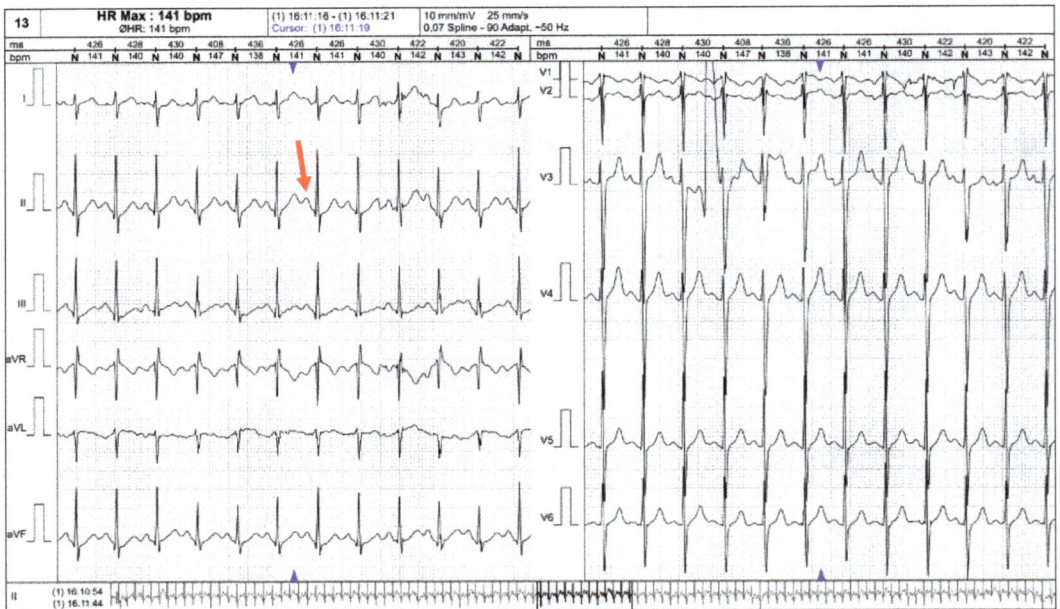

Figure 28.6 The tracing shows sinus rhythm, 141 bpm with normal P wave.

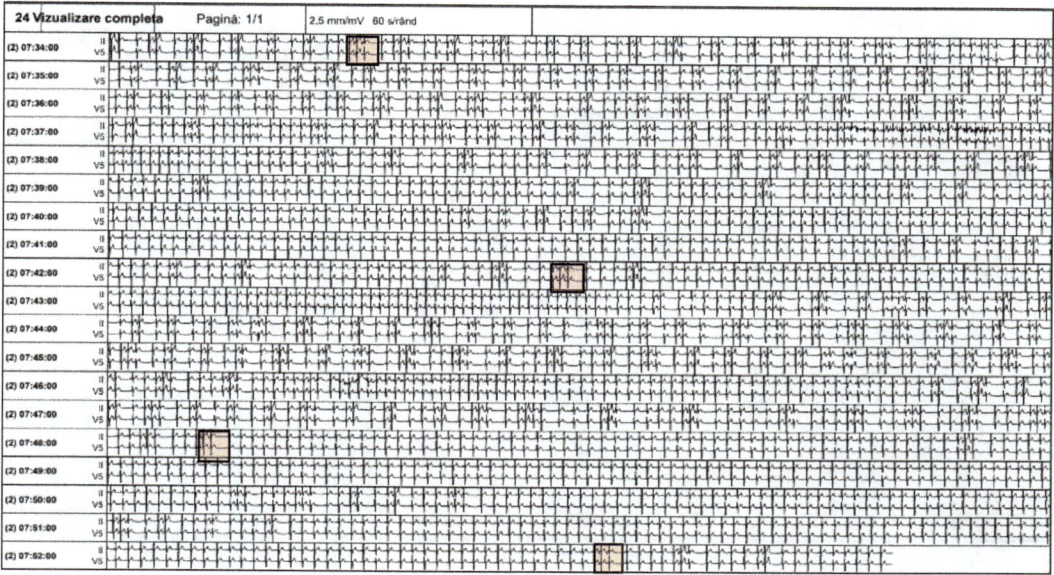

Figure 28.7 The summary tracing shows frequent salvos of PACs.

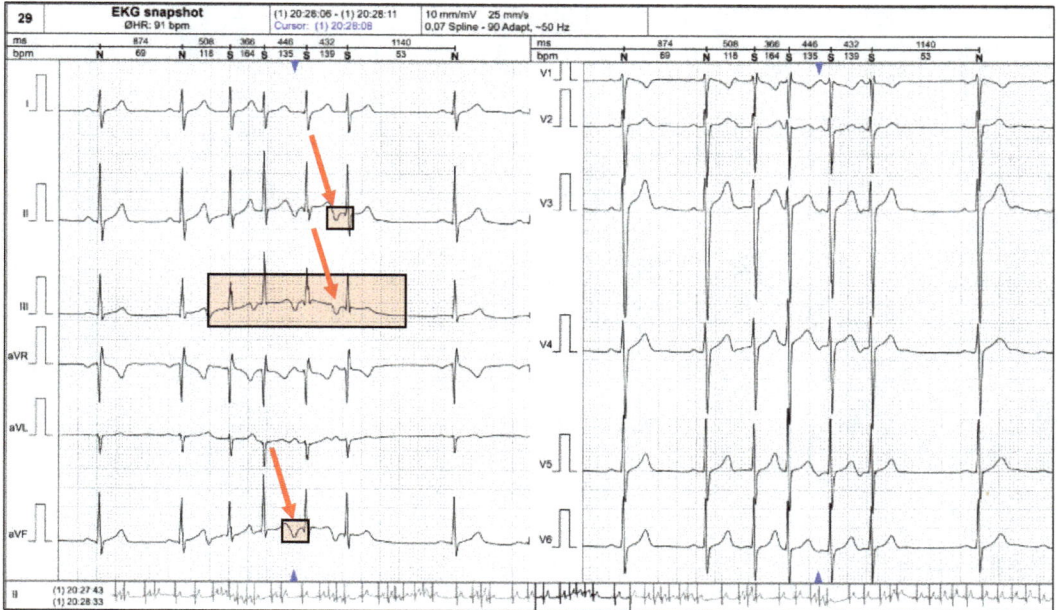

Figure 28.8 The tracing shows a salvo of 4 PACs with narrow QRS complexes. The P wave is negative in inferior leads.

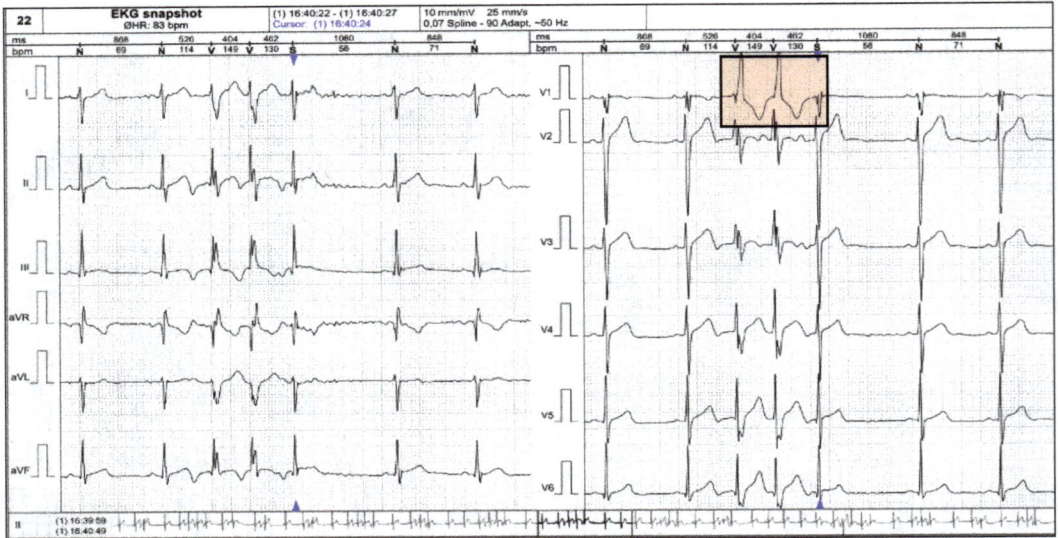

Figure 28.9 The tracing shows a salvo of 3 PACs with 2 large QRS complexes due to RBBB aberrancy. The P wave is negative in inferior leads.

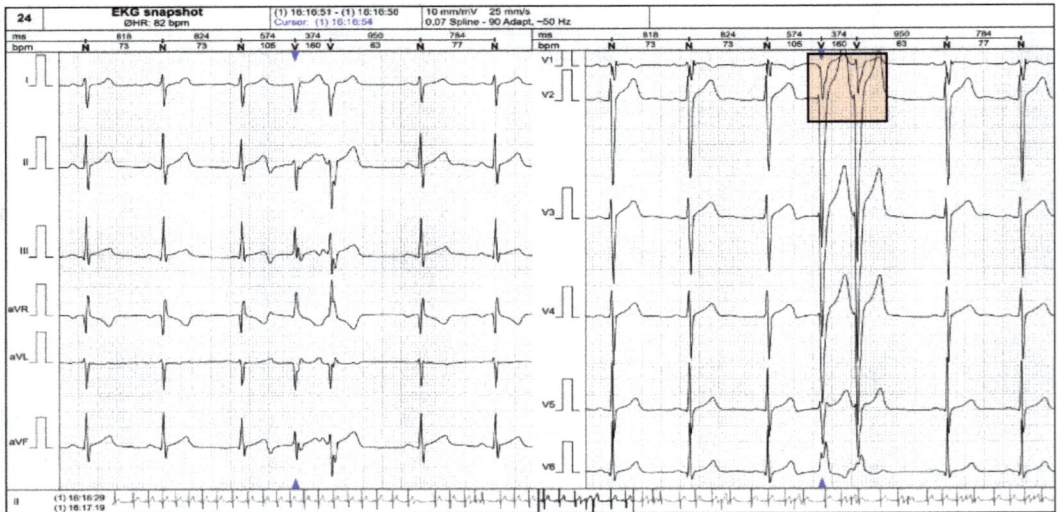

Figure 28.10 The tracing shows 2 PACs with large QRS complexes due to LBBB aberrancy. The P wave is negative in inferior leads and the PR interval is different from that of sinus rhythm.

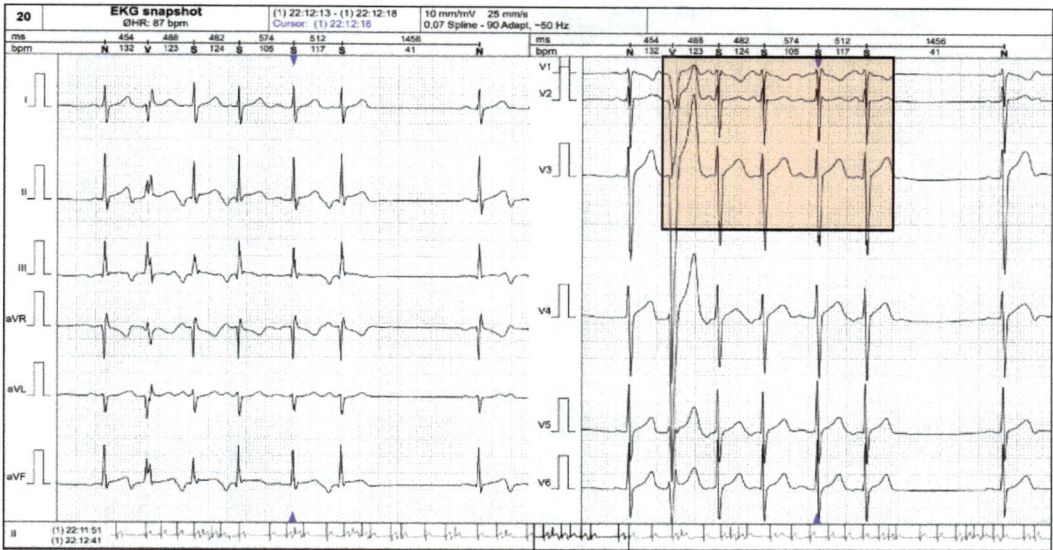

Figure 28.11   The tracing shows a salvo of 5 PACs with 1 large QRS complex due to LBBB aberrancy. The P wave is negative in inferior leads.

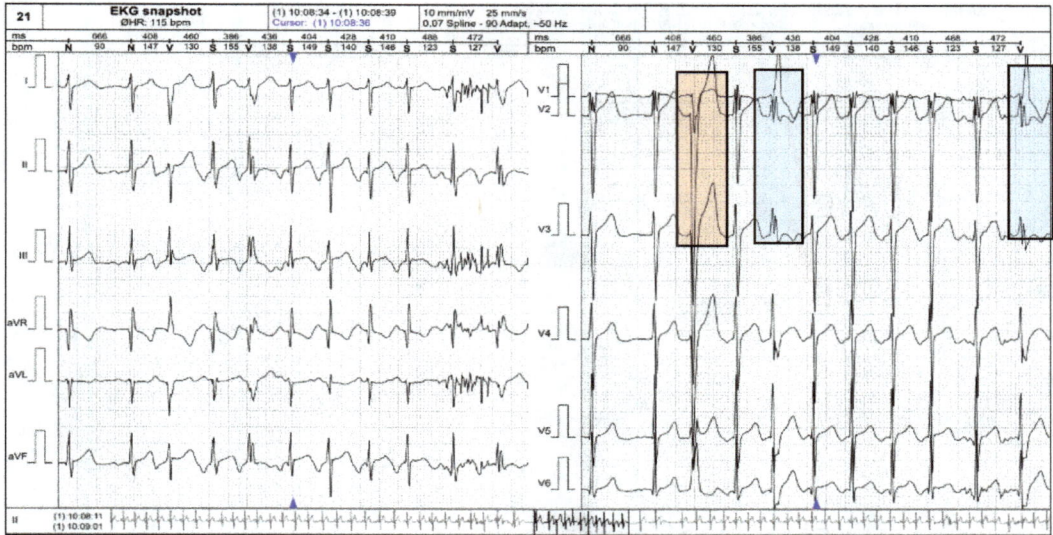

Figure 28.12   The tracing shows a salvo of 10 PACs with LBBB (red square) and RBBB aberrancy (blue square).

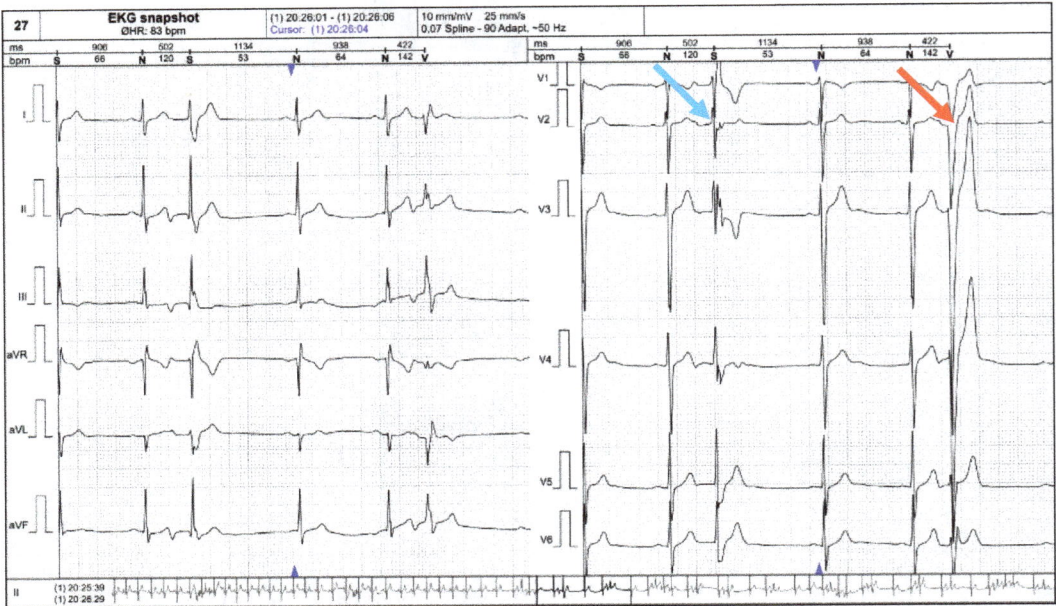

Figure 28.13 The tracing shows PACs with LBBB and RBBB aberrancy.

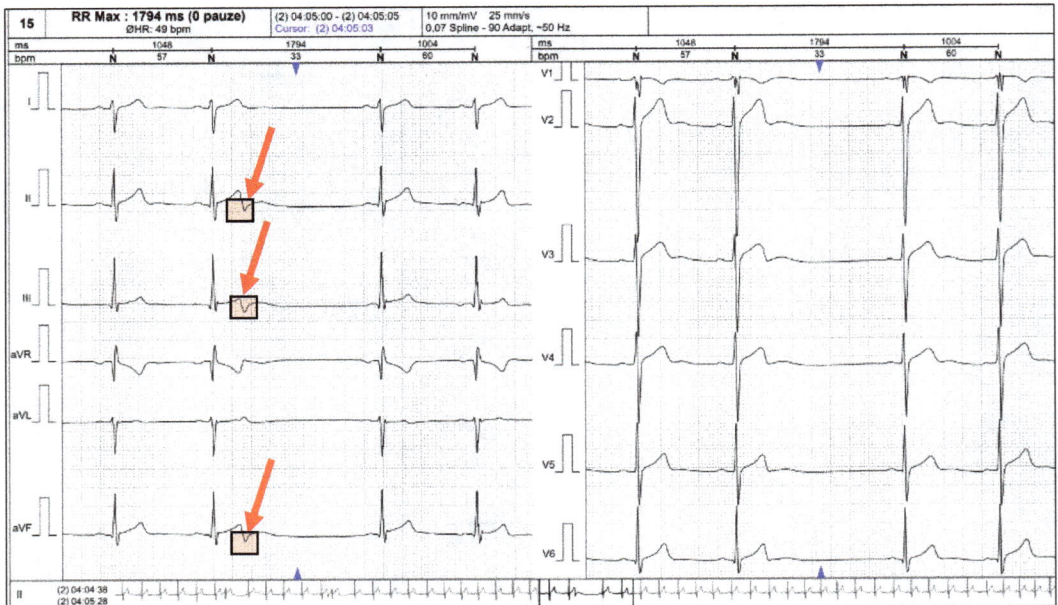

Figure 28.14 The tracing shows one blocked PAC which is non-conducted to the ventricles.

HOLTER SUMMARY

This Holter ECG shows 4 types of PACs: conducted to the ventricles with a narrow QRS complex, conducted to the ventricles with RBBB aberrancy, conducted to the ventricles with LBBB aberrancy and non-conducted to the ventricles. The total number of PACs was 3703 on 24 hours which is a low to moderate burden of 4%. The longest atrial salvo had 3 seconds duration with a rate of 137 bpm.

DISCUSSION

Premature atrial contractions (PAC) are abnormal beats originating in the atria. A PAC produces an electrical impulse that occurs prematurely, before the normal sinus beat. The majority of children do not perceive premature atrial contractions; however, a minority may experience symptoms as a missed heartbeat or a sudden jolt in the chest. The sinoatrial node usually controls the heartbeat in normal sinus rhythm; however, PACs arise as alternative atrial depolarization prior to the sinoatrial node, resulting in a premature beat. PACs are identified by an atypical P wave morphology succeeded by a normal narrow QRS complex. However, if the atrial contraction occurs prematurely, it may arrive to the atrioventricular node during its refractory phase, resulting in non-conducted beat to the ventricle and the absence of a QRS complex after. These are referred to as blocked premature atrial contractions.

Sometimes the premature atrial contraction arrives to the bundle branch during its refractory period and is conducted with a right bundle branch block or a left bundle branch block. These are referred to as conduction aberrancy. The term "aberration," originally defined by Lewis as an aberrant distribution of a supraventricular impulse to the ventricle, was first described in the context of atrial fibrillation by Gouaux and Ashman in 1947. The Ashman phenomenon, or the aberrant conduction, is applicable to both atrial fibrillation and atrial ectopics. QRS widening occurs due to functional right bundle branch block (RBBB) or left bundle branch block (LBBB). Right bundle branch aberrancy is more common than the left one, typically presenting in lead V1 of the ECG with an unusual premature P wave succeeded by a moderately enlarged QRS exhibiting a rSR' or rsR' morphology, referred to as "rabbit ears." The QRS complexes in the other precordial leads are frequently narrower than those observed with a left ventricular premature contraction, indicating that the bundle branch block is incomplete and the QRS duration is dependent on the prematurity of the PAC and on the coupling interval of the atrial ectopic beat.

Two consecutive PACs are termed a couplet, whereas three consecutive PACs are designated a triplet. When > 3 PACs are encountered, the correct term is salvo, or non-sustained atrial tachycardia.

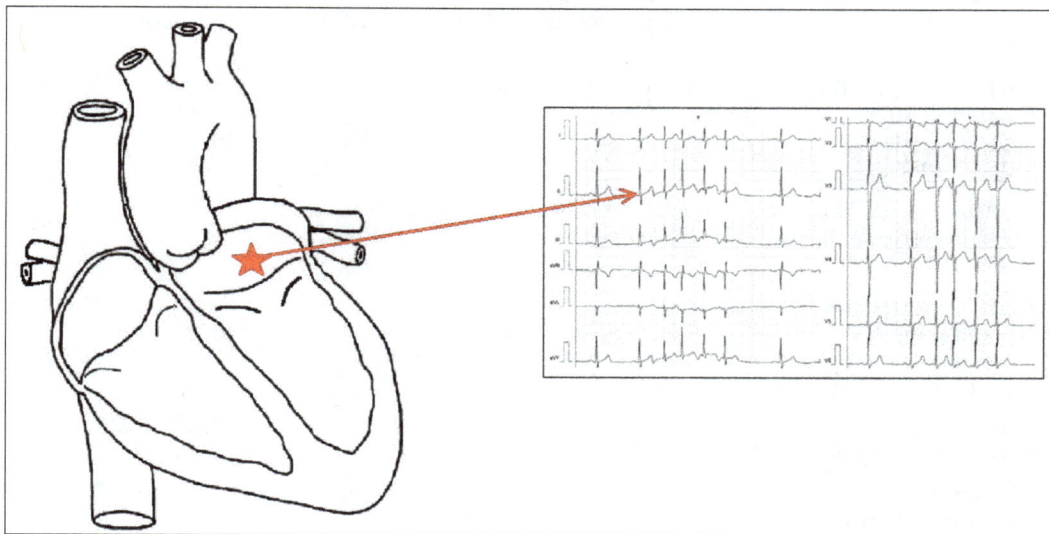

Figure 28.15 Premature atrial contractions. They are characterized by: 1) a premature atrial complex compared to sinus rhythm; 2) different P wave morphology; 3) different PR interval compared to sinus rhythm; and 4) normal or aberrantly conducted QRS.

Escape beats must be differentiated from PACs. When the sinus cycle stops or decelerates significantly, additional escape pacemaker foci from atria or AV node take over the control of heart rhythm. The most rapid among these are supposed atrial escape foci, characterized by their later onset compared to the basic sinus cycle and displaying a distinct P wave morphology compared to sinus beats. The defining characteristic of atrial ectopy is its premature occurrence. An escape beat is, by definition, not premature. It may occur late and immediately preceding the subsequent planned sinus beat.

Premature atrial contractions are mostly benign and do not necessitate therapy. Occasionally, antiarrhythmic medications may be necessary in the presence of symptoms. A beta blocker is frequently recommended for symptomatic PACs. In more severe instances, a class I antiarrhythmic agent may be administered, such as Propafenone or Flecainide. In the presence of structural heart disease, a class III antiarrhythmic agent such as Amiodarone is preferred.

The prognosis of PACs is generally good. In children with no congenital heart disease, PACs usually disappear with adolescence. In the presence of high-burden PACs, tachycardia-induced cardiomyopathy may develop, necessitating catheter ablation as a therapeutic intervention.

BIBLIOGRAPHY

1. Mond HG, Haqqani HM. The electrocardiographic footprints of atrial ectopy. *Heart Lung Circ.* 2019 Oct; 28(10):1463–1471. doi:10.1016/j.hlc.2019.03.005. Epub 2019 Apr 26. PMID: 31076238.

2. Bagliani G, Della Rocca DG, De Ponti R, Capucci A, Padeletti M, Natale A. Ectopic beats: Insights from timing and morphology. *Card Electrophysiol Clin.* 2018 Jun; 10(2): 257–275. doi:10.1016/j.ccep.2018.02.013. PMID: 29784483.

3. Teuwen CP, Kik C, van der Does LJME, Lanters EAH, Knops P, Mouws EMJP, Bogers AJJC, de Groot NMS. Quantification of the arrhythmogenic effects of spontaneous atrial extrasystole using high-resolution epicardial mapping. *Circ Arrhythm Electrophysiol.* 2018 Jan; 11(1): e005745. doi:10.1161/CIRCEP.117.005745. PMID: 29269560.

4. Rodríguez-Sotelo JL, Cuesta-Frau D, Castellanos-Dominguez G. Unsupervised classification of atrial heartbeats using a prematurity index and wave morphology features. *Med Biol Eng Comput.* 2009 Jul; 47(7): 731–741. doi:10.1007/s11517-009-0435-2. Epub 2009 Jan 31. PMID: 19184158.

5. Grigg WS, Pearlman JD, Nagalli S. Ashman phenomenon. 2024 Sep 11. In: *StatPearls* [Internet]. Treasure Island (FL): StatPearls Publishing; 2025 Jan–. PMID: 32965982.

6. Morton MB, Morton JB, Mond HG. Aberrant ventricular conduction: Revisiting an old concept. *Heart Lung Circ.* 2023 May; 32(5): 555–566. doi:10.1016/j.hlc.2023.03.001. Epub 2023 Mar 24. PMID: 36967303.

7. Hongliang Y, Ming Y, Qini Z, Daoyuan S, Yaliang T, Ying W, Yuquan H. A confused ECG with multiple rhythms caused by atrial premature contractions: A case report. *Medicine (Baltimore).* 2017 Dec; 96(50): e6997. doi:10.1097/MD.0000000000006997. PMID: 29390251; PMCID: PMC5815663.

8. Massumi RA, Mason DT, Fabregas RA, Vismara LA, Miller RR, Amsterdam EA, Vera Z. Intraventricular aberrancy versus ventricular ectopy. *Cardiovasc Clin.* 1973; 5(3): 35–86. PMID: 4135233.

9. Folli G, Libretti A, Vitolo E. Extrasistoli atriali con complessi ventricolari aberranti; considera-zioni su un particolare quadro di aberranza ventricolare [Atrial extrasystole with aberrant ventricular complexes; special aspects of aberrant ventricular complexes]. *Cuore Circ.* 1955 Dec; 39(6): 362–373. Italian. PMID: 13317469.

10. Ranjan P. Premature atrial contractions: "Are they really harmless?" *Am J Cardiol.* 2023 Aug 1; 200: 188–189. doi:10.1016/j.amjcard.2023.05.018. Epub 2023 Jun 20. PMID: 37348271.

11. Leeper BB. Are premature atrial contractions benign? *AACN Adv Crit Care.* 2023 Sep 15; 34(3): 263–265. doi:10.4037/aacnacc2023145. PMID: 37644628.

12. Farinha JM, Gupta D, Lip GYH. Frequent premature atrial contractions as a signalling marker of atrial cardiomyopathy, incident atrial fibrillation, and stroke. *Cardiovasc Res.* 2023 Mar 31; 119(2): 429–439. doi:10.1093/cvr/cvac054. PMID: 35388889; PMCID: PMC10064848.

13. Thompson C, Tsiperfal A. Are premature atrial contractions clinically significant? *Prog Cardiovasc Nurs*. 2006 Winter; 21(1): 53–54. doi:10.1111/j.0197-3118.2006.04978.x. PMID: 16522972.

14. Marcus GM, Dewland TA. Premature atrial contractions: A wolf in sheep's clothing? *J Am Coll Cardiol*. 2015 Jul 21; 66(3): 242–244. doi:10.1016/j.jacc.2015.04.069. PMID: 26184617.

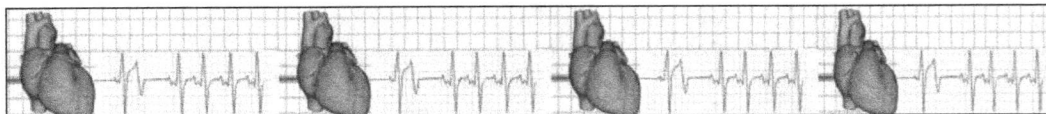

Case 29 Atrial Tachycardia with Bundle Branch Aberrancy

Andrei Mihordea, Gabriel Cismaru, and Andrei Cismaru

CLINICAL CASE

A 16-year-old female patient experienced multiple episodes of brief palpitations that lasted between 10 and 30 seconds. They were present during both periods of relaxation and exertion. She experienced palpitations on a daily basis during the past year.

Her ECG was normal and her echocardiography showed normal ejection fraction without any sign of structural heart disease. A Holter ECG was conducted, revealing episodes of palpitations.

Figure 29.1 The summary page shows a maximum heart rate of 190 bpm and a minimum rate of 20 bpm. This last value should be verified as it may be just an electrical artifact. There were 197 PVCs and numerous PACs with a burden of 19%/24 hours. There were 131 episodes of supraventricular arrhythmia with a duration of up to 8 seconds and a rate of up to 190 bpm.

DOI: 10.1201/9781003545040-29

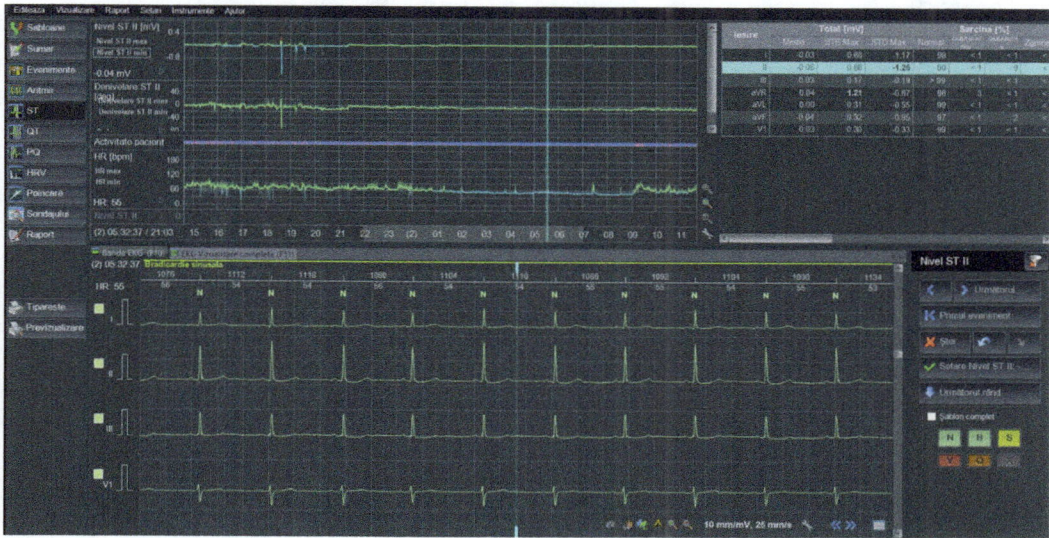

Figure 29.2 The tracing shows normal sinus rhythm with a rate of 55 bpm.

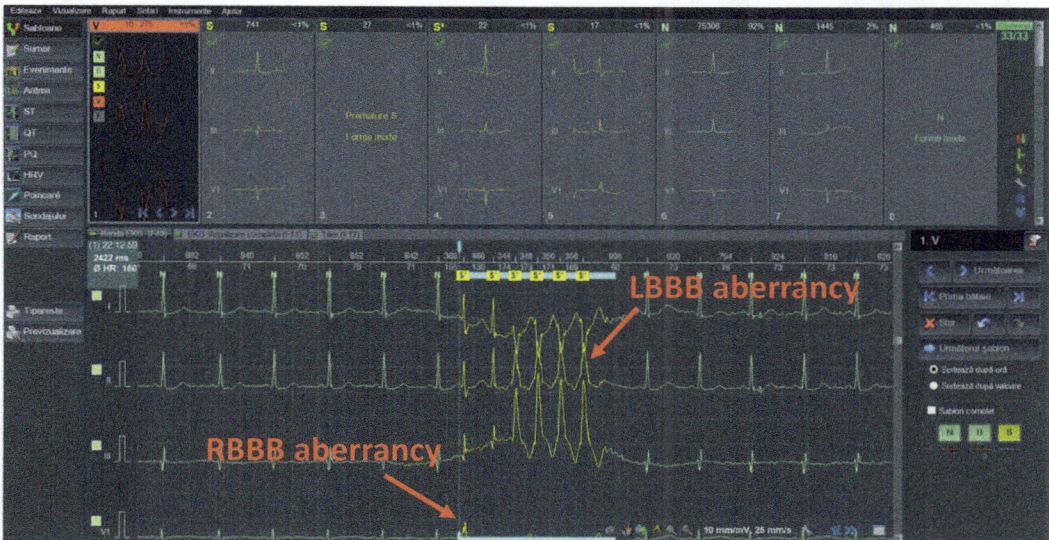

Figure 29.3 The tracing shows an episode of paroxysmal supraventricular tachycardia comprising 6 consecutive beats: The first has an RBBB aberrancy as it follows a long-short sequence, the second beat is narrow and the following 4 beats have a LBBB aberrancy.

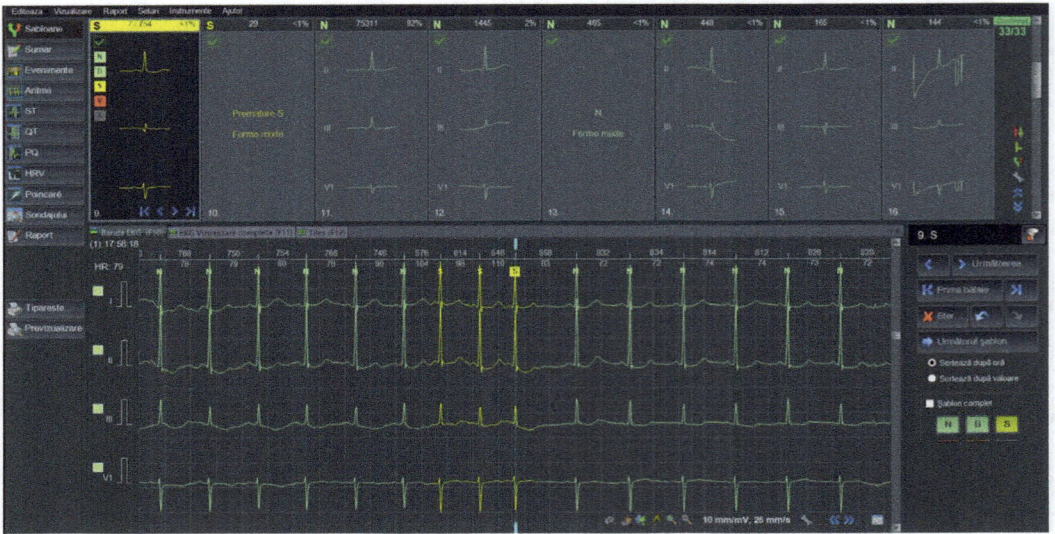

Figure 29.4   The tracing shows 3 atrial premature beats marked with yellow color.

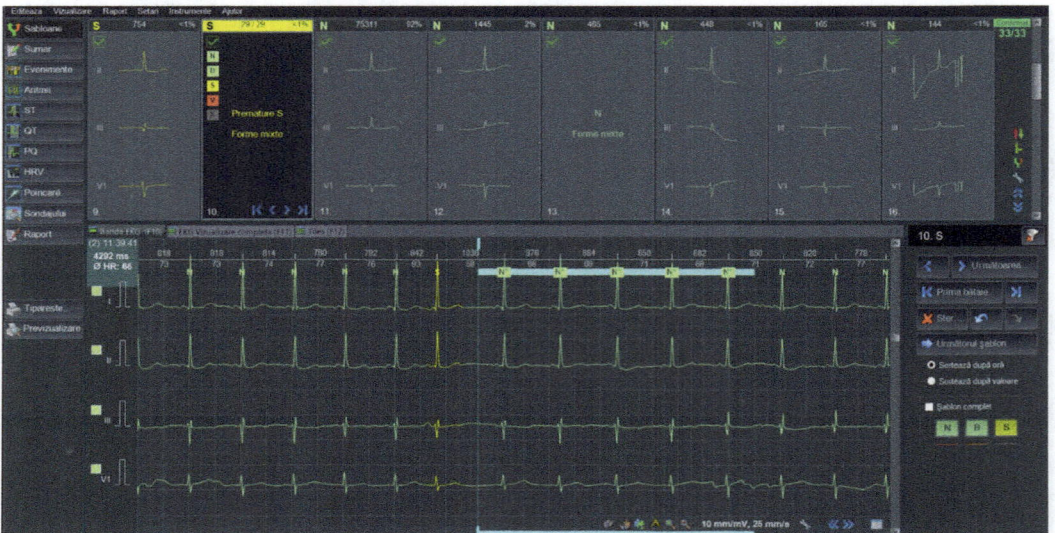

Figure 29.5   Shows 1 premature atrial beat marked with yellow color.

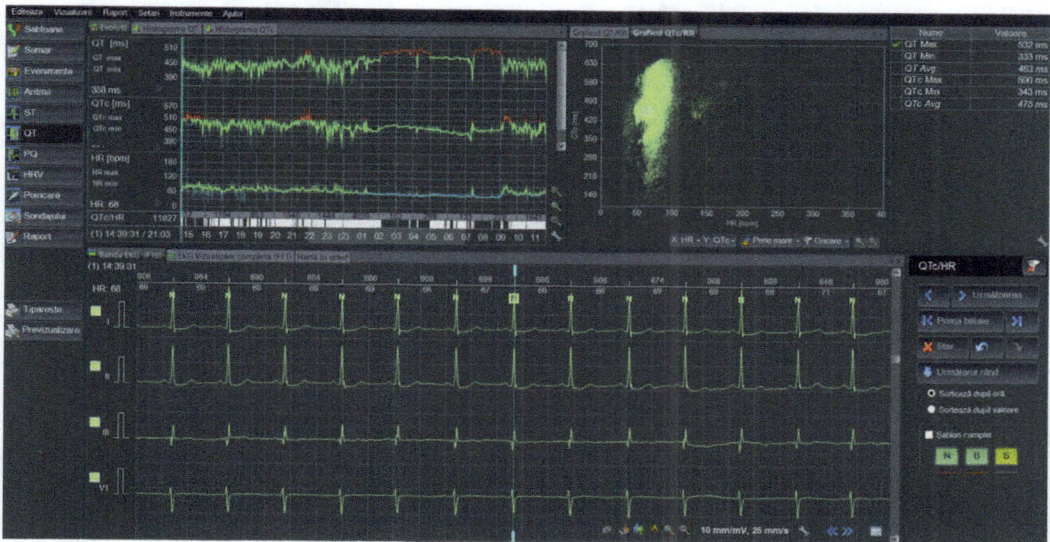

Figure 29.6   Shows normal sinus rhythm with a rate of 68 bpm.

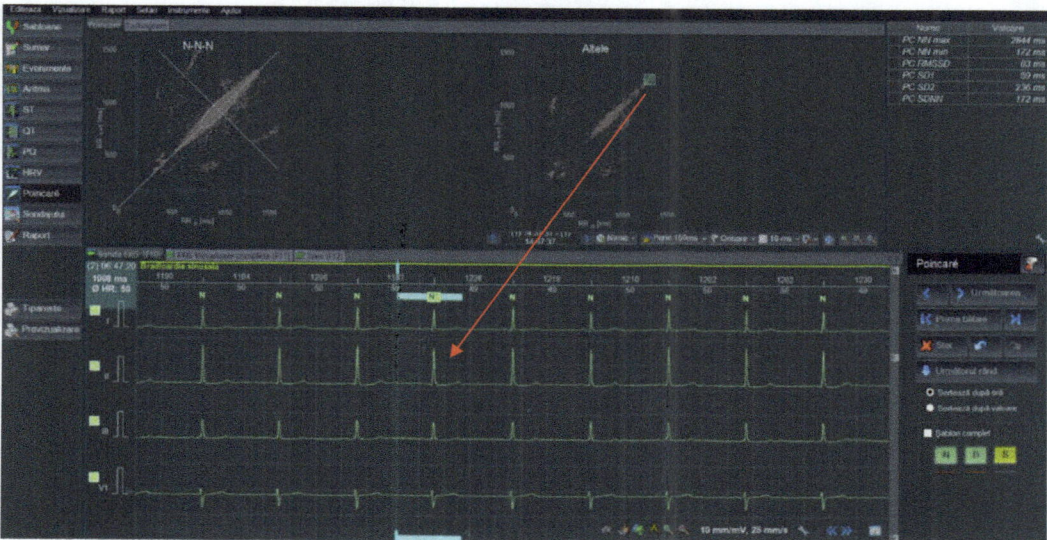

Figure 29.7   Shows 2 Poincaré graphs of heart rate variability in the upper panels and a point from the oblique line of normal RR intervals.

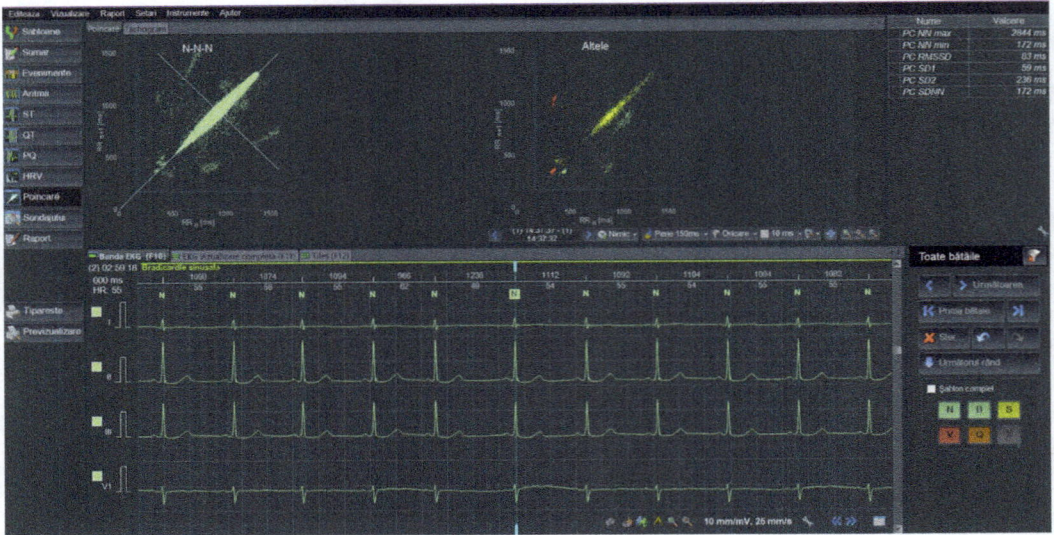

Figure 29.8 Shows 2 Poincaré graphs of heart rate variability in the upper panels and normal sinus rhythm in the lower panel.

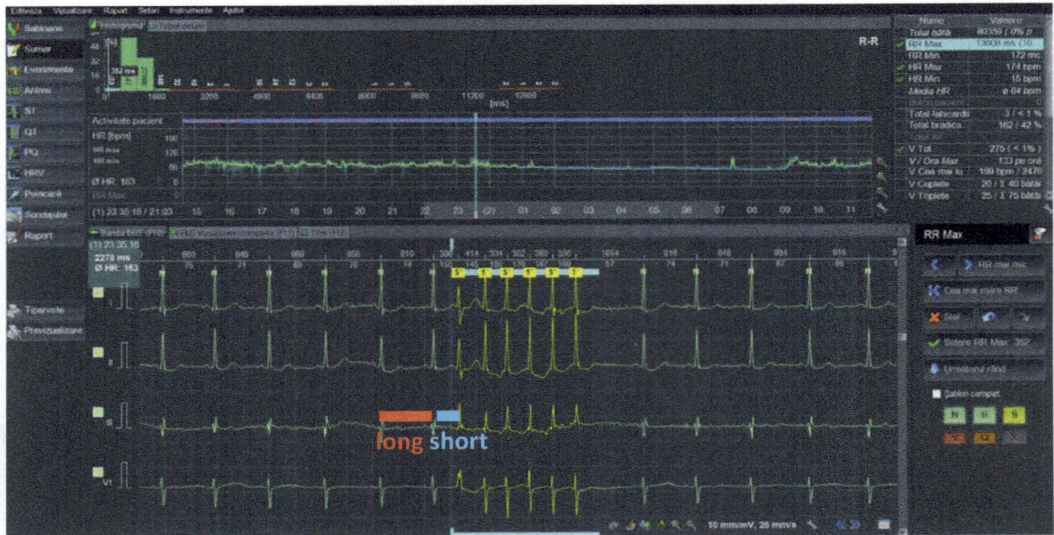

Figure 29.9 The tracing shows an episode of paroxysmal atrial tachycardia. The first beat shows RBBB aberrancy which occurs after a long-short sequence. The subsequent beats have a narrow QRS complex.

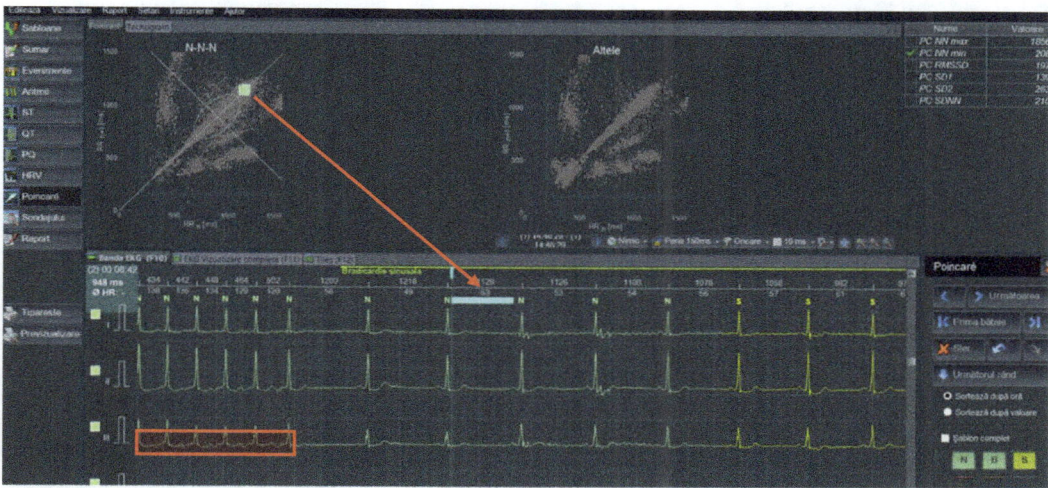

Figure 29.10   Heart rate variability with Poincaré graphs. The marked point situated on the 45° reference line shows normal RR interval preceded by normal RR interval. The bottom image shows an ECG and in the beginning of the trancing there is an episode of tachycardia followed by normal sinus rhythm.

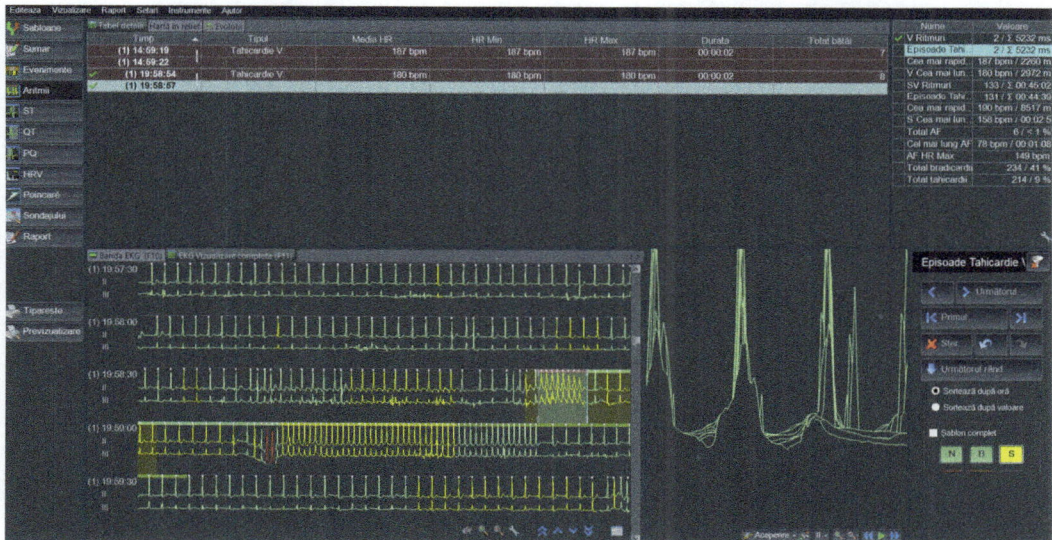

Figure 29.11   The arrhythmia column shows 3 episodes of atrial tachycardia, at 19:58:40, 19:58:50, and 19:59:10.

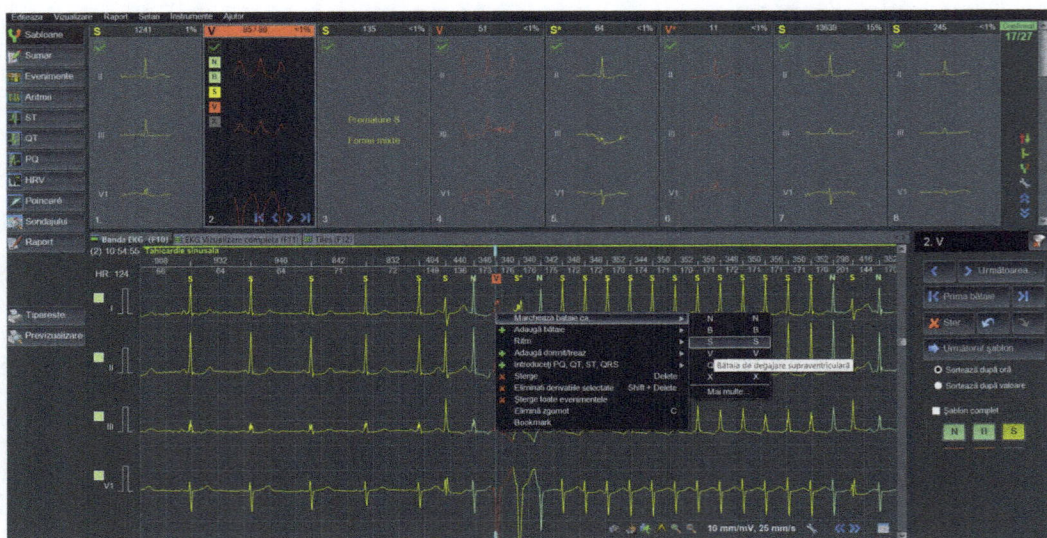

Figure 29.12 Shows an episode of atrial tachycardia with RBBB aberrancy of the first beat and LBBB aberrancy of the third and fourth beats. It also shows the way the software redefines the third beat from ventricular (red color) to supraventricular (yellow color).

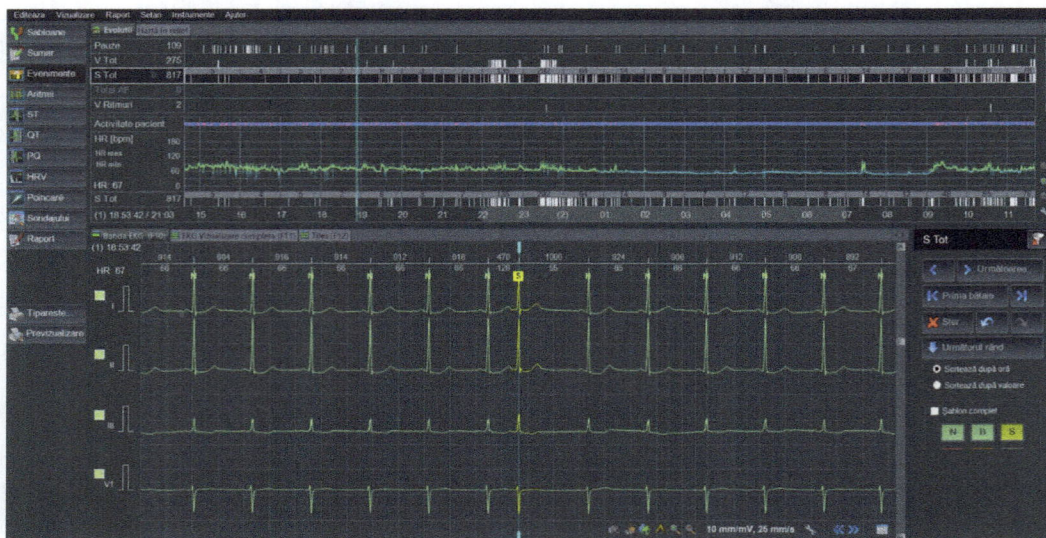

Figure 29.13 The tracing shows a supraventricular premature contraction with narrow QRS complex followed by a normal T wave. In the upper panel, S Tot represents the total number of supraventricular premature contractions, and a white line is used to indicate the occurrence of PACs in a chronological order.

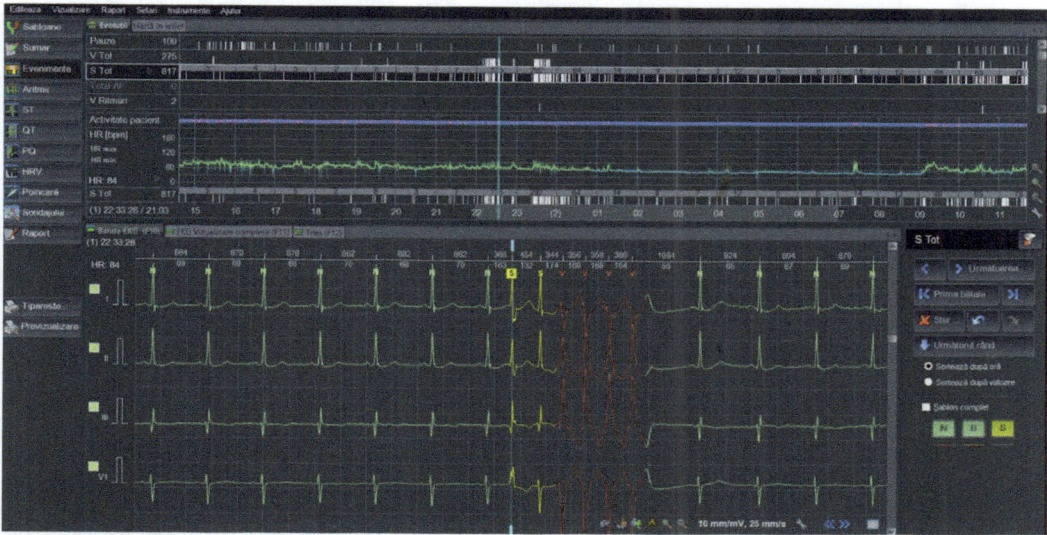

Figure 29.14   Shows an episode of atrial tachycardia made of 6 beats, with RBBB aberrancy of the first beat and LBBB aberrancy of the third, fourth, fifth and sixth beats.

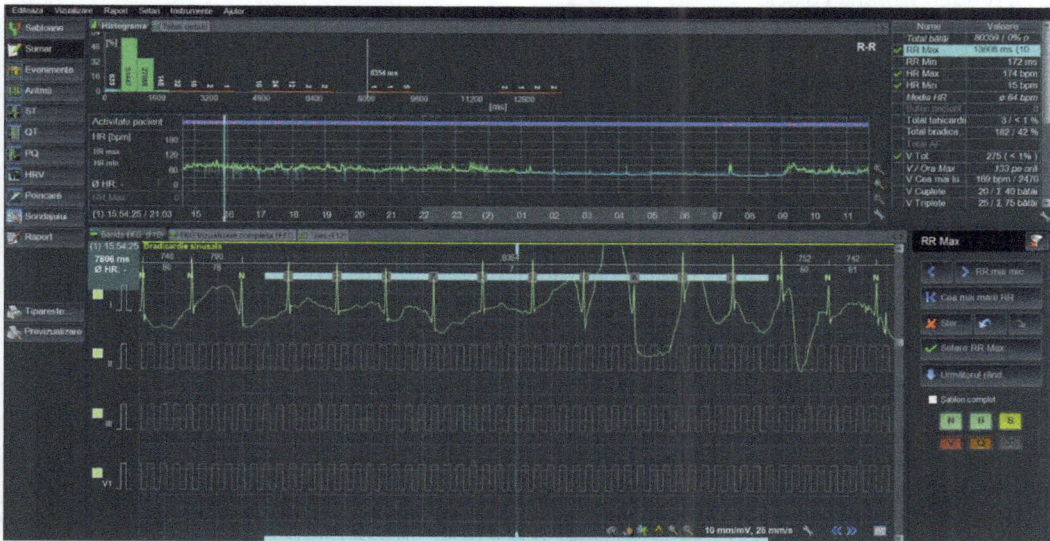

Figure 29.15   Shows electrical artifacts on leads II, III and V1 mimicking asystole of 7.8 seconds. However, lead I demonstrates normal sinus rhythm with a rate of 88 bpm.

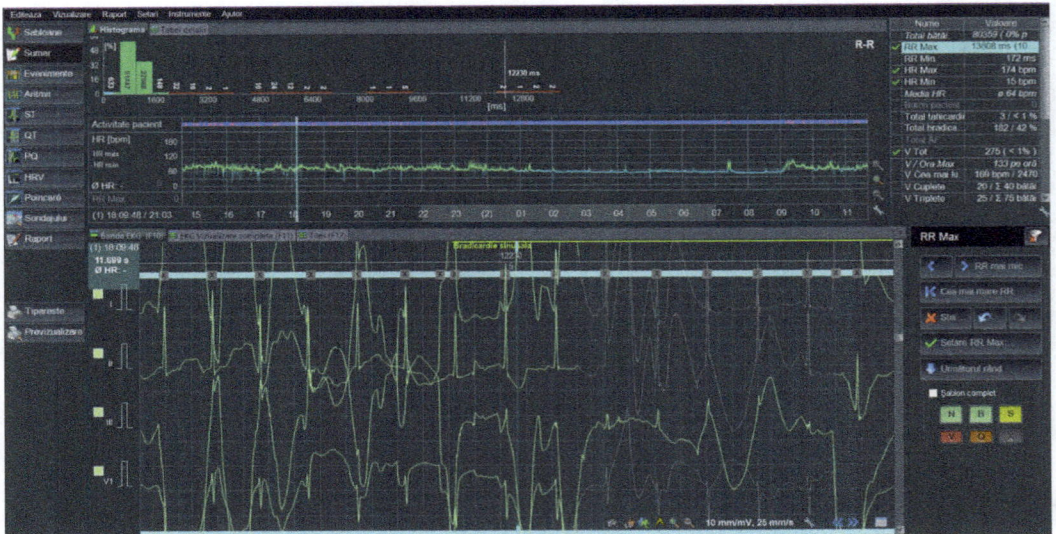

Figure 29.16 Shows electrical artifacts on all leads, mimicking asystole of 11.7 seconds. However, the rhythm is sinus with a rate of 80 bpm.

HOLTER SUMMARY

The monitoring indicates 18% PACs and episodes of atrial tachycardia. The longest episode had a duration of 8 seconds with a rate of 190 bpm. The tachycardia has narrow QRS complexes; nonetheless, ventricular aberrancy with a right bundle branch block is intermittently observed, as well as left bundle branch block.

DISCUSSION

Focal atrial tachycardia is a rare cause of tachycardia in pediatric patients, originating from an atrial focus with increased automaticity. Our patient had an abnormal atrial focus situated at the ostium of the coronary sinus. The mechanism included automaticity or a small reentry which disappeared after one RF application.

ECG characteristics of focal atrial tachycardia are:

- Atrial rate above 100 bpm;

- Abnormal P wave morphology and axis with normal or shorter PR segment;

- Unifocal, identical P wave morphology;

- Isoelectric line between P waves (as opposed to atrial flutter);

- Narrow QRS morphology, except in cases of aberrant ventricular conduction.

Aberrant ventricular conduction is defined as the enlargement of the QRS complex as a result of a delayed or blocked bundle branch conduction. The right bundle branch block is more prevalent due to the prolonged refractory period of the right branch. The right-bundle-branch refractory period will be increased by a relatively long R–R interval. Conversely, the right bundle branch may be refractory if the next impulse is conducted after a shortened R–R interval. This leads to Asman's phenomenon of aberrancy. The Ashman phenomenon was first reported in 1947 by Gouaux and Ashman. Only approximately one-third of the cases are attributed to the left bundle branch block as the left branch has a shorter refractory period than the right branch. The R–R interval of the preceding cycle influences the action potential duration of the following beat.

The mechanism of aberrancy in our case can be either phase 3 aberration or acceleration-dependent aberration or retrograde concealed conduction. When a new impulse is received by conduction fibers before they have entirely repolarized, phase 3 aberration occurs. The refractory period of the bundle branch is being invaded by a premature impulse. This is a physiological

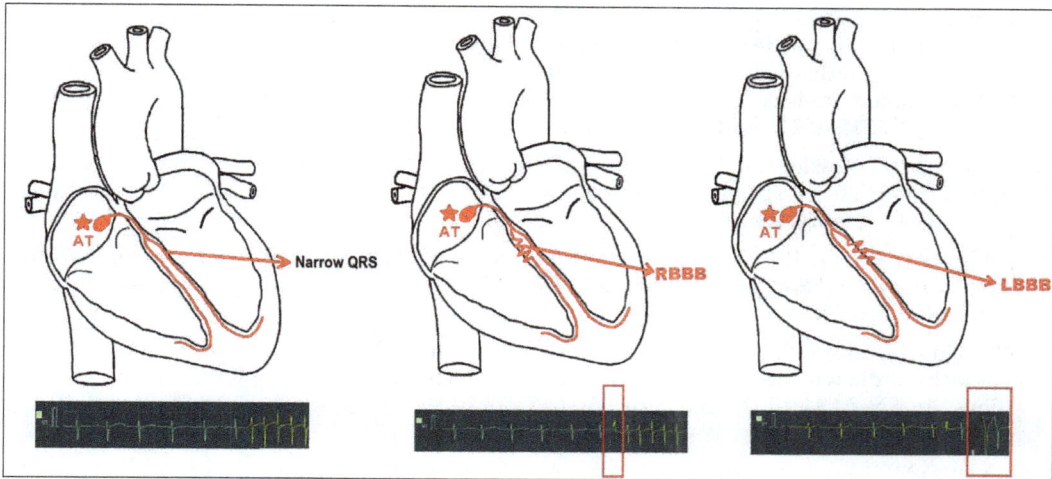

Figure 29.17 Focal atrial tachycardia may be conducted to the ventricles with narrow QRS complex or with bundle branch block in the case of refractoriness. In the first image lead V1 shows a narrow QRS, in the second image a large positive QRS, and in the third image a large negative QRS complex.

phenomenon which may occasionally be observed at the onset of paroxysmal supraventricular tachycardias or in case of a long-short sequence in which the refractory period of the long sequence is prolonged. This phenomenon is also known as the Ashman phenomenon. A minor increase in rhythm that leads to aberrancy as a result of an abnormal response of tissue that has reduced excitability is called acceleration dependent aberrancy. The most prevalent mechanism for sustained aberrancy in tachycardia is concealed retrograde conduction. After a QRS widening due to a phase 3 aberration in the initial premature beat with LBBB, the right bundle conducts the subsequent impulse to the apex and then retrogradely through the left bundle, giving the LBBB pattern. This can persist until a new premature ventricular complex induces a compensatory pause and 'resets' the mechanism, leading to a narrow QRS complex.

Figures 29.12 and 29.14 show LBBB aberrancy but the first beat of tachycardia in Figure 29.12 shows RBBB aberrancy. The RBBB occurs as a result of a sudden shortening of the R–R interval due to a short-coupled atrial extrasystole, with the right branch of the specific conduction system remaining refractory (the so-called "Ashman phenomenon"). Additionally, aberrancy may occur when the cycle length of the atrial tachycardia drops below the refractory period of the left branch of the conduction system, which leads to LBBB aberrancy during focal atrial tachycardia.

BIBLIOGRAPHY

1. Singla V, Singh B, Singh Y, Manjunath CN. Ashman phenomenon: A physiological aberration. *BMJ Case Rep*. 2013 May 24; 2013: bcr2013009660. doi:10.1136/bcr-2013-009660. PMID: 23709552; PMCID: PMC3669876.

2. Chenevert M, Lewis RJ. Ashman's phenomenon—A source of nonsustained wide-complex tachycardia: Case report and discussion. *J Emerg Med*. 1992 Mar.–Apr.; 10(2): 179–183. doi:10.1016/0736-4679(92)90213-d. PMID: 1376740.

3. Gulamhusein S, Yee R, Ko PT, Klein GJ. Electrocardiographic criteria for differentiating aberrancy and ventricular extrasystole in chronic atrial fibrillation: Validation by intracardiac recordings. *J Electrocardiol* 1985 Jan.; 18(1): 41–50. doi:10.1016/s0022-0736(85)80033-9. PMID: 2579180.

4. Carbone V, Carerj S, Calabrò MP. Bundle branch block on alternate beats during atrial fibrillation. *J Electrocardiol*. 2004 Jan.; 37(1): 67–72. doi:10.1016/j.jelectrocard.2003.11.002. PMID: 15132372.

5. Antunes E, Brugada J, Steurer G, Andries E, Brugada P. The differential diagnosis of a regular tachycardia with a wide QRS complex on the 12-lead ECG: Ventricular tachycardia, supraventricular tachycardia with aberrant intraventricular conduction, and supraventricular tachycardia with anterograde conduction over an accessory pathway. *Pacing Clin Electrophysiol*. 1994 Sep.; 17(9): 1515–1524. doi:10.1111/j.1540-8159.1994.tb01517.x. PMID: 7991423.

6. Trohman RG, Kessler KM, Williams D, Maloney JD. Atrial fibrillation and flutter with left bundle branch block aberration referred as ventricular tachycardia. *Cleve Clin J Med*. 1991 Jul.– Aug.; 58(4): 325–330. doi:10.3949/ccjm.58.4.325. PMID: 1889115.

7. Miles WM, George P. Physiologic variants of cardiac conduction (aberration, gap, supernormal conduction). *Card Electrophysiol Clin*. 2021 Dec.; 13(4): 607–624. doi:10.1016/j.ccep.2021.07.002. Epub 2021 Sep 25. PMID: 34689890.

8. Tonkin AM, Tornos P, Heddle WF. Atrial pacing in ventricular tachycardia and supraventricular tachycardia with aberrant intraventricular conduction: Diagnostic and therapeutic implications. *Aust N Z J Med* 1979 Dec.; 9(6): 661–666. doi:10.1111/j.1445-5994.1979.tb04196.x. PMID: 294923.

9. Calabrò MP, Cerrito M, Luzza F, Oreto G. Alternating right and left bundle branch block aberration during atrial tachycardia. *J Electrocardiol*. 2009 Nov.–Dec.; 42(6): 633–635. doi:10.1016/j.jelectrocard.2009.03.013. Epub 2009 Apr. 18. PMID: 19376525.

10. Oreto G, Luzza F, Satullo G, Donato A, Carbone V, Calabrò MP. TachiCardia a QRS larghi: un problema antico e nuovo [Wide QRS complex tachycardia: An old and new problem]. *G Ital Cardiol (Rome)*. 2009 Sep.; 10(9): 580–595. Italian. PMID: 19891250.

11. Costantini M. Conduzione supernormale e alternante nel blocco di branca intermittente e nella preeccitazione ventricolare intermittente o occulta. Studio elettrofisiologico, meccanismi coinvolti e considerazioni cliniche [Supernormal and alternating conduction in intermittent bundle branch block and intermittent or concealed ventricular preexcitation. Electrophysiological study, mechanisms and clinical considerations]. *G Ital Cardiol (Rome)*. 2016 May; 17(5): 370–376. Italian. doi: 10.1714/2252.24266. PMID: 27310911.

12. Kennedy LB, Leefe W, Leslie BR. The Ashman phenomenon. *J La State Med Soc*. 2004 May–Jun.; 156(3): 159–162. PMID: 15233390.

13. Guo H, Hecker S, Lévy S, Olshansky B. Ventricular tachycardia with QRS configuration similar to that in sinus rhythm and a myocardial origin: Differential diagnosis with bundle branch reentry. *Europace*. 2001 Apr; 3(2): 115–123. doi:10.1053/eupc.2001.0151. PMID: 11333048.

14. Langendorf R, Pick A. Concealed intraventricular conduction in the human heart. *Adv Cardiol*. 1975; 14: 40–50. doi:10.1159/000397637. PMID: 1136891.

15. Morton MB, Morton JB, Mond HG. Aberrant ventricular conduction: Revisiting an old concept. *Heart Lung Circ*. 2023 May; 32(5): 555–566. doi:10.1016/j.hlc.2023.03.001. Epub 2023 Mar 24. PMID: 36967303.

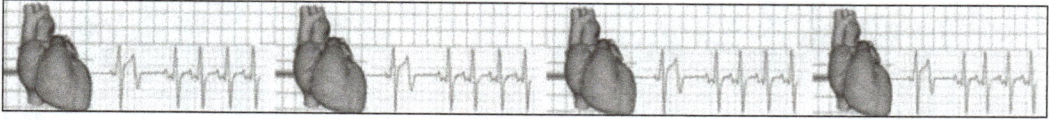

Case 30 Accelerated Idioventricular Rhythm

Nikola Krmek

CLINICAL CASE

An 11-year-old child was referred to our cardiology center for evaluation of an accidentally discovered wide QRS arrhythmia. He had no symptoms and had no underlying heart disease. Continuous heart rate monitoring identified accelerated idioventricular rhythm across the majority of the monitoring period. In a 24-hour Holter ECG, wide QRS complexes consisted of 73% of all complexes. An electrophysiological study was performed which identified the source of origin and radiofrequency ablation of the ectopic focus was performed, resulting in an immediate restoration of sinus rhythm with no other recurrence of the arrhythmia.

Figure 30.1 The summary page shows a high burden PVC with episodes of ventricular tachycardia.

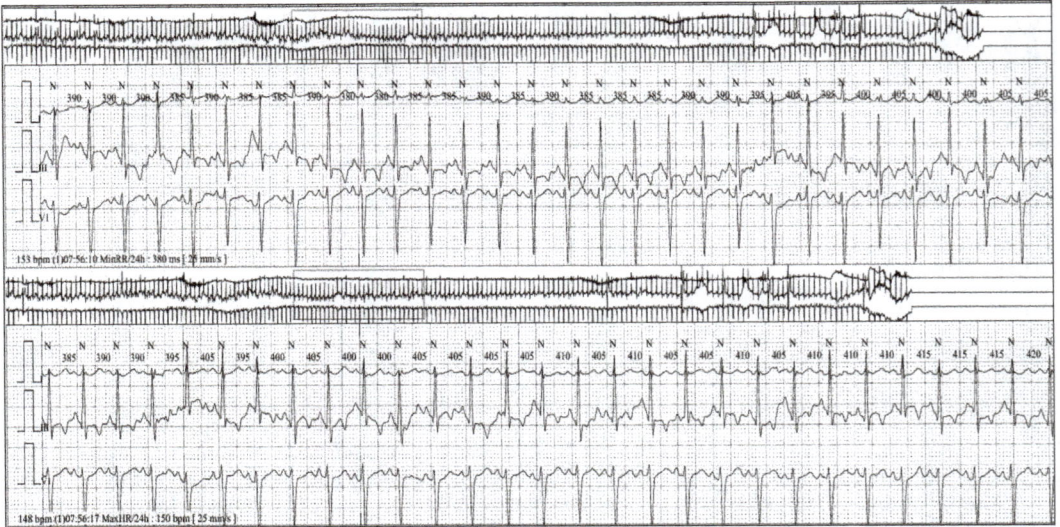

Figure 30.2 Sinus rhythm with a rate of 153 bpm.

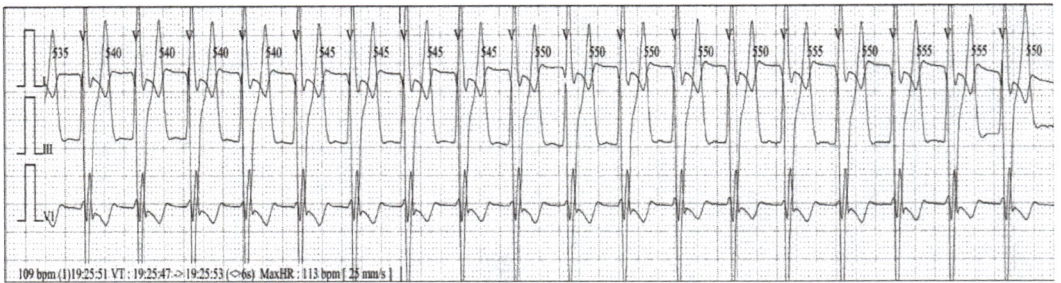

Figure 30.3 Accelerated idioventricular rhythm with a rate of 113 bpm. Compared to Figure 30.2, the rate is slower than the sinus rate.

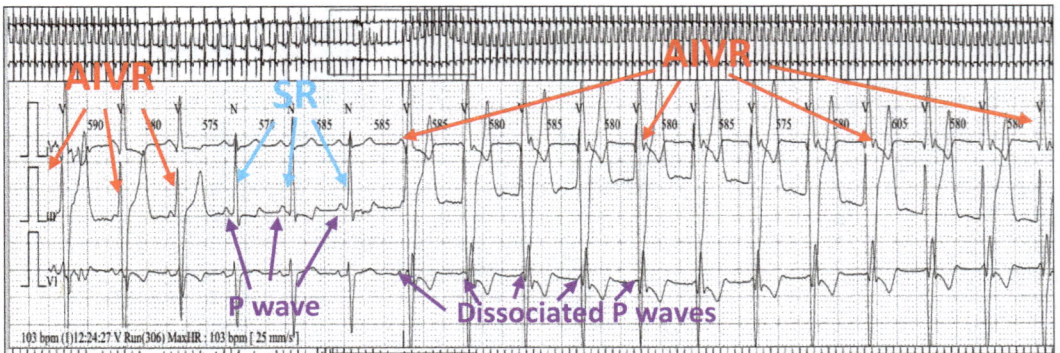

Figure 30.4 The rate of the sinus rhythm is close to the rate of the accelerated idioventricular rhythm. AIVR is recognized by the large QRS and the dissociated P wave.

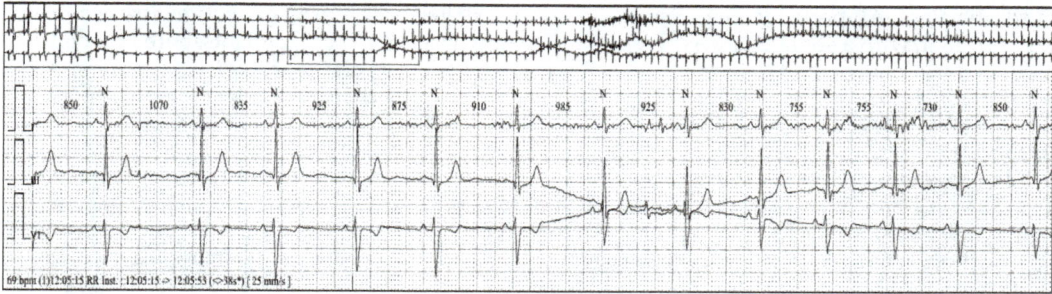

Figure 30.5 Sinus rhythm without PVCs.

HOLTER SUMMARY

Accelerated idioventricular rhythm was detected during Holter monitoring with a heart rate lower than the sinus rate. The arrhythmia had wide QRS complexes, suggesting a ventricular origin and P wave were dissociated from the QRS complexes.

DISCUSSION

Accelerated idioventricular rhythm (AIVR) is a benign arrhythmia characterized by wide QRS complexes with a minimum of three successive ventricular complexes. It can occur in both adults and children. In adults, it is defined by a cut-off rate ranging from 50 to 120 beats per minute, whereas in children, the rate is defined by a percentage of the normal sinus rhythm (usually 10–15% lower than the sinus rhythm). In the event of wide QRS tachycardia with a rate exceeding 15% relative to the sinus rhythm, it should be designated as ventricular tachycardia.

In the pediatric population, it is typically observed in children with congenital heart disease and is relatively uncommon in the absence of underlying heart diseases. Usually it is asymptomatic, and it is frequently an accidental finding on a routine electrocardiogram. It is believed to be associated with increased automaticity in His-Purkinje fibers or the functioning contractile ventricular cells.

An extensive cohort of patients was presented by MacLellan-Tobert in her 1995 publication. Twelve pediatric patients were reported, including two infants and four children with congenital heart disease. The ECG spontaneously normalized in eight cases during the follow-up period. No patient reported symptoms or clinical signs of hemodynamic instability. The follow-up period was 68 months. Wang et al. reported on 19 children with AIVR, including six neonates. All children were hemodynamically stable; fewer than half exhibited symptoms, with palpitations being the

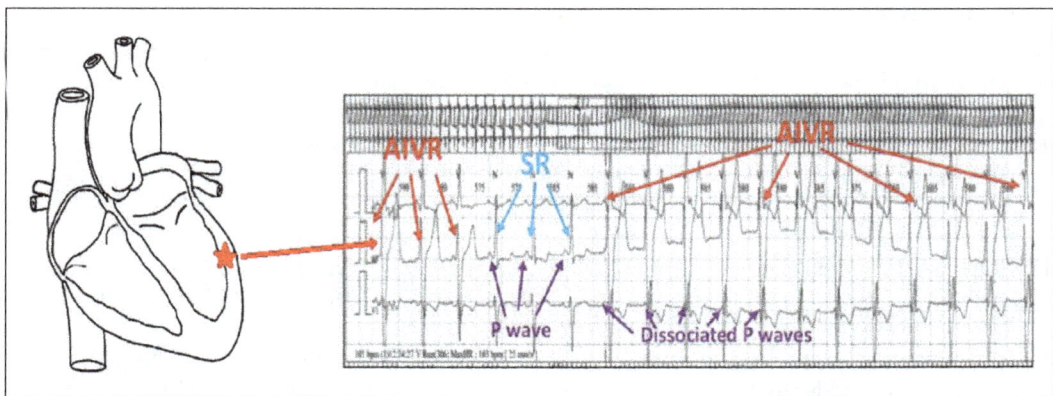

Figure 30.6 In accelerated idioventricular rhythm, the arrhythmia originates from the Purkinje network or ventricular myocardium. The QRS complexes are large and P waves are dissociated.

most prevalent. All participants performed a 24-hour Holter ECG. Cardiac function assessments were normal, with a slight decrease in ejection fraction observed in two patients, both of whom exhibited spontaneous regression of AVIR. Six children received pharmacological treatment, resulting in arrhythmia resolution. However, the authors argue that it is unclear whether this outcome was attributable to the medication or to spontaneous resolution, which occurred in 13 untreated individuals. No EPS has been conducted in this cohort of patients.

Recommendations for the management of this dysrhythmia in pediatric patients are limited. The 2014 HRS consensus statement indicates that if the patient is asymptomatic, has no hemodynamic repercussions, lacks an arrhythmogenic cardiac disease, and has no preexisting myocardial dysfunction, there are no reasons for treatment. However, the literature supporting these suggestions does not address patients with frequent and recurrent episodes AIVR. If therapy is necessary, however, it may involve antiarrhythmic drugs, typically beta blockers, or ablation if arrhythmia is not sufficiently managed with antiarrhythmic drugs.

BIBLIOGRAPHY

1. Crosson JE, Callans DJ, Bradley DJ, Dubin A, Epstein M, Etheridge S, et al. PACES/HRS expert consensus statement on the evaluation and management of ventricular arrhythmias in the child with a structurally normal heart. *Hear Rhythm* 2014; 11(9): 55–78.

2. Chen M, Gu K, Yang B, Chen H, Ju W, Zhang F, et al. Idiopathic accelerated idioventricular rhythm or ventricular tachycardia originating from the right bundle branch: Unusual type of ventricular arrhythmia. *Circ Arrhyth mia Electrophysiol*. 2014; 7(6): 1159–1167.

3. Errahmouni A, Bun SS, Latcu DG, Tazi-Mezalek A, Saoudi N. Accelerated idioventricular rhythm requiring catheter ablation in a child: The dark side of a benign arrhythmia. *Ann Cardiol Angeiol (Paris)*. 2017; 66(5): 323–325.

4. Ergul Y, Kafali HC, Uysal F. Accelerated idioventricular rhythm resulting in torsades de pointes and cardiac arrest in a child: Successfully cryoablated in left coronary cusp. *Cardiol Young*. 2020; 30(3): 410–413.

5. Grimm W, Marchlinski FE. Accelerated idioventricular rhythm and bidirectional ventricular tachycardia. In: *Cardiac Electrophysiology*. Elsevier; 2004. pp. 700–704.

6. MacLellan-Tobert SG, Porter CJ. Accelerated idioventricular rhythm: A benign arrhythmia in childhood. *Pediatrics*. 1995; 96(1):122–125.

7. Wang L, Liu H, Zhu C, Gu K, Yang G, Chen H, et al. Clinical characteristics and therapeutic strategy of frequent accelerated idioventricular rhythm. *BMC Cardiovasc Disord*. 2021; (1): 1–9.

8. Bisset GS, Janos GG, Gaum WE. Accelerated ventricular rhythm in the newborn infant. *J Pediatr*. 1984; 104(2): 247–249.

9. Van Hare GF, Stanger P. Ventricular tachycardia and accelerated ventricular rhythm presenting in the first month of life. *Am J Cardiol*. 1991; 67(1): 42–45.

10. Anatoliotaki M, Papagiannis J, Stefanaki S, Koropouli M, Tsilimigaki A. Accelerated ventricular rhythm in the neonatal period: A review and two new cases in asymptomatic infants with an apparently normal heart. *Acta Paediatr Int J Paediatr*. 2004; 93(10): 1397–1400.

11. Ljubas Perčić D, Krmek N, Benko I, Kniewald H, Bitanga S, Katavić M, Perčić M. Frequent accelerated idioventricular rhythm in an otherwise healthy child: a case report and review of literature. *BMC Cardiovasc Disord*. 2023 Jan. 20; 23(1):37. doi: 10.1186/s12872-023-03074-5. PMID: 36670379; PMCID: PMC9862554.

12. Kappy B, Johnson L, Brown T, Czosek RJ. Accelerated idioventricular rhythm: A rare case of wide-complex dysrhythmia in a teenager. *J Emerg Med*. 2021 Apr; 60(4):e89–e94. doi: 10.1016/j.jemermed.2020.12.011. Epub 2021 Jan. 21. PMID: 33485745.

13. Curtis TM, Sady KM, Randall JT, Kervin P, Mosher DM, Dailey MW. 18-month-old with lethargy and accelerated idioventricular rhythm in prehospital setting: A case report. *Prehosp Emerg Care*. 2024; 28(7):961–964. doi: 10.1080/10903127.2024.2337755. Epub 2024 Apr. 5. PMID: 38551813.

14. Beach C, Marcuccio E, Beerman L, Arora G. Accelerated idioventricular rhythm in a child With status asthmaticus. *Pediatrics.* 2015 Aug; 136(2):e527–e529. doi: 10.1542/peds.2015-0449. Epub 2015 Jul. 13. PMID: 26169431.

15. Fouron JC, McNeal-Davidson A, Abadir S, Fournier A, Bigras JL, Boutin C, Brassard M, Raboisson MJ, van Doesburg N, Berger A, Brisebois S, Gendron R. Prenatal diagnosis and prognosis of accelerated idioventricular rhythm. *Ultrasound Obstet Gynecol.* 2017 Nov.; 50(5):624–631. doi: 10.1002/uog.17382. PMID: 27943499.

Index

Pages in *italics* refer to figures and pages in **bold** refer to tables.

For Product Safety Concerns and Information please contact our EU
representative GPSR@taylorandfrancis.com
Taylor & Francis Verlag GmbH, Kaufingerstraße 24, 80331 München, Germany